D0385729

PSYCHIATRIC NURSING AS A HUMAN EXPERIENCE

Lisa Robinson, R.N., Ph.D.

Associate Professor of Psychiatric Nursing,
School of Nursing;
Instructor of Psychiatry,
School of Medicine,
University of Maryland

W. B. SAUNDERS COMPANY

PHILADELPHIA   LONDON   TORONTO

W. B. Saunders Company: West Washington Square
Philadelphia, Pa. 19105

12 Dyott Street
London, WC1A 1DB

833 Oxford Street
Toronto 18, Ontario

Pyschiatric Nursing as a Human Experience   ISBN 0-7216-7620-0

Print No.:   9   8   7   6   5   4   3

For
Esther G. Robinson
1911-1970

PREFACE

Many decades ago the nurse ruled the sick room. She ministered to her patient in an effort to meet all his needs: she cleaned his room, cooked his meals and performed all his treatments. Preparations for the attending physician's daily visit were similar to those of the field officer awaiting the colonel's inspection. Except for the physician, the nurse was the final authority and without peer.

The Age of Technology, with its array of drugs, monitors and computers, as well as health workers with highly specialized education, has all but eradicated the all-giving bedside nurse. Comprehensive care is still the goal of the nurse, but responsibility for it is now divided among many workers. The nurse is often a coordinator. He or she guides others as they administer a multitude of drugs, monitor life-maintaining machines and perform complex procedures.

Unlike many others, the psychiatric nurse still has concerns which keep her at the bedside. Psychotherapy, through interpersonal relating, remains an infinitely human process. Drugs and machines do not take the place of people. Though theory has expanded the basis of psychiatric nursing, in clinical practice the patient and the nurse still interact. The work they do together evolves from their humanness: the patient—from his fears, his anxieties and his inability to cope; the psychiatric nurse—from understanding, self-confidence and an ability to facilitate learning.

This book is about human beings—their problems, their expressiveness and their capacity to help one another. In writing this text, I have been concerned with keeping awareness of self and others in the forefront of the reader's mind. In the main I have tried repeatedly to demonstrate that the student knows much about his or her patient because patient and nurse share many human qualities. Thus, much of their relationship is predictable and need not be a source of anxiety for the student. The latter may draw from his or her reservoirs of warmth, empathy and caring to support patients with emotional problems.

The early chapters of the text depict the psychiatric nurse as a caring person who encounters patients with psychological problems in many settings. The interpersonal relationship is presented as a vehicle for support. The next group of chapters is concerned with the meaning of mental illness. Anxiety is presented as both a function of self-maintenance and a signal of illness.

As the material moves into clinical problems, the human being is again emphasized. In these chapters he is seen in states of depression and withdrawal. The psychiatric patient is often a person who is too sad to care for himself or to cherish his own existence. He is sometimes so terrified of others that he cannot reach beyond his bonds of loneliness.

The reader will also find some material that focuses less on people and more on differences in clinical settings. Problems of the large state institution, such as overwhelming numbers of patients, chronic illness and staff members with vested interests, are discussed. Intervention through environmental manipulation, behavior modification and re-motivation techniques is described. In the latter third of the text emphasis is once more on the human being in distress. For the most part, the problems presented involve a social matrix. With the exception of the material on children, the later chapters focus on such social issues as drugs, alcohol and mental retardation. A chapter on organic disorders focuses primarily on the nurse's and the patient's feelings about irreversible organic disease.

This book is directed to those who are learning about people who experience human agony. It is for readers who cannot "turn off" the scenes they react to, but feel compelled to help. It is my hope that the readers of this text will find useful suggestions herein for bringing comfort to people in pain.

Though one writes basically in solitude, there have been friends, colleagues and family who have helped me. For their invaluable suggestions concerning the chapter on community mental health, I thank Evelyn McElroy and Barbara Blaha. For his commentary on chemotherapy and other somatic therapies, I am indebted to Dr. Frank Ayd, Jr. For their countless ideas, I thank Marilyn Kandlbinder, Doris Scott and Florence Schubert, who talked, debated and argued with me about the ethics of psychiatric nursing and the assumptions underlying its practice. Anna Holmes provided me with many resources in my study of mental retardation. The thoughts and suggestions of all these people have strengthened the book.

Evalyn and Walter Swartz, my parents, listened with patience verging on masochism to the countless revisions that were made. My husband and children tolerated more than their share of grouchiness as the work went through various stages of ups and downs. To all of them I am grateful. Finally, I wish to thank my steadfast editors, Helen Dietz and Robert Wright, of the W. B. Saunders Company, who surely have the greatest patience of all.

LISA ROBINSON

CONTENTS

chapter 1

PSYCHIATRIC NURSING— WHAT IS IT? WHY STUDY IT?

"I'm so afraid. . . . It's not that I'm going to die. It's, . . . it's
that all the people I know are still going to be here. I'm going to
cease to be. They are all out there. I am alone. Nobody can know
how it feels, but me. It's just all alone. My friends would not know
me anymore. I have lived centuries since I last saw them. The people
who care for me in the hospital are strangers to me. My dying does
not *really* matter to them. They know what is going to happen to me
and after I don't exist any more, they will go on as if I never was.
I feel like I'm about to be engulfed by a huge wave."

The speaker was an 18 year old girl dying from leukemia. She
spoke haltingly, but with immense feeling. Her companion was another
young girl, a nursing student who sat in the hushed room of the leukemic
patient sharing her profound thoughts in the middle of the night. The
student had entered the room because she had heard stifled sobs as
she made her rounds. Once there, she was committed to hearing the
message of this dying girl and to making a meaningful reply.

What does one say to another human being as that person faces
the pressing imminence of death? How does a nurse communicate to
one who is dying that she will not allow that dying person to leave
life anonymously? Is there a need to share the agony of separation?

"I don't believe there is no orange juice in the kitchen. You
really don't like me, do you? That is why you won't bring me the

1

juice. What is it that you hate about me? Why have you been trying
to hurt me since I came here?"

The speaker is a middle-aged woman who has Parkinson's disease.
She has been on the neurological service for evaluation and for treatment with drugs. Though her physical symptoms have been alleviated,
psychological problems have taken their toll; and they are growing
steadily worse. The patient seems to believe firmly that the day nurse
dislikes her to the point of planning vengeful acts against her. What
can the health team do? Will a categoric denial be helpful? Should
the specific nurse be kept away from this patient? Should the patient
be told that her thoughts are not valid, but rather a symptom of
another problem?

> "You know, you are the first person who ever took time to listen
> to me. I feel like you really want to help me. I believe you when
> you say you care about me and so I'm going to give you a chance
> to really help. I need a fix. . . . I need it bad. My guts are on fire."

How can the nurse hearing this drug-addicted youth help him
to realize that she is worthy of his trust even though she does not satisfy
his need for drugs? In what way can she show her willingness to be
of help without actually meeting his felt need?

All these situations require the skills of a sensitive individual who
is capable of hearing both the overt messages and their covert meanings.
Such a knowledgeable person must be able, in turn, to offer replies
that communicate understanding and, hopefully, comfort. To do this,
the nursing student studies the art and science of psychiatric nursing.
In this segment of her education she becomes aware of some of the
bases for her own perceptions of life's experiences; she acquires the
knowledge to understand that all behavior has meaning and that all
human beings are basically more similar than dissimilar. The student
increases her skill in setting realistic goals for herself and in moving
in the direction of her long-term objectives.

As a more skilled observer of her own behavior and its inherent
meaning, the student is able to appreciate the factors that lead others
to perceive life differently than she does. Instances of gross disturbances
in perception lose their mystery and give way to formulations that indicate *why* disturbed people have needed to distort what they perceive.
From her awareness of the meaning of behavior, the nursing student
evolves skills to help others alter their dysfunctional behavior.

Thus, the study of psychiatric nursing has two major foci: The
first is the nursing student herself; the student focuses on herself in
order to better understand those factors which influence her perceptions of self and the world around her. Second, she focuses on patients,
their problems, and the means to modify those problems. Through
the first focus the nursing student gains some of the tools needed for

development of her own potential; through the second she helps others develop their potential.

THE NURSE FOCUSES ON HERSELF

People are very complex. We cannot hope to understand every facet of our own beings even if we undertake extensive analytic therapy; however, some awareness of those forces that make up our personalities is important for nurses who work with patients. A good jumping off point for the voyage into self-exploration might be, "Why did I decide to become a nurse?" or "Why am I feeling frightened about encountering patients with psychiatric problems?" If one is ready to answer such questions honestly, the quest should be interesting and enlightening. Once the beginning is made, further exploration will come naturally. One will quickly see that many things that have been simply *assumed* really have interesting roots. Let us say, for instance, that a nurse realizes that she became a member of the profession because she enjoys caring for human beings; she likes planning and directly administering the type of care that involves touching and comforting—much the same as the attention she received as a child. Perhaps this nurse chose nursing in order to keep alive those warm, secure feelings that she had when others cared for her; only now she is the doer, rather than the recipient.

Let us suppose further that this nurse finds it ungratifying, or even irritating, to care for those patients who are well enough to be relatively independent. Such patients are those who can get out of bed, take tub baths, and ambulate. It may be that this nurse feels inadequate and frustrated when she cannot give total care, when she cannot foster the dependence of her patients upon her. For such a nurse, it would be highly useful to have some knowledge of her difficulty in working with those patients who can assume some responsibility for their own care. Perhaps she would never bother to trace the exact reason for her frustration and resultant irritation; however, if she could become conscious of the difficulty itself, the nurse could make special efforts to work out her problem.

It is only through conscious awareness of a problem that one can begin to study it and attempt to work it out. If one can label a particular set of issues as perplexing, or at least unsatisfying, then one can begin the work of resolution by identifying the components of the problem and trying to manipulate them into a more advantageous pattern.

Let us look at a not unusual situation in which a nursing student is afraid of working with psychiatric patients. What might her reasons be? There are numerous ones offered. Some students are afraid that they will be hurt emotionally. This is not an impossibility, but its like-lihood is small. Could the nurse's underlying reason be fear that she might hurt her patient? Again, this is unlikely because we are more alike than dissimilar, and our words are likely to be heard as friendly or, at worst, fumbling attempts to reach out and make someone feel that our effort to help is sincere.

Perhaps on this quest for self-understanding, the nurse comes to the conclusion that the fear of psychiatric nursing actually represents a fear of the unknown; it is a fear that she will not be able to perform in the new type of setting. Such a feeling is understandable, but again there are other considerations. The individuals that she will encounter who are called "psychiatric patients" are not unique. They are people with emotional problems. They are people who feel disturbed. They are not very different from the emotionally disturbed patients whom the student has cared for in the labor suite and the delivery room undergoing their first experience of childbirth, or the frightened busi-ness men regaining consciousness in intensive or coronary care units after sudden myocardial infarcts. Psychiatric patients are sometimes like the elderly patients who become confused and climb over their bed rails. A few of the psychiatric patients will be people who misinterpret what they hear, feel and see, and, as a result, react inappropriately. In short, "psychiatric" patients are seen in many settings. The nurse com-ing into a psychiatric setting will not be seeing her first psychiatric patient. She will have encountered them in other hospital settings and health agencies.

The nurse who is entering a psychiatric affiliation should have some awareness of her own problems, anxieties and hang-ups. With such knowledge plus an awareness that the patients she is about to encounter will be similar to others she has cared for, and her understanding that the psychiatric patients' problems are not vastly different from her own and those of people close to her, the nurse can try to respond to her psychiatric patients thoughtfully. She will approach her patients as human beings who need help.

It is natural to decide, consciously or otherwise, to defend oneself against pain, and the majority of human beings do this without think-ing or planning. For instance, when one has learned that fire burns, it is a rare instance when a finger or limb is placed in contact with a substance that is burning. We act similarly in terms of psychological pain. For instance, most nurses come into contact with families who are experiencing grief in preparation for, or immediately after, the death of a loved one. As nurses, we try to comfort members of the family. We bring prescribed sedation, we find a room where the family can be alone, we sometimes hold a crying person, trying by our physical presence to be comforting. As we do these things we partially gird our-selves, so that we will not feel the full extent of the family's suffering.

This is good. Were we to permit ourselves the same degree of barrenness, grief and depression as the families involved, we could hardly hope to keep practicing. Our natural defenses are called into play with good reason; they act to blunt our reactions just a bit, to protect us just enough that we are not incapacitatingly injured by what we encounter.

It is important that the nurse "keep in touch." It must be kept in the forefront of her thinking and acting that we human beings are more alike than dissimilar. Thus, when we are being somewhat protective of self by saying about those we care for, "I am different from them" or "Poor things" or "They don't realize what they are doing," we are behaving defensively. Such defensive maneuvering can be antitherapeutic, for if we deny the possibility of being in similar straits ourselves we shut off a useful and spontaneous avenue to understanding. It is quite possible that were the nurse less able to withstand the assaults of daily life, she too might require professional help.

Though such realizations may be frightening at times, they are also potentially helpful to us because we can then approach others with more understanding. If the individual is crying and afraid, we can draw upon our memories of times when we were afraid and cried. We can assume that some of our sensations were similar to those of the person we are now helping. Because of our knowledge of the feelings of fright, we can understand and find useful things to do and say. Thus, the nurse uses herself to begin to search for commonalities that will lead to a more precise understanding of her patient.

THE NURSE FOCUSES ON HER TASK

It cannot be disputed that the practice of nursing has changed radically since its historical beginnings prior to the fifteenth century. Social and economic conditions, as well as medical research and, more recently, nursing research, have combined to influence "eras" of nursing, very much as they have influenced other historical events.

In the last 20 years our knowledge of disease processes has grown at a remarkable rate. New drugs and nonchemical therapies have been developed as a result of painstaking clinical investigation. At the same time, nursing practices have been influenced by the quantities of research data engendered; thus, nursing perspectives have broadened, and new and exciting nursing techniques for delivery of care have been developed.

Psychiatric nursing is no exception to this. Though basic interpersonal skills have not changed, their focus and the responsibilities of the nurse utilizing them have broadened. Therapeutic interaction with sick individuals and their families has been accepted as a nursing function. The nurse today has taken her legitimate place among the other health team members. She is now recognized as an agent of positive value in the planning for and the care of the mentally ill. The nurse is utilized in many settings today in the prevention of mental illness, that is, in the practice of mental hygiene. Nurses have moved far and wide since the days of dungeon-like seclusion cells and camisoles. Nurses have every right to look with pride upon their progress in the historical unfolding of psychiatric nursing; they can regard their membership on the therapeutic team with realistic pleasure and a sense of accomplishment.

The task of the psychiatric nurse has not changed as much in the last two decades as has her freedom to practice and the respect in which her efforts and therapeutic accomplishments are held. Basically the task is, as it always was, to support the patient in the healthy aspect of his personality and to provide a setting in which he can learn healthier or more effective adjustments, thereby altering the pathological elements of his personality. The nurse acts to assist the patient in learning to deal more effectively with the problems of his daily life. She views, as a long-range goal, helping the patient to find the kinds of behavioral patterns that will enable him to act and interact in his community so that he is optimally effective in his working and his social life. This objective is more easily stated than it is described, for it will differ for each individual encountered: the problem of deciding what is "optimally effective" in the social and working spheres for any individual is a difficult and challenging task. It requires becoming familiar with the life of the person being studied. It is not a decision that can be made simply by reading a chart or looking at an agency's records.

The nursing assessment should represent an intimate knowledge of the individual, his community, his talents and his aspirations. It is an evaluation that is made *with* the individual in question and probably with his family, as well. It is a kind of profile that is best arrived at through the help of others on the health team, such as the doctor, psychologist, social worker and others who contribute to the pool of information on the patient. When one is working in an agency, such resource people may be available. Sometimes the nurse must work alone. In such instances she will have to rely on the best rounded picture she can formulate with her patient's help.

The nurse is in a position to make a valuable contribution. She needs to be constantly aware that each patient she encounters in her work is unique. Though the stories she hears and the faces she observes may seem superficially similar, just below the surfaces are a multitude of factors that separate one person from the next. It is these factors that the nurse must seek to clarify. In this way she will soon begin to sketch in the outlines of the individual with whom she works, and the real problems of that person can begin to emerge. The work is exciting and challenging and the nurse can anticipate with pride the outcome of her endeavors.

Psychiatric nursing can be relatively simple; it can become quite complex. An important element of the work is to be able to state goals that are helpful to the patient *and* to define objectives that are appropriate to the nurse's level of preparedness.

At the master's level of preparation the psychiatric nurse will be able to assist her patient by seeking information from and about him in order to develop a working composite of *how* the patient tends to perceive his world. From this the nurse can better understand *why* the patient responds and interacts as he does. The nurse can use herself and groups of whom her patient is a member to demonstrate when the patient has misinterpreted the world around him or when he has not reacted in a manner that adequately communicates his wants, needs or expectations. The psychiatric nurse with advanced preparation can, in selected instances, manipulate her patient's environment so that more effective behaviors are likely to be learned by him.

The nurse prepared at this level has evolved a philosophy of nursing as well as a definition of mental illness which confers upon her a frame of reference within which to work. She has developed these concepts out of a conglomerate of theoretical and clinical knowledge. Such a practitioner has the tools to enable her to act with some independence in the therapeutic relationship; that is, she does not require consistently close supervision.

The nurse in a psychiatric setting who has not had advanced training can also make substantial contributions. She, too, gathers information from and about the patient in order to better understand him. She works under close supervision to identify more effective means for her patient to communicate and interact. She uses herself and groups of patients to this end. The student nurse does not have the fund of knowledge and experience to enable her to choose from a variety of treatment modalities and approaches, but with good supervision she can identify appropriate goals for her patient. She can implement plans to guide the patient in meeting the goals of treatment. Such a nurse is likely to focus the majority of her efforts on augmentation of the psychiatrist's therapy. The nurse with advanced psychiatric training is apt to devote more time to pursuing goals which she identifies as enabling the expansion of the patient's repertoire of behavior.

In the following chapters nurses will find useful suggestions for assisting in the implementation of their nursing objectives. The majority of goals will be reached by talking with patients. It is this simple. Listening carefully to what the patient says, and responding, is the heart of psychiatric nursing. These are the activities that we are all familiar with from an early age; they are a part of communication. We can all perform these tasks. There is little harm we can do by listening and talking. For this reason the beginning psychiatric nurse need have little anxiety. She is using communication skills that were developed long ago. It is these very skills of giving information and receiving other information that will enable her to help people with psychiatric illnesses begin the return to psychological health and useful, effective lives.

UNIQUENESS OF THE PSYCHIATRIC NURSE

In this era when there are so many disciplines represented on the mental health team, such as the psychiatrist, social worker, psychologist, psychiatric aide, and occupational therapist, it is sometimes difficult to find a role that is unique to the nurse. In some settings, work does not seem to be assigned according to levels of competency or role. In such places it is difficult to say "I am a nurse" and have any definite feeling about just what "nurse" is. Again, in other settings, the nurse's role is well differentiated.

In the past 10 years the psychiatric nurse and the social worker have found themselves doing tasks that seem strikingly similar. Some representatives of both groups have begun to explore the possibility that they actually *are do*ing the same kinds of things. There are others who disagree. One study designed to explore this question demonstrated that in the psychiatric setting, when the social worker and the nurse worked as a team, the social worker functioned best with the families of patients; the nurse seemed more comfortable dealing with patients themselves. This indicated that social workers coped best with healthy elements of families; nurses were better prepared to deal with illness.[1]

It is easier to see differences between the roles of the psychiatrist and the nurse. The former is prepared through long years of training to diagnose disease processes, to prescribe chemotherapy and to administer various types of long-range and short-term psychotherapy; the nurse is equipped to assist the patient in finding more effective means of meeting his needs, for attaining his goals in life. Often the nurse, seeing the patient on a daily basis, is in the best position to provide a milieu in which new behavior can be tried. In this way the nurse is nurturing. She is practicing, in a psychiatric setting and in the community, what nurses of the past have always done: the nurse is promoting good mental health by providing a setting in which the patient can experiment with more effective styles of living. However, she is utilizing the most modern, up-to-date nursing techniques as she provides services to her patients in the hospital and in the community.

The nurse has an impressive array of resources to utilize in her efforts to aid the patient. She can call upon the doctor for chemotherapy; she can ask the social worker for help in tapping family and community resources. When the nurse is fortunate enough to be attached to a hospital or agency that utilizes occupational therapy and psychologists, she can expect guidance and assistance in designing a program to promote mental health in her patients. Nonetheless, the nurse remains central in the picture; she is a constant nurturing force in the patient's life.

REFERENCE

1. Anderson, M. M., Glasser, B., and Manning, M. J.: Nursing and Social Work Roles in Cooperative Home Care and Treatment of the Mentally Ill. *Nursing Outlook*, 2 (No. 2) : 112, February, 1963.

SUGGESTED READING

Bettelheim, B.: To Nurse and Nurture. *Nursing Forum*, 1:60-76, Summer, 1962.

Though the writer's primary concern is with pediatric patients, he writes with such fluidity that it is easy to apply his philosophy of nursing to the adult patient. His basic premise is that the nurse is in a position to care for the whole patient, rather than solely attending to his physical problem. Through a clinical example he illustrates the mental agony patients suffer and how they can be helped by the perceptive nurse.

Bojar, S.: The Psychotherapeutic Function of the General Hospital Nurse. *Nursing Outlook*, 6 (No. 3) :151-153, March, 1958.

The visible patient is not the whole patient. The parts we cannot see are the fears and the anxiety due to hospitalization itself, pain, the unknowns of surgery, unconsciousness, and the fear of death. The nurse can help the patient to accept dependency and passivity in order to recover physically. She can give him the mothering care he needs to stop his inner turmoil.

Brill, N.: The Importance of Understanding Yourself. *Am. J. Nursing*, 57 (No. 10) : 1325-1326, 1957.

This is a delightful treatise that discusses the nurse as a human being. The author, a psychiatrist, suggests that nurses' behavior, like patients', is influenced by unconscious motivation and by reality factors. It is well for the nurse to have as firm a grip as she can on these factors, through insight, before she attempts to help patients.

Gregg, D.: The Psychiatric Nurse's Role. *Am. J. Nursing*, 54 (No. 7) :848-851, July, 1954.

This article is certainly a classic for its era. It proposes the role of the psychiatric nurse to be that of creator of an interpersonal environment in which the patient can experience freedom to talk out and, if necessary, act out his problems. The article points out ways that the nurse works towards or hinders this end. It further discusses the necessity of teamwork and how this is accomplished. The article provides a good basis for the beginning student who is primarily concerned with promoting helping relationships on the ward. It is useful historically because the reader can see how far we have come in two decades in movement into the community.

Jacobs, L.: Beginning Practitioner's Adjustment to a Psychiatric Unit. *Nursing Outlook*, 18 (No. 10) :28-31, October, 1970.

Impatience and insecurity are hallmarks of the beginning practitioner's experience. Self-understanding is therapeutic. When this process is underway the nurse can begin to help others. In the early phases of her clinical experience, the nurse uses "coping devices." This is a pertinent and useful article for the new student of psychiatric nursing. The author's description of "coping mechanisms" strikes the reader as real because the author is "telling it like it really is."

Maloney, E.: Does the Psychiatric Nurse have Independent Functions? *Am. J. Nursing,* 62:61-63, June, 1962.

This is an article which discusses from a philosophic point of view the roles of the psychiatric nurse. The article does not purport to enumerate "correct answers," and for the inexperienced nurse it is a poor choice to use for reference material. For the reader who can tolerate uncertainty and the fun of exploration, the material is pleasurable to peruse.

Sinkler, G.: Identity and Role. *Nursing Outlook,* 18 (No. 22):22-24, October, 1970.

This article presents a challenge to the reader to make more congruent her identity and her role. The author, a graduate student in psychiatric nursing, utilizes her observations on a psychiatric ward to illustrate the theme. The article is very interesting, exceedingly valid, but difficult reading for the student who is not clearly interested in the analysis of dynamics.

Tuteur, W.: As You Enter Psychiatric Nursing. *Am. J. Nursing,* 56 (No. 1):72-74, January, 1956.

For the neophyte in psychiatric nursing this article provides a written "guided tour" of the situation about to be embarked upon. It gives a good, basic overview of the world of the psychiatric patient in the typical psychiatric hospital setting. Armed with this information, a new student might feel more comfortable entering the psychiatric affiliation.

Worth, B.: Reflections of a Psychiatric Nurse-Patient. *Perspectives in Psychiatric Nursing,* 7 (No. 2):73-75, 1969.

This is a unique article because it points out how we are more similar than dissimilar. The article does this through the words of a psychiatric nurse who has also been a psychiatric patient. The view of "patienthood" is well described.

BOOKS

Robinson, L.: *Psychological Aspects of the Care of Hospitalized Patients.* Philadelphia, F. A. Davis, 1968.

This very small collection of papers covers many of the problems that the nurse must deal with in her care of patients in the general hospital. It offers some solutions that have been of use to the author in her work as a psychiatric nurse in the general hospital setting.

Skipper, J., and Leonard, R.: *Social Interaction and Patient Care.* Philadelphia, Lippincott Company, 1965.

This is an unusually fine collection of articles dealing with the social and psychological aspects of the nurse's role in the general hospital, the patient's view of his situation, and doctor-nurse-patient relationships. The material in this group of papers tends to be sophisticated but offers the basic student a new and different type of appraisal of her role and position as a nurse.

chapter 2

THE THERAPEUTIC
NURSE-PATIENT
RELATIONSHIP

A human relationship involves people who have something in common: that is, there is an element which is mutual and which draws two or more persons together. In all nurse-patient relationships, it is the patient's problems and the nurse's interest in alleviating the suffering associated with these problems that draws both parties together.

The therapeutic relationship between the psychiatric nurse and the patient is one in which both must work to bring about changes that are deemed appropriate in the patient. Sometimes the nurse changes as well, and the changes in her are regarded as growth. The means of bringing about change is through communication, which is the major component of the working relationship. The therapeutic nurse-patient relationship is the most important tool at the disposal of the psychiatric nurse. In order to use it, however, other elements must be present. These elements include: caring, trust, love and empathy. In a very specific manner, even anxiety is utilized. It is important that the nurse understand the role and functions of each of these elements because they are necessary to the establishment and maintenance of the therapeutic relationship. The quality of this relationship will determine the effectiveness of the therapeutic work done.

One cannot guarantee that the patient will always desire the nurse-patient relationship. People who have been lonely or rejected by others over long periods of time or during their formative years are not always brave enough to risk the possible pain of new human relationships. In such instances, helping the patient to accept another person's concern is a major part of the therapeutic work.

CARING AND PATIENCE

The nurse who enters into a working relationship with a patient must care about the patient if change is to occur. The patient must know that the nurse cares; that she is really interested. There is no standard formula for the communication of caring. Obviously a prerequisite is that the nurse really *does care*. Next, she needs creativity and perseverance in order to devise many ways of communicating her caring; she needs much patience so that she can state and restate her feelings many times. There is probably no field of nursing that can be more frustrating than psychiatric nursing. In this specialty one must be willing to repeat a theme many times, for patterns of psychological illness are learned through repetition, just as are healthy patterns. The· pathological patterns must be, in a sense, *unlearned* before more effective adaptations can be made. Time is usually a big factor in improvement. The nurse cannot afford to look for desired responses immediately. To communicate a sense of caring, to teach another person that he is the object of the nurse's caring, can be a slow, painful, time-consuming process.

Caring is communicated by the genuine interest shown in the patient. It is not difficult to show that one cares in the hospital setting. The visit in which the nurse takes time to sit down in the patient's room indicates that the nurse cares. Sharing a cigarette, a coffee break, or a snack with the patient in a mental hospital shows caring, as does accompanying the patient to activities or going with him for a walk. In the community, caring is shown by meeting with the patient at a designated location. It may be demonstrated by visiting a harried mother in her home on Monday morning and helping her as she begins to do the weekly wash. Caring might mean seeing a working client on his lunch break. Caring is taking time, making an effort for the other person.

Miles was a 22 year old boy diagnosed as paranoid schizophrenic. The graduate student in psychiatric nursing who chose to work with him for 16 weeks was enthusiastic as she launched her effort. She saw Miles twice a week for the first month. At each visit the young man would describe to her, conversationally, the events that had led up to his illness. He spoke easily and repeated his tale effortlessly. Occasionally Miles asked the nurse about her interests and her goals. It was almost one month before the student realized that her patient was really talking *at* her and that little was being accomplished in the time they spent together.

The second month progressed like the first until the third week, when Miles ran away. On coming to the hospital, the nurse was informed that her patient had disappeared. The nurse, truly surprised and concerned, called her patient's home. Miles answered the phone and in response to the nurse's inquiries said that he would very much like to talk to her. She went to his home several days later and met his mother; the three people spent several hours together.

Miles returned to the hospital. When the nurse next saw him there his discussion with her was different. Among other things that he shared with her that reflected great feeling was the statement that he "didn't know she cared." This realization, apparently brought about by the nurse's telephone call and visit, led to the boy's willingness to finally enter into a meaningful relationship with the student, a relationship in which he was able to share many of his painful feelings of rejection, rage and loneliness. The work could not go on, however, until the boy realized that his nurse "really cared."

The nurse can show her interest in a patient, can show that she cares, by meeting with her patient at a *regular, predictable* time. Emotionally ill patients benefit from the security gained from a stable, fixed schedule. Knowing "my nurse" will be at a given place at a given time is highly supportive. Through the patience and caring, the interest shown, and the predictability of one person, the patient can learn to *trust*.

TRUST

One can examine the concept of trust from many vantage points. The baby trusts the mothering one because she does not drop him. She decreases his discomfort when he cries by either offering nourishment or making him warm and dry again. The fortunate child trusts his parents because he is secure in their affections. Additionally, he knows that he can depend on predictable behaviors from them. If mother says she will pick him up at school, the child knows to expect the family car to appear at the appointed hour. The child trusts his parents because they have demonstrated their honesty. When the child angers his parents, as all children do from time to time, he knows that his parents will indicate their feelings to him. Their responses are predictable for him. The trusting child knows that his parents will tell him the truth.

These same expectations must be met by the psychiatric nurse before she can expect her patient to trust her. She must tell the truth; she must do the things she says she will; most basically, she must not violate the being of her patient. The psychiatric nurse must regard her patient as a unique composite of spirit, intellect and feelings that must be nurtured and allowed to grow. Violation of this ethic through neglect, aggression or misguided commitment is sufficient grounds for the stifling of trust.

Learning to trust in the therapeutic relationship is often a difficult lesson. The most effective teachers are those who can be infinitely patient and predictable in their movements. They are the nurses who are not hasty in judgments or the making of decisions.

The nurse who hopes to establish an effective working relationship with her patient tries to promote trust. An important element in a trusting relationship is one's knowledge that the other person will permit exploration and growth. As a nursing student, the reader may recall that a comfortable milieu for learning was evident when an instructor permitted the student to question and to experiment with various approaches to nursing problems. The student may also recall that the effective teacher was one who was not overly critical. She permitted the student sufficient latitude in her thoughts and activities so that the student could "digest" new material at a speed that was comfortable and appropriate for her.

The learning situation for the patient is similar. The nurse who attempts to be therapeutic is, in part, teaching the patient new behavior patterns. She permits the patient to learn because she provides an environment in which learning can occur. Such an environment is created when the patient recognizes that he can "be"; that is, the patient may behave as he feels necessary in order to express himself as he experiences self at that point in time. For one patient that may mean being able to lie curled up on the floor, nude, behind a wooden bench; for another, it may be telling the nurse that he questions the usefulness of their therapeutic relationship because he questions the nurse's motives in choosing to work with him. For a third patient, the freedom to express self could be sitting outside alone, just thinking, or perhaps drawing, in preference to attending a scheduled activity.

The role of the nurse in establishing trust is one of acceptance. If the nurse can permit the patient to express himself through verbal and nonverbal language, if she can acknowledge that she has received and understood the message and, most important, if she can respond *nonjudgmentally* to that message, she will be demonstrating her acceptance of the patient. This process fosters trust. The patient can then examine other areas of his self that have been unacceptable to him or to significant others.[1, 2] With the support of a nurse who will tolerate even "intolerable" facets of his personality, the patient can take a more candid look at himself. Because he has the luxury of time, and a helpmate who, though reactive, will not respond automatically to him (as the significant others in his past life may have), he can decide which of the identifiable parts of himself he finds acceptable, and which facets of self he will commit his efforts to altering.

The work of the nurse-patient relationship cannot commence until the element of trust has been established. It is only then that the patient can safely divulge himself.

LOVE

The nurse who is effective in working with patients must be able to *feel* a variety of emotions. One of them is that positive, warm feeling that is generally called *love*. It is a feeling that does not necessarily signify the emotion that one feels toward a lover; nor does it have to be that emotion one feels for a parent, or one's child. Love is a difficult feeling to define. Human beings feel it in response to many different people in a variety of situations. The feeling of love is a positive one in regard to the love object. It can be sexual, or not, depending again on the love object. In the nurse-patient relationship the feeling of love usually involves a warm, positive regard for the patient. It enables the nurse to respond to the needs of the patient in a consistent, interested, helpful manner. Warm positive feelings motivate the nurse to assist the patient in moving from a dependent position to an independent one in which he, having acquired new behavioral skills such as trust, can function without the nurse's support.

EMPATHY

The ability to empathize involves skill in reaching out and trying to understand the thoughts and feelings of others. It is the ability to feel *with* the patient. Though empathic feelings are necessary in effective nursing, it must be understood that the nurse may easily misunderstand her intuitive feelings regarding the patient and really be responding to her own feelings. Such a situation is called projecting. It is a common problem for people who try to help others and it is one that can create great difficulties.

> Mrs. Winthrop, a second year nursing student in a community college, had had poliomyelitis as a child. She remembered vividly her own feelings of frustration and anger when her mother had put on her leg brace every morning. As Mrs. Winthrop helped her patient, a 30 year old mother of four children, into her leg brace, the nursing student relived her own feelings of the past and she sympathized with the woman before her. Mrs. Winthrop felt, again, the childhood pangs of rejection as the neighborhood youngsters stole quick glances at her steel and leather "prison." She knew again the childhood shame she had felt because in her fantasies she had leaped and twirled for an appreciative father, but when he actually appeared, she could only limp and drag her weakened limb toward him.
> Reliving these memories, Mrs. Winthrop wondered how to comfort the young mother before her. The nurse was so involved in her own feelings that she was unaware that the patient's real concerns were for her children and their care while she was hospitalized.

In this case, the nursing student missed an opportunity to help her patient. She projected her own feelings into the situation and onto the patient so that she did not maintain the open communications that would have given her access to the patient's true concerns.

> In the following situation, Mary, a high school student, and Miss Brown, the school nurse, are observed as they meet after Mary's classes end. They are talking together in the nurse's office.

"Some mornings I just can hardly get out of bed. I don't understand what is wrong with me. I just feel sort of tired and heavy. It's
a strange feeling. It's like I've done a day's wash and cleaned the
house for grandmother and then gone out with the gang. I'm just
beat before I even start."

Miss Brown listened carefully. She did not speak immediately.
Finally, she said, "You sound tired and discouraged. The heaviness
you described sounds like you must feel like you're carrying the
weight of the world around with you."

Mary nodded. Her shoulders were hunched and she slumped
dejectedly in the chair. "It's awful. I just feel so low."

The nurse could almost feel Mary's discouragement; she was
aware of a weighty, oppressive quality in the room. She recognized
that Mary's words and feelings created this sensation. The nurse
said, "You must be very depressed."

In this case, Miss Brown had listened carefully. As Mary described
her feelings, the nurse could appreciate them, and she was aware of
the oppressiveness of the girl's condition. Because Miss Brown could
understand and feel with the high school student, she could identify
the feelings of her patient. Now they were ready to explore why Mary
experienced these uncomfortable feelings. Miss Brown had utilized her
empathic skills wisely.

Empathy is an invaluable tool in nursing. It is like a powerful
drug; to be useful, the dosage must be regulated carefully—too much
can harm the patient, too little is ineffectual. The nurse must be aware
of her feelings so that she can recognize whether they reflect those of
the patient, or are reactions of the nurse herself and stem from experiences outside the current situation. Also, the nurse needs to be sufficiently in control of her feelings so that she can continue to help
the patient.

FEELINGS OF ANGER, ANNOYANCE OR DISLIKE

Like other human beings, nurses have feelings. At times they
experience anger, jealousy, outrage, indignation or repugnance. As
with the nurse's positive feelings, her negative ones cannot be evaluated;
they simply exist.

Sometimes the nurse will choose to communicate her feeling to
the patient. She should do so when she is certain that her response
is to *him* and not to others in her own past whom the patient may
resemble. She communicates her feelings when she is certain that they
do not stem from her own anxiety. Above all, the nurse does not
communicate her negative feeling unless she thinks the patient is sufficiently mature to understand that the feeling is in response to one
aspect of his behavior, not to *him* as a total person.

The writer recalls a fifty year old syphilitic male who resided on
a ward in one of the chronic cottages of the state hospital. This

patient was short, very fat, and had no neck to speak of. He waddled about and embraced any females he could catch. As he embraced them, he put his hands under their skirts and began reaching toward their genitals. "Thunderbird," as he was known, was extremely psychotic, and communication with him was all but impossible. The majority of the staff were repelled by this hapless man with tertiary syphilis. Such feelings are easily understood, and one does not have to analyze in depth to identify the origins of the feelings. In cases like this, it would be without meaning to communicate one's reaction to the patient. Nonetheless, the nurse's feeling is a valid one.

The nurse communicates her negative feeling to the patient because she has a therapeutic objective in mind. It is generally one of providing feedback to the patient concerning the effect of his behavior. In any such transaction, basic trust in the therapeutic relationship is reinforced because the nurse indulges in the same, sometimes painful, self-disclosure that she asks of her patient and she enables him to perceive her more adequately. Hopefully, the patient sees, also, that "socially unacceptable" feelings can actually be handled within the relationship.

ANXIETY AS A PART OF THE THERAPEUTIC NURSE-PATIENT RELATIONSHIP

Anxiety is an interesting phenomenon. At times it causes one to feel mild unrest. In some instances the anxious person experiences feelings bordering on panic. Anxiety is a feeling of unrest that is experienced without a clear point of reference; this is to say, the individual is not clearly aware of the cause of his feeling. Put another way, anxiety is triggered from internal danger; fear arises in response to danger external to the individual.

Internal danger is a threat to the identity of the individual. It is difficult to recognize the source because it comes from within each person and is peculiar to him. Thus, for one person, anxiety might be engendered in the face of an examination. The true source of the anxiety, i.e., the internal danger, might be the student's possible loss of self-esteem if he did not do well. For him a great value is placed on intelligence and achievement.

For a socially oriented girl, anxiety might be aroused if acne appeared suddenly just prior to a dance. Such a person might be threatened by the presence of skin blemishes which, to her, would indicate a loss of beauty. In both instances it is the individual's own values and the threats to them that represent the internal danger.

External danger which causes fear is more easily recognized. The sight of a fast-moving car bearing down on a pedestrian creates fear in him. He is responding to the danger of being hit by the car. Such an outcome represents disaster to his physical self. In this case, the danger (the car) is external.

It is clear that both nurse and patient bring many feelings to the relationship that they share. The fun, the challenge, is to understand as well as possible the complex set of feelings that are present between nurse and patient at any time as they interact. The nurse aids the patient in using these feeling interactions to change his behavior patterns. At any time during the relationship, anxiety is likely to be felt by one member or the other, or both.

The nurse who understands herself in terms of her own major problems and who is sufficiently "in touch" with her feelings can use herself as an instrument to detect the presence of anxiety. It may happen that the nurse is comfortable and content within herself. Then she initiates some activity with a patient. Suddenly the same nurse is aware of feelings of vague restlessness and discomfort; she identifies her experience as anxiety.

In the nurse-patient relationship, the nurse's awareness of the sudden presence of anxiety in herself is useful since it provides a clue. The nurse may then wonder what these new feelings represent. Why did they arise? Are they symptomatic of the patient's feelings? Are they anxious feelings that have spread contagiously? If the patient cannot identify feelings of anxiety within himself, is it possible that the nurse is responding to something more personal, to some element within herself? Often the nurse will not be able to identify the source of her anxiety. At times she and the patient will not be able to arrive at a meaningful conclusion regarding the patient's anxiety. This should not disappoint either nurse or patient. Frequently time is needed to work through the exploration of feelings. It is likely that eventually one party or the other will say: "Remember last week when we were talking about feeling so uncomfortable. I think I know why. . . ." And often the explanation will be correct. It is valuable to understand the sources of anxiety; however, it is not always possible. Being aware that one's feelings represent anxiety is a very valuable step, for without the ability to identify one's feelings, one cannot be aware that a problem exists, and therefore the steps one should undertake to explore the problem would not be initiated.

SUPPORTING THE PATIENT

One hears over and over that the appropriate nursing therapy is to "support" the patient. More often than not the term is used in the vaguest sense. It is not indicated *what* is to be supported exactly, or *how* the nurse should go about the task. The nurse can perform very adequately in giving "support" to the patient. It is only necessary to define what facet of the patient has to be supported. Usually support is given to the effective, productive parts of a personality. This means that those techniques a person has developed for getting along in the world, the mechanisms that effectively enable him to live his daily life comfortably, are to be encouraged. Thus, the young, yet distrustful drug addict, making his first tentative steps toward a constructive relationship, must have his efforts encouraged. He will need to see that the nurse really wants to respond to him because she finds him worthy of her attention and respect. Doubtless it will be difficult for him to comprehend her attitude, especially because she does not totally gratify his needs. The nurse will indicate her interest in him as a person. At the same time she will let him know that she cannot supply him with drugs because she does not think this will ultimately be of value to him. The nurse supports this patient by communicating her interest in him. She encourages his tentative movement toward another human being by listening and being receptive to the information he gives about himself. She might support this new trend in his behavior even further by offering, in turn, some information about herself. Such a message might communicate her awareness that her refusal to supply a "fix" will be frustrating and anger-provoking, but that she hopes he can ultimately approach her again and share more of his thoughts and feelings.

MEETING THE PATIENT'S NEEDS

The nurse is involved eight hours a day in meeting the needs of others. Very likely she is meeting some of her own at the same time. Every person has needs all the time. The age, phase of development, and life situation of an individual influence his needs and the route of their attainment. The infant needs warmth, food and security. The adult also has needs. In addition to his basic biological needs he needs self-esteem, recognition, a sense of belonging. The adult needs license to depend on others and to be independent. He may need the gratification of one position at a point in time and shortly thereafter require the other stance. Dependence-independence needs are determined by the life situation and the individual's physical and mental resources. The infant must depend on his environment to meet his needs. The adult is likely to be able to provide for some of his own needs; others will be met by his spouse, his children and his business and social acquaintances. It is evident that human "needs" are physical and psychological entities that help to keep the individual alive and in balance. The term "to meet needs" means to provide these factors which are necessary to the organism's well-being.

It will be heard often by the nurse that "all behavior is meaningful." This fact is related to human needs, for the active individual utilizes behavior to communicate a need to others, or to meet the need himself. Thus, much of the nurse's time will be spent attempting to understand behavior, to decipher the communication, to "get the message." It is an indication of mental health when an individual can clearly communicate his needs to others.

Any nurse who has worked in a general hospital setting is familiar with the patient who uses the call signal constantly. What is the patient saying? She asks for water, the bedpan, or something for pain; she may request help in changing positions. Her light is on most of the observing nurse's shift. Each demand is met. Yet the nurse still senses a definite restlessness in this patient. Here is a typical situation in which communication is not open and effective. The nurse must try to understand her patient's behavior. In the numerous demands and the constant bell cord activity will be found the "real" message. It says, "I am afraid, stay with me" or "I am lonely; comfort me." Perhaps the patient cannot make these statements aloud. She may not be totally aware of her real feelings; if she is aware of them, it is likely that she considers them, and thinks others will consider them, childish and unacceptable. Thus, it is the responsibility of the nurse to understand the patient's hidden message if she is really to be of service. This is not always an easy assignment, but it is fun and challenging.

PHASES OF THE NURSE-PATIENT RELATIONSHIP

Various factors which contribute to the effective nurse-patient relationship have been described. The actual process of establishing the relationship cannot be taught, for this process is a dynamic one which cannot occur according to rules. The process involves people, and human beings do not act and react in a prescribed manner that can be described, as, for instance, a chemical reaction. However, we can attempt to portray the nurse-patient relationship as a three-phase process.

The first phase occurs as the people involved become acquainted. This is the time when the nurse tells the patient who she is and what she hopes to accomplish with him. In this phase, which can be quite long, depending on how trusting and how ready the patient is for help, the nurse tries to get to know her patient; the patient also begins to get acquainted with the nurse. Factors such as open communication, acceptance and caring are important for the establishment of a trusting relationship.

Mr. James, a nursing student, was on his psychiatric affiliation for three months at State Hospital. With his instructor he selected a patient with whom he wished to work. He visited the patient's ward for several hours every day and joined the patient at activities.

Mr. James talked with many other patients but tried to spend some part of every visit with the patient he had chosen. At the end of the second week, the nursing student joined the patient outside to smoke a cigarette. He said, "Miss T., I have been here for several weeks now. I think you probably remember that I am Mr. James, a nursing student. I am going to be here for three months and I'd like to spend part of every day with you."

Miss T. smiled vaguely. She flicked the ashes from her cigarette and focused her gaze in space. Mr. James watched her closely. "I shall be here until December 13th, Miss T., and I hope to spend the time between 9 and 10 A.M. with you on Monday, Wednesday and Friday. We can talk about whatever you want. We can take walks or go to the gym or perhaps to other places on the grounds."

Miss T. nodded almost imperceptibly and moved away. Mr. James did not follow her, for he knew that she had heard him and was fearful. He would return in two days and begin again.

Mr. James initiated his relationship with thoughtfulness and care. He told the patient *who* he was, *what* he hoped to do, and *when* he planned to do it, including the date that he would have to leave. The nursing student knew that his patient probably was aware of his identity, but Mr. James did not leave this to chance. He also recognized that his statements were overwhelming and frightening for Miss T. to cope with, so he did not press the matter, but left her with only as many details as she seemed able to handle. It is likely that with a frightened patient like Miss T., who is very ill, attaining the goals of the first phase of the nurse-patient relationship will require all of the time permitted Mr. James in his psychiatric affili-ation. The main objective, creating a trusting relationship, is thera-peutic in itself for this kind of patient, whose illness is, in part, her inability to trust others. Therefore, while Mr. James will probably not get into the areas of *why* his patient cannot trust others, which would be the second phase of the relationship, he deserves much credit and should feel a great sense of accomplishment if, when he leaves his psychiatric affiliation, he has provided Miss T. with a situa-tion in which she can begin to explore the possible behavior involved in trusting another person.

When the first phase is completed, the nurse and patient begin the next or "working" phase of their relationship. This is an exciting time for both. As the name implies, this is the period when the patient's problems can best be discussed and, hopefully, modified. If the first phase has been effective, the second is likely to progress well. The initial phase is like the carefully poured cement foundation of a house. It is likely that a strong "house" can be built if the foundation is strong and the "bricks" of knowledge are placed upon it with care.

The reader may recall the interaction between Mary and the school nurse. When Mary began meeting with the nurse on a regular basis, this represented the beginning of the second or working phase. In this period, nurse and patient discussed many of Mary's concerns.

The third phase, the period of terminating the relationship, occurs when nurse and patient decide together that their work is ready to end and they begin planning for this goal. The third phase is usually not so long as the first or second. When possible, it is good to prepare for it from the very beginning.

THE OBJECTIVES OR END RESULTS OF THE NURSE-PATIENT RELATIONSHIP

Just as the steps for establishing the nurse-patient relationship cannot be described with precision because the principals are human beings rather than chemicals which interact and react in a predictable manner, so the end results of any relationship cannot be prescribed in any manner that can be guaranteed to be complete. The reason, again, is that the nurse is working with other human beings whose health problems are similar in some ways and uniquely dissimilar in others. This factor is one that makes psychiatric nursing exciting and challenging for the creative nurse. Each patient must be approached as an individual.

Within the uniqueness of the therapeutic relationship that the nurse and the patient create, the latter will be helped to acquire more effective behavior patterns to replace those representing the pathological aspects of his personality. For some patients such behavior patterns might be represented by the ability to speak directly to another, to make his needs known through literal speech, or to request to be left alone. All these behaviors indicate that the patient has sufficient self-esteem that he feels comfortable communicating to others about his inner self. For some patients such behavior patterns might be represented by the ability to eat with others, to take part in group activities, or even to act as spokesman for a group in ward meetings. These behaviors indicate that the patient is aware of his need to belong and can take action to meet that need.

The outcomes of the therapeutic nurse-patient relationship are as varied as the people who take part in it. All that can be identified as universal is that the therapeutic relationship will bring about constructive change and growth in the participants.

REFERENCES

1. Pearce, J., and Newton, S.: *Conditions of Human Growth*. New York, Citadel Press, Inc., 1963.
2. Sullivan, H. S.: *The Interpersonal Theory of Psychiatry*. New York, W. W. Norton and Company, Inc., 1953.

SUGGESTED READING

Hoffman, G.: The Concept of Love. *Nurs. Clin. N. Amer.*, 4 (No. 4) :663-672, December, 1969.

This article is a "must" for practicing nurses or those who plan to become professional nurses. It discusses the undeniable need of both patient and nurse to feel the powerful, positive responses that we call love.

Holmes, M. J.: What's Wrong with Getting Involved? *Nursing Outlook*, 8:250-251, 1960.

Much psychiatric jargon is confusing and even contradictory. Student are told to "communicate with patients, understand their needs, don't get involved. Get close but stay away." The author advocates a professional relationship that is warm and gentle and tender, one in which the nurse maintains an awareness of her own emotions and involvement in the situation.

Jensen, H., and Tillotson, G.: Dependency in the Nurse-Patient Relationship. *Am. J. Nursing*, 61 (No. 2) :81-84, 1961.

Three patients are described. Each case illustrates a need communicated by the patient through, seemingly, inappropriate behavior. As long as the nurse did not understand the patient's communication, a nontherapeutic atmosphere prevailed. When the nurse accepted the patient's behavior, understood his need, and met it, positive changes were noted in the patient's behavior.

Kachelski, M. A.: The Nurse-Patient Relationship. *Am. J. Nursing,* 61 (No. 5) :76-81, 1961.

A detailed report is presented of 10 days' work involving a psychiatric nurse and her patient, a 23 year old girl. The article permits the reader to observe a skilled interviewer as she works to decrease the patient's anxiety and to encourage her communication.

Rohweder, A.: Can Love, Compassion, and Involvement Be Scientific? *Nurs. Clin. N. Amer.,* 4 (No. 4) :701-708, December, 1969.

This is "must" reading for every student of psychiatric nursing, as well as every thinking practitioner. The author, using well chosen words, coupled with her incisive philosophy, cuts through the mountain of words at the clinician's disposal and leads us to the core of the nursing problem. She is helpful. She is optimistic. Her article should not be missed.

Schmahl, J.: The Psychiatric Nurse and Psychotherapy. *Nursing Outlook,* 10 (No. 7) : 460-465, July, 1962.

In a rather lengthy and erudite presentation, Schmahl explores the role and functions of the psychiatric nurse. Her conclusion is that the nurse can conduct herself in a therapeutic situation without losing her identity as a nurse. The article is particularly interesting, but may be a difficult one for the casual reader.

Zderad, L.: Empathic Nursing—Realization of a Human Capacity. *Nurs. Clin. N. Amer.,* 4 (No. 4) :655-662, December, 1969.

This presentation provides a very detailed analysis of the concept, empathy. The content of the article is excellent; however, for the unsophisticated reader the material may be awesome.

BOOK

Schwing, G.: *A Way to the Soul of the Mentally Ill.* (Translated by Rudolf Ekstein and Bernard Hall.) New York, International Universities Press, 1954.

This small, unimposing looking volume will stand out in the novice's memory as one of the literary experiences that really presented psychiatric nursing. The author is a psychiatric nurse with a background in analysis. She discusses her approaches to severely disturbed patients. The book is not a text. It does not advocate any particular "procedure" or "therapeutic approach." Rather, it is a tender message describing how one caring, empathic individual has reached "the soul of the mentally ill." It is "must" reading.

chapter 3

COMMUNICATION AND INTERVIEWING

Human beings relieve their basic state of aloneness by communicating, and this process results in relatedness. One might envision relatedness as the solid facing of a brick wall: communication would be represented by the mortar that holds the bricks together. It is not possible to have relatedness without some form of communication. Human beings come closer together by expressing to one another what their "beings" are. This is done by sharing perceptions of self and the mutual world. All these communications affect both the persons expressing themselves—the senders of messages—and the persons hearing them—the receivers.

Talking and listening are not the only means of communication. Messages are given through body movements, posture and tonal quality. According to Ruesch, "Communication embraces all the modes of behavior (verbal and nonverbal) that one individual employs, consciously or unconsciously, to affect another."[1]

The art of communication is initiated early in life. The newborn infant begins to express himself when he cries out, releasing his tensions, which are generated by hunger or other painful stimuli. In crying he communicates his state of distress to a mothering one who responds by taking measures to decrease his discomfort. In this way the infant, unknowingly, protects himself from physical distress. The young child, adept at communicating his physical needs, learns to express his desire and need for security by behaving in such a way that attention is turned toward him. Thus, he is protected from both physical and psychological danger. The adult, though more mature than the child, still needs security. He shuns psychological danger, i.e., isolation, by finding some means of communicating his needs and wishes to other human beings.

Communication, the art of sending messages from one person to another or to and from groups of people, is the very heart of psychiatric nursing therapy. It is the task of the nurse to understand the patient's communications and to make sure that the patient understands the message that is returned to him. This is not always easy, because the words used to communicate with, or the body language, may have different meanings for the person sending and the person receiving the message.

Consider the word "flag." One individual hearing the word may think of a piece of cloth flying from a pole. Another person may think of a long-stemmed purple flower, otherwise known as an iris. Still a third person might hear "flag" and immediately think of his native country and patriotism. Consider the shrug of a shoulder. To one observer, the action might represent a message of not caring. To another, it might communicate a snub, and to still a third person, such a body motion might indicate one of the involuntary muscular movements that all experience periodically. Communication, verbal or nonverbal, that is, spoken or not spoken, is complex. People involved in social relationships tend to assume that their messages are understood, i.e., that sender and receiver agree on the meaning of a particular message. For those at a party, in the dormitory, or casually at play, this is sufficient. In a therapeutic relationship, such an assumption is not enough. One of the differences between a social and a therapeutic relationship is that in the latter, attention is paid to making the understanding of all communication mutual; such understanding is not left to chance.

The psychiatric nurse sends her message to the patient in verbal or body language by using symbols (words or behavior) that she has reason to believe the patient will understand. She does not consider the communication cycle complete until she receives feedback from her patient indicating that the message has been understood. (The reader should be aware that understanding and acceptance are not synonymous. Thus, the patient can *understand without accepting* and, conversely, may *accept without truly understanding.*)

ELEMENTS OF COMMUNICATION

OPENNESS

An important factor in the sending and receiving of messages between nurse and patient is that the parties involved should feel free to communicate that which is important to them. This is called "open communication." The nurse working in a community agency sees examples of this when she greets a young mother in a well-baby clinic. During the time allotted to weighing the infant and discussing problems associated with the child's care, the alert and empathic nurse may hear about mother's fears that another pregnancy may start too soon, or of the need for contraceptive advice. The nurse who creates an environment in which the patient can speak of the *real concerns* of the moment is providing a setting in which comprehensive care can be a reality. The need for open communication is not confined to the psychiatric patient.

Consider the preoperative patient who is being prepared for surgery the following morning. The nurse who is promoting open communication will not chatter at length about topics that the patient has not initiated. She will present herself as Mrs. B., a nurse who will help to prepare the patient for his operation. The nurse need not appear somber, but a neutral or friendly demeanor is preferable to a gay, bubbling attitude that does not permit the patient to express his true feelings. He may feel obligated to maintain a cheerful social facade such as the nurse has presented.

Given the opportunity, the preoperative patient will frequently ask questions regarding his surgery, describe his fantasies, and express his fears. Permitting open communication allows the patient to learn about his anticipated experience. It allows him to identify his feelings about it and to attempt to cope with them.

> Mrs. R. a 45 year old housewife was admitted to General Hospital for a breast biopsy. She had noticed the mass in her breast two weeks prior to admission and had made an appointment with her family physician, who had referred her to a surgeon.
>
> When the evening nurse came into Mrs. R's room to "prep" her for the operation, she found Mrs. R. curled up in bed with her back to the door.
>
> "Hello, Mrs. R. I'm your nurse, Miss Walters, and I'm going to get you ready for your operation," she said, as she put the prep tray on the dresser.
>
> Mrs. R. turned over. She looked at the nurse and smiled. "Oh, hello. How are you?"
>
> Miss Walters smiled and said, "Fine, thank you. I'm going to roll the bed down flat and ask you to lie on your back." The patient complied. "Good. Now what I'm going to do is wash your breast with this green soap. It's cold. . . . Then I'm going to shave your breast with a safety razor."
>
> Mrs. R. looked apprehensive. While the nurse did not scrutinize her patient's expression minutely, she did notice that Mrs. R. looked worried. The nurse said nothing as she swabbed the patient's breast. Several minutes passed. The nurse was mindful of the value of silences and so she did not initiate a conversation. Mrs. R. asked hesitantly, "Is my operation dangerous?"

"No," said the nurse. "It is really a diagnostic procedure to help the doctor to determine what is in your breast tissue."

"Do you think I could die?" asked Mrs. R., trying to control her quivering jaw.

The nurse knew that she was faced with a difficult problem. Her patient was anxious and asking the kind of question that required a careful answer; the patient was asking for reassurance. Miss Walters knew that she needed to reassure her patient, but to do so in an honest way and in a manner that allowed the communication to continue. She stopped shaving the patient's breast and looked at Mrs. R's face as she spoke quietly.

"I don't think it is likely, Mrs. R. The operation you will have tomorrow is not life threatening; but I can understand your fears. Can you tell me more about your feelings?"

Mrs. R. began to cry. She sobbed as she told the nurse about her fear of not waking up. She talked about the possibility that she might have cancer. Miss Walters listened quietly. She did not interrupt the patient or try to stop her crying. When Mrs. R. had become quieter the nurse said, "I can understand your fears and anxieties. Many patients feel as you do about their operations. Perhaps I can tell you a bit concerning what will happen tomorrow and this will relieve some of your fears."

The patient nodded and tried to smile as Miss Walters handed her a tissue and began to tell her of the routine events which occur on the day of one's operation.

Miss Walter's care of her patient was very good. She prepared Mrs. R. both physically and mentally for her operation. The nurse was able to give psychological care because she was sensitive to her patient's distress. She allowed Mrs. R. to verbalize, that is, to talk about her fears. The nurse permitted communications to remain open. She gave Mrs. R. the opportunity to say what was really on her mind. Once this was done, the nurse was in a position to know how Mrs. R. felt. She could reassure her because she was able to respond to the patient's real concerns. Miss Walters was able to help this patient by describing to her the course that events would take the following day. While this information could not allay all the patient's anxieties, it did make her feel more in control of the situation because she knew what to expect. Thus, one can see that open communications is important in many areas of nursing.

In the following example the nurse again creates an environment in which important issues can be explored.

"Hello, Miss S. I have a few minutes and thought I'd like to spend them with you. May I rub your back?"

"I'd love it," said the patient, "but I know how busy you are."

"Not at all. I really want to." The nurse got the alcohol and powder from the bathroom. Miss S. did not speak as the nurse began to slowly knead the skin around her shoulders. "You've been here a while. How are things coming?"

The patient mumbled into her pillow. "O.K." Again, a long silence followed. The nurse continued quietly with the back rub.

"Do you think I can ever have a baby with only one ovary?"
The nurse asked, "Is this a concern of yours?"
"Yes."
"What information have you gathered about it?"
The patient said that she had asked the surgeon and he had said she could become pregnant. There was another silence which was finally broken by the patient. "What man is going to marry me when he discovers I've had all this surgery and have only one ovary?"
"How do you feel about it?" asked the nurse quietly.
"I feel like half a woman. I'm a freak. No man is going to want me."
"It sounds to me as if you feel very bad about yourself in relation to your operation. . . . Do you suppose everyone else will feel the same way you do?"

In this situation, the nurse provided a milieu in which the patient felt comfortable blurting out her hidden feelings. The nurse's readiness to spend time, her quietness and perhaps the calming effect of her touch motivated the patient to talk concerning her fears.

FLEXIBILITY

Flexibility is important in the nurse's communication. She must be able to send her messages in a form that the patient can understand. For one patient the best form may be speech. For another, body language may be more understandable. The nurse in a general hospital setting is likely to find that she can most often convey warmth and caring through touch.

TIMING

Another aspect of communication is timing. In a social relationship the speaker is apt to send messages without much thought as to timing, unless he is attempting to be dramatic or amusing. Both the actor and the comedienne use timing to enhance their communications. The nurse in a therapeutic relationship should pace her communications. This means that she sends her message slowly if she knows that her patient (the receiver) must think or take in (receive) stimuli slowly. This means, also, that she gives the patient plenty of time to understand the message and to make a response to it. Conversely, a rapid expletive may emphasize a necessary message most effectively.

APPROPRIATENESS

In order for communication to be appropriate, it must be understandable, it must say what the sender means, it must fit the circumstance, and it must reflect the sender's chronological level of development. To be understandable, communication must utilize language which has meaning to both sender and receiver. For the patient, this means using words and body movements which are understandable to him. For the nurse the utilization of meaningful language requires close observation of the receiver to find out the kinds of words or actions that have meaning for him. Thus the nurse might normally request a newly admitted patient to please urinate in the proffered receptacle so that she might collect an admission specimen. If she listened to the way her patient expressed himself, however, she might conclude that the word "urinate" would not be understood, as would be the phrase "pass your water." Likewise, the nurse might be tempted to point out to an increasingly agitated patient that he "appeared to be becoming more anxious"; however, if that patient had referred to the process as being "possessed by the demons," it would be more understandable to that patient if the nurse used similar language.

In the following example the patient is sending an inappropriate message because the verbal content is belied in the nonverbal message.

> The patient greeted the nurse at the opened front door. "I'm so glad that you could come today." The patient stood with her arms extended, blocking entry. One hand was on the door knob, the other leaned against the door frame. She smiled through tightly clenched teeth.

In the next example, inappropriateness is again demonstrated.

> The nurse has come to visit her patient in the latter's home. The patient is on leave from the hospital because her mother has died unexpectedly.
> Nurse: I wanted to visit you, Joann, because I have been thinking about you and wondering how you are doing in this very sad and trying time.
> Joann: Gee, I am glad you came. It's been so cool out and the autumn leaves are gorgeous.

In this exchange the patient's statements do not fit the circumstances. In addition, they are not relevant to the initial comments made by the nurse.

> In the last example, the patient, an eight year old boy who is in traction because of a fractured femur, has just thrown his lunch tray to the floor. The nurse had entered the room after hearing the clang and clatter.
> "What happened, Tommy?"
> "I hate peas. I told the aide not to bring me peas. I won't eat them. I won't."
> The nurse stoops over and begins to pick up the tray and its contents.
> "Well, . . . what are you going to do?" asks the boy.
> "Nothing. What is there to do?"
> The little boy looks concerned. "Are you angry at me?"
> "I am rather disappointed in you, Tommy. I think you can behave better than this and make your wants known without throwing your tray around this way."

In this example, a frustrated eight year old boy has expressed his feelings in a regressed manner. His behavior has been more typical of a one to two year old who often plays with his food and displays his pleasure and displeasure in it by throwing or smearing it. The nurse has indicated that she understands Tommy's message and that she is confident of his ability to communicate at a higher level, i.e., that his mode of expression has been inappropriate for his age. She has also been careful to indicate that, though she believes he can communicate his frustrations more appropriately, she will not punish him for the behavior he has utilized.

INTERVIEWING

Interviewing is a goal-directed method of communication. It is a process that is used in the nurse-patient relationship to give and to gain information. Because the nurse-patient relationship may extend for some time, the goals which the nurse has originally formulated may be modified. Therefore, the purposes of the interview will vary from time to time. At one time the interview may be used to elicit pertinent historical data or to give orienting information. This is the case in the first phase of the relationship when the nurse is focusing on getting to know her patient and on having him become acquainted with her in order to establish a trusting relationship.

In the second, or working, phase of the relationship, it is most common to find the nurse using interviewing to provide an opportunity for the patient to talk about his feelings, that is, to *ventilate*. This is helpful because it releases tension. Another purpose for the interview is often demonstrated in the third, or terminating, phase of the nurse-patient relationship in which interviewing is utilized to help the patient in understanding and resolving his own problems and feelings. Interviewing techniques assist the patient in becoming more independent and consequently more able to live effectively without professional help.

Interviewing is communication through the mode of speech. While the meaning of the sender's message is important in terms of his choice of words, the receiver does gather additional data through the sender's tone of voice, facial expression and body movements. In the following example, note both the verbal message and the interviewee's body position and gestures.

> The scene is the dayroom of a state hospital ward. A boy sits on a couch. Beside him, in a chair, sits the nurse.
>
> Nurse: I'd like to spend a half hour with you today, Jim. Would that be okay?
>
> Patient: (After some silence.) Why not? (He does not look at the nurse, but shrugs his shoulders as he speaks.)
>
> Nurse: You've looked pretty down in the dumps since the weekend. . . . Did your visitors upset you?

Patient: Nope. (He edges a bit farther from the nurse. His shoulders are rounded. His neck is slightly flexed.)

Nurse: You really look so sad.

Patient: You're wrong. I'm very happy. Why don't you leave me alone?

The nurse hears that her patient is "very happy." She sees, however, that he says little and that his body is slumped over on the couch. Additionally, the boy requests to be left alone. The patient's subjective perception of his mood is at variance with that which can be objectively observed.

THE INITIAL GREETING

When the patient is well enough to come to conferences without undue assistance or encouragement, the nurse should keep her greeting brief, indicating interest, warmth and respect, but without conveying a particular mood. This is important because the patient needs to have the freedom to express his own feelings. If the nurse sets the feeling tone for the interview, the patient is likely to try to reflect her example. This is a habit which human beings acquire in their social relationships. One cannot hope to re-educate the patient in this respect, nor would it be appropriate. Rather, it is up to the nurse, as part of her responsibility in the interview, to provide a neutral setting so that the patient can take the lead in setting the feeling tone. Therefore, the nurse should not greet her patient with "Hi, Mr. J. I'm glad to see you," accompanied by a wide grin and sparkling eyes. She should save this greeting for a social occasion and substitute for the therapeutic interview a more somber approach. She need not look like the stock market has just crashed; however, her warmth can be communicated through her direct gaze into the patient's eyes. Her words, "I'm glad to see you" or "I'm glad that you could come," will convey her interest in and respect for the patient.

This approach will seem difficult and even alien to most nurses when they first try it, for it is extremely hard to give up the social habits that have been learned over a long period of time. This is part of the nurse's responsibility in the communicating process. She "sets the stage" so that the patient can proceed to describe his problem. The nurse's greeting is the open door through which the patient enters the communicative process. When the nurse finds her own particular style (and this requires some effort and experimentation) she will then cease to feel out of place and unnatural. Finding this style is part of gaining skill in the communicative process, and as skill is acquired, the nurse will see that her patients progress more rapidly. This will be reward enough for the work the nurse has put into developing this highly important skill!

THE BODY OF THE INTERVIEW

Once greetings have been exchanged and nurse and patient have taken the positions that they are likely to maintain for the interview, the work of the conference is ready to begin. It is unusual for a patient to jump into the discussion with mention of an emotionally charged subject. More likely he will initiate the interview with a discussion of something neutral or even lacking in apparent relevance to the purpose of the interview. This is not to be discouraged by the nurse. She may look upon this exchange as a "warming up." It is not unlike the first turning over of a car's motor on a cold morning; the wise driver allows the car to warm up for a few minutes before releasing the brake and driving away. So it is in the interview; the nurse allows the patient to warm up by talking about things that don't require much thought or intense emotional activity. This is a protective device; it allows the patient to watch the nurse, once more, to reassure himself that she really will permit him to say what he wants. This exchange reaffirms the patient's belief that the nurse is ready to accept him. Thus, this seemingly unimportant exchange really does have therapeutic value, for it reinforces one of the elements that the nurse has tried to communicate. The exchange permits the patient to see that the nurse "really means it."

If the nurse listens very carefully, as she must in order to use the tool of communication, she will eventually hear the patient mention something that she recognizes to be important to him and probably central to one or several of his problems. This is a point to recognize and a place where the nurse can begin to take a lead in structuring the interview if the patient begins to ramble in his discussion.

The following is an interview between a public health nurse and a pediatric patient's mother in the latter's home.

> Mother: Let me see. . . . He was 7 pounds, 4 ounces at birth. He was a one. You wouldn't have believed the fuss my husband made. You know, first boy and all that. Why the toys and the plans and all, . . . you know.
>
> Nurse: (Smiling slightly.) You were telling me about Jimmy. Let's see, you mentioned his birth weight. How about his development? When did Jimmy first sit up with support?
>
> Mother: Oh, I guess we were propping him a lot by the time he was three months old. He sat pretty good by himself 'fore he was six months old. . . . We got a puppy for him round about then. My mother used to come over and see that baby and the dog on the floor together and she'd just about have a heart attack.
>
> Nurse: When did Jimmy walk and talk?
>
> Mother: Well, as I can remember he was walking by 10 months and he talked okay when he was about three. He was a funny

one. Used to run to his room and hide whenever company came. Sometimes I'd have to just drag him out, but he got over that after a while. Yes, siree, Jimmy's been a pretty healthy boy.

Nurse: How old was he when the company scared him?
Mother: Gee, I don't rightly remember, . . . guess four or five.
Nurse: Has anything else frightened him particularly?
Mother: I guess he still gets pretty upset when company stops in. Jimmy kind of disappears until I call him.

In this example the public health nurse utilized good interviewing techniques. She used a broad statement initially in order to permit the mother to focus the conversation. Such a move offers the interviewer an opportunity to observe what the interviewee considers important. Such information can be very helpful when the interviewer is gathering data about a patient.

When the mother digressed, the nurse refocused on the topic. When the mother inadvertently described a behavior which might have been symptomatic of a psychological problem, the nurse sought further clarification.

The following excerpt is taken from a conference between a nurse and a very sick young woman in a mental hospital. The patient was sitting with other patients out of doors. She was wringing her hands and mouthing words to herself.

Nurse: Good morning, Sue.
Patient: Oh God, Miss W., give me a cigarette.
Nurse: You will be smoking in five minutes in our meeting together in the conference room.
Patient: Will Miss T. be there?
Nurse: No, Sue, not today. But she will be coming to some of our other meetings together.
Patient: Oh God, I like Miss T.
Nurse: I like her too. Sue, I'll be waiting for you in the conference room. I'll get your cigarettes.

Sue comes into the conference room wringing her hands. She stands looking at the walls, mumbling and making hitting gestures toward the wall. She frequently looks out the open conference room door.

Nurse: Sue, I'm going to close the door because of all the noise in the corridor. Why don't you sit down?

Sue walks slowly to the chair near the nurse and lowers herself into it.

Patient: I sure do miss that other nurse. I like it when she comes. . . . I like it when you give me cigarettes. . . . The patient then is silent. The nurse waits quietly. She continues to watch the patient with an expression of interest and caring. After several seconds the nurse speaks.
Nurse: Can you tell me something about your thoughts, Sue?
Patient: In a minute. I'm talking to Charles. Yes, Charles. I know, Charles. (She strikes out toward the wall.)
Nurse: What are your thoughts about Charles?

Before this conference between the nurse and the sick patient the nurse greeted the patient and indicated that they would meet together. This was necessary because of the severity of the patient's illness. The nurse, in evaluating her patient's condition, recognized that she would have to structure the situation so that the patient would know when and where the meeting would take place. In addition, the nurse used another valuable technique. She explained that the patient could smoke in the meeting. Many patients enjoy smoking, and the anticipation of it allows them to feel more comfortable in the interviewing situation. Thus, the nurse very skillfully communicated to her patient in a few simple sentences her expectations for the interview. The patient, though she was very ill, still followed the pattern of most individuals by discussing less important topics before she allowed the nurse to share what was really uppermost in her thoughts. This was, of course, Charles. When she mentioned this name, the nurse recognized that they had come to an emotionally charged area and she attempted to get the patient to discuss it more fully.

At this point in the interview the nurse is ready to employ other means at her disposal for continuing toward the goals of the interview. Up to this point she has given the patient the initiative. The patient has led and the nurse has followed, interrupting only to seek clarification or to make statements that indicate her understanding. Now the nurse's task will be to keep communications open, to encourage spontaneity, but also to focus on the problem(s) that the patient brings up and to encourage the expression of feelings. The movement of the interview depends on the nurse's being an excellent listener. She must pick up the patient's verbal and nonverbal leads, and she must recognize clues or signals from the patient. The nurse, as a good listener, hears the words that are spoken, but she also sees the body gestures that accompany those words. In addition, she categorizes the patient's statements into themes. This type of thinking on the nurse's part is like finding pigeon holes for storing information. It is a "shorthand" method of thinking which is necessary because no one can store vast numbers of words in his memory. Instead, we memorize ideas that can later be recalled. This is an important skill for the nurse who attempts to help a patient through use of the interview. She looks for recurring themes in the many conferences that take place between nurse and patient. Thus, in the example used, if the patient speaks several times of Charles and accompanies her words with angry gestures toward the wall, the nurse can safely categorize this as an important theme of this patient and one which probably involves angry feelings. The nurse may not remember each of Sue's statements about Charles, but she will recall that the patient's feelings toward him are intense and, at this time, angry.

The nurse will use various means to keep the interview moving. This does not necessarily mean she will keep the patient talking, but it means she will continue the thought process and the sharing of ideas and feelings. The nurse tries to use as few words as possible in order that her words do not interrupt the patient's or that her thoughts influence those of the patient unduly. Such statements as "Tell me more about it," "Go on in that area," and "That interests me" are useful for encouraging the patient. They also indicate that the nurse is listening. The words indicate that the nurse needs more information if she is to understand more fully. It is useful to say, "I don't understand. Could you tell me again?" or "Could you tell me more?" if the nurse really is unsure of the meaning of her patient's statements.

Another means of encouraging the patient is by *reflection*. This is an interviewing technique which involves repeating carefully selected words that the patient has said. In the example used, the patient said, "I am talking to Charles." The nurse would have used reflection if her comment had been "Charles?" Reflection is a useful means of encouraging the patient to share his ideas; however, if it is overused and done without sensitivity, it is most disagreeable to the individual who listens. This technique is often used to the exclusion of others by inexperienced interviewers. In this case, it sounds mechanical. Everything that the nurse is trying to communicate to her patient in terms of her interest, warmth and caring is decreased or negated, for the patient becomes aware that the nurse is merely repeating his words rather than listening carefully and responding in a spontaneous but thoughtful way, reflecting the character of the listener. It is better to use a large variety of comments to encourage the patient than to use only one means over and over again. The nurse must not lose track of the fact that she is dealing with another human being who is similar to herself in many respects; the patient is a thinking, reacting individual who will soon realize whether the nurse truly cares and is trying to understand or whether she employs techniques mechanically and does not have the ability to empathize. The patient will "feel" the nurse's effort to speak directly to him, even though he has camouflaged his real feelings behind his many words. Techniques, by themselves, are without warmth and sincerity. To use them wisely, the nurse must use them sparingly. They are like seasoning on a salad; too much is distasteful. The right amount highlights flavor and brings out the best in the mixture.

The nurse may at times make observations concerning what she sees. Thus, in the example used, the nurse noted that Sue seemed angry as she gestured at the wall while mentioning Charles. This observation is one which the nurse might choose to share with her patient. Perhaps she will withhold her observation until another time if she feels the patient is not ready to admit that she appears angry. In another interviewing situation, the nurse might witness other non-verbal cues. Useful statements such as "You appear tense, are you uncomfortable?" or "You seem very sad today" may permit the patient to describe his true feelings.

Often the nurse will recognize when communication is disorganized. This is a sign that the patient's thinking is also disordered and this, in turn, is part of the patient's illness. Therefore, it is of genuine benefit to the patient when the nurse asks for clarification in terms of placing an event described in time or in sequence. In this category also is the seeking of clarification when the patient uses indefinite pronouns like "they." Often the nurse will hear a patient speak of people or events in terms of "they" or "it." Unless the nurse is really certain of the identity of "they" or "it," she should ask the patient to explain, for then she can be sure that they both understand what has been shared.

It is useful for the nurse to encourage descriptions of the patient's perceptions. This process is often one from which inexperienced nurses shy away. Thus, if the patient says he sees things, the nurse is apt to deny that "things" exist; or the nurse feels more comfortable pretending she did not even hear the statement. Neither event is useful to the patient. As the patient mentions his perceptions, the nurse should seek more information about them. Thus, the patient who says he feels warm may be describing feelings associated with an overheated room. On the other hand, if the room feels cool or drafty to the nurse, she might seek more information from the patient concerning his warmth. It might indicate embarrassment, excitement, fever or even anger. The point is, *the nurse will not know unless she questions the patient* about it.

If the patient reports seeing or hearing things which are not obvious to the nurse, it is a disservice to the patient if the nurse explains that these things do not exist, because in the patient's world they *do* exist. It is beneficial to the nurse-patient relationship for the nurse to seek further descriptions of the patient's perceptions. Through such questioning on the nurse's part, and description on the patient's part, the two parties can further their mutual understanding of the patient and his world. Therefore, the nurse should respond to the patient's report by asking such questions as "What is happening to you right now?" or "Can you tell me more about what you see?"

When the patient has had time to discuss his perceptions, it may be useful for the nurse to present reality as she sees it. The nurse may indicate that she does not see someone else in the room, or that she does not hear what the patient is hearing. In the case of a patient who is misidentifying the nurse, it is certainly necessary for the nurse to clarify her identity. Thus, the nurse might say, "I am not your sister.

I'm Miss W., your nurse." It is comforting to the patient and indicates the nurse's interest in him and her concern for him if she can make some statement about her awareness of his feelings as he misidentifies her. The nurse can communicate her concern by such statements as "It must be frightening to think that people are not who they say they are" or "You must miss your sister very much."

Statements of this kind lead into another area of extreme importance to nurse and patient—the area of mutual agreement on the meaning of words and actions. Both parties may assume that they are understanding the other's communications, but it is only through direct questioning that this knowledge can be had. When the nurse suggests that her patient is frightened, she is actually saying something about her own feelings if the roles were reversed. Therefore, it is wise to seek the patient's opinion. The nurse might follow her statement about misidentification with a question, "Is this your feeling?" or "Do you agree?" Through these means the nurse and patient move closer to mutual understanding.

At the end of the time allotted for a conference, the nurse should indicate this to the patient. She should time her remark so that she does not cut into statements of the patient if he is speaking of something important to him. In addition, she should time her comment so that it is not made at the end of a group of statements from the patient that represent an emotionally charged area. Thus, the nurse should have at her disposal a means of noting the time. When she sees that the allotted time is coming to an end, she should take the lead in beginning to summarize the information and the feelings shared during the interview. This allows both nurse and patient to leave the conference with similar ideas about what has been said. In addition, it gives the patient a few moments to gather his feelings and get them under control. If possible, the last few seconds should be reserved for comments of a lighter nature to help the patient to move away from particularly sad or anxiety-provoking statements or ideas that might have arisen during the interview. This is an appropriate time also to make plans for the next meeting, such as time and place. In addition, the nurse can indicate her interest in discussing further a topic that has been initiated during the conference just past.

SUMMARY OF THE INTERVIEWING PROCESS

Useful means of furthering the purposes of an interview are: allowing the patient to take the initiative, encouraging open ended communication, and spontaneity. Focusing on emotionally charged areas is important, providing the patient can do so without being shattered by the experience. It is important that the patient be encouraged to focus on his feelings. The nurse's responsibility in the interviewing process is to use minimal verbal activity, but to maintain movement by listening for themes and picking up verbal leads, clues or signals from the patient. She must seek clarification if there is any doubt as to the meaning of the patient's message.

Communication is likely to continue in the interview unless the nurse changes the subject, jumps to conclusions or gives inappropriate reassurance. These events are likely to occur if the nurse is anxious and attempts to lessen her own tension. Thus, it is seen again that the nurse must be aware of her own feelings. If she decides to interrupt the patient's thoughts, it should be because she judges the situation to be too difficult for the patient to handle, not too difficult for herself.

REFERENCE

1. Davis, A. J.: The Skills of Communication. *Am. J. Nursing,* 63 (No. 1):66-70, January, 1963.

SUGGESTED READING

Arteberry, J.: The Disturbed Communication of a Schizophrenic Patient: An Approach to a Clinical Nursing Problem. *Perspectives in Psychiatric Care,* 3:24-37, 1965.

This article is quite detailed and takes a long, analytic look at communication. The material is more detailed than the reader of this text will find necessary, but it is suggested because of the perspective that reading it will afford.

Davis, A.: The Skills of Communication. *Am. J. Nursing,* 63 (No. 1):66-70, January, 1963.

An excellent discussion of communication, this article presents much necessary content. It is very readable and will enrich the student's experience.

Jones, E.: The Use of Speech as a Security Operation. *Perspectives in Psychiatric Care,* 3:18-21, 1965.

Like the Arteberry contribution, this too is more detailed than necessary for the basic student. The content is interesting, however, and the overall subject matter is relevant at all levels of study.

Nelson, A.: How Can You Stand the Crying? *Am. J. Nursing,* 70 (No. 1):66-69, January, 1970.

How unusual to find an article on communication wrapped in the confines of the pediatric milieu. How very appropriate, however, to consider communication at its less articulate levels. This article is excellent in its presentation of the nurse's response to crying children. The author points out graphically that crying means varying things to each child at the time he communicates in this manner. The skilled nurse hears the message and responds accordingly.

Peplau, H.: Talking with Patients. *Am. J. Nursing,* 60 (No. 7):964-966, July, 1960.

An excellent summary is provided for the basic student of communication. The material affords an easily comprehended matrix for understanding the importance of communication with the psychiatric patient.

Robinson, A.: Communicating with Schizophrenic Patients. *Am. J. Nursing,* 60 (No. 8):1120-1123, August, 1960.

The writer presents her own concepts of psychiatric nursing. Though the frame of reference is communication, the author says much more. She allows the reader to see why she has become well known for her consummate skill in patient care. This article is well worth reading by all.

BOOKS

Hays, J., and Larson, K.: *Interaction with Patients*. New York, The Macmillan Co., 1963.

The material is quite basic and focuses entirely on communication. Though it is written in a very detailed manner and is sometimes laborious, it is an excellent source for the student who feels some inadequacies in communication skills.

Reusch, J.: *Therapeutic Communication*. New York, W. W. Norton and Company, Inc., 1961.

This compendium, written by one of the most widely recognized authorities in communication, is not addressed to basic psychiatric nursing students. It is, however, extremely readable and so may be of use to the average student who is particularly interested in this area. The book is regarded as a classic in the field, and for any discerning student who aspires to understand communication with the psychiatric patient the book is without peer.

Spiegel, R.: Specific Problems of Communication in Psychiatric Conditions. *In* Arieti, S. (ed.) : *American Handbook of Psychiatry*. Vol. I. New York, Basic Books, Inc., 1958.

This paper is at a high level, and will be useful for advanced undergraduate students, graduate students, or those readers who are interested in studying communications in depth.

chapter 4

THE MENTAL HEALTH–
MENTAL ILLNESS
CONTINUUM

Psychiatric nursing in the latter half of the twentieth century has broadened its scope. The patient is no longer found sequestered in a "back room" of the family home, nor is he sentenced to the confines of a locked ward in the state institution. The nurse may care for patients who come to a psychiatric setting during the day and go home at night; she may work in an institution in which patients remain for the entire 24-hour period; she may find her patients in the community.

In the community setting diagnostic labels do not abound, nor are treatment regimens prescribed. Though medical supervision is usually available, the psychiatric nurse may be employed in a setting in which she is expected to identify potential patients in the community (case finding) and to initiate therapeutic interventions in their behalf. To this end, the nurse must be able to categorize patients according to rough criteria. The criteria in psychiatry are behavioral patterns. When the nurse can observe behavior and make judgments about individuals and their level of functioning based on their behavior, she then can assign them positions along a mental health–mental illness continuum. From such a rough approximation the nurse can begin to plan for the care of those individuals for whom she takes responsibility.

MENTAL HEALTH

Those who attempt to create definitions of mental health do so on theoretical constructs and symptoms reflected in behavior. No researcher can yet demonstrate mental health at the cellular level; the mind remains, for the most part, a mystery to its investigators. This is not to say, however, that there is a scarcity of theories regarding the nature of mental health; the literature abounds with theories and descriptive phrases, but none states unequivocally that "mental health is: . . ."[13] For the sake of simplicity and brevity, mental health will be considered in this text as *the best adjustment an individual can make at a given time, based on his internal and external resources.* The definition implies that mental health is like physical equilibrium. The individual experiencing it is constantly correcting to retain it. Mental health, like equilibrium, requires continuous effort to cope with new situations. It is like the heading of a sailboat into the wind: the helmsman must constantly work with sail and rudder to keep the craft on a predetermined course; adjustment is made continuously to changes in the wind and the current.

Such is mental health in the human being. The individual maintains his "course" and lives productively and without undue discomfort as he comes upon those vicissitudes that make up a lifetime. The mentally healthy individual is able to maintain his equilibrium because he is able to select from among his talents, skills, thoughts and feelings, as well as whatever tangible resources he possesses, and utilize these components of self in order to maintain whatever direction he assumes for himself in a particular situation.

In order for an individual to choose his useful assets he must be able to evaluate himself realistically. Such a process can only follow from an awareness of one's identity. The healthy mature individual has evolved an identity through his years of development. The hallmark of this achievement is finding meaning in life by setting and moving toward self-imposed goals which are congruent with his identity. Frankl has stated the following proposition, indicating the individual's responsibility for defining his own course of action:

> Everyone has his own specific vocation or mission in life; everyone must carry out a concrete assignment that demands fulfillment. Therein he can't be replaced, nor can his life be repeated. Thus, everyone's task is as unique as is his specific opportunity to implement it.[6]

MENTAL ILLNESS

For the majority of mental illnesses there are no tissue biopsies nor other laboratory studies which indicate the presence of pathology. It is not possible to get a stat "blood level for schizophrenia." Psychosis cannot be observed on a brain scan. There is no known mass to palpate; inflammation cannot be diagnosed at the cellular level. Instead, the presence of mental illness is inferred through symptomatology. The person who feels the illness might say that mental illness is the experiencing of painful, irrational anxiety, sadness or terror. Members of the patient's community and family might recognize the presence of mental illness when an individual is unable or reluctant to respond appropriately in his network of relationships. Members of the health professions recognize psychopathology, or mental disease, in terms of symptoms such as poor interpersonal relationships, delusions, hallucinations, and distortions of mood which are reflected in behavioral manifestations.

Because there is no clearly identified definition of mental illness, the student of psychiatry must develop a concept based on evidence and argument. Upon this tentative frame of reference, a philosophy of treatment can be built. In order to guide the reader in this difficult task, such a concept is offered. It does not represent all the thinking in the field; it does not purport to be unassailable. It is a concept based on behavioral terms because the nursing care of the mentally ill requires efforts to change behavior. Mental illness, for purposes of this textbook, is defined as *the inability to effectively adjust to life as demonstrated by the use of multiple coping mechanisms which do not buffer the individual from profound psychic insults.*

The mentally ill patient is sometimes so acutely disturbed that he is unaware of his real self, disguised as it is by layer upon layer of protective behavior. These kinds of behavior, called defense mechanisms, when utilized effectively, buffer individuals from anxiety. They defend the individual by helping him to remain unaware of his uncomfortable feelings. Some people, however, use many mechanisms without achieving release from psychic pain or anxiety; the mechanisms simply becloud feelings to the point that the individuals utilizing them become totally estranged from themselves. These people, termed psychotic, are usually unable to perceive reality sufficiently to interact with others in their communities on a day-to-day basis. Their behavior indicates gross problems in perception, memory and judgment. Psychotics tend to exhibit such symptoms as delusions, which are fixed ideas that are not based in reality. They also describe hallucinations, which are phenomena that are seen or heard by the patient but do not actually originate external to him. Hallucinations, except those caused by physiologic abnormalities, arise from the patient's own ideas, but they are unacceptable to him and are attributed to the world around him. The hallucinations that accompany delirium tremens, fever or drug reactions may be due to irritation or stimulation of the areas of the brain that cause misperceptions or perceptions for which there are no external stimuli.

For the *neurotic,* security may be purchased through the expenditure of great amounts of energy which are utilized in maintaining defense mechanisms. The felt security is not a settled constant one, but a continuously tenuous sense of peace which threatens to deteriorate if the person is not vigilant in the maintenance of his defenses. Neurotics have less severe personality disorders than psychotics. Adjustments to life are impaired, but not totally absent. Severe symptoms, such as hallucinations and delusions, are not seen in neurotic behavior. The neurotic is usually able to identify conditions of reality which are compatible with those perceived by others. The degree of disability, or the amount of difficulty the individual experiences in coping with daily living, will determine the position chosen by the nurse for his placement along the mental health–mental illness continuum. This placement cannot be an accurate one based on true quantitative measures but must be an approximation based upon the frequency of the coping maneuvers needed and the kind evolved by that individual to feel secure.

From such a frame of reference the nurse can better understand the philosophy behind the task of the psychiatric nurse. She supports the patient in his search to find real identity and a life style that is congruent with his identity. This concept offers clarification of the previously discussed nurse-patient relationship, in which the nurse helps to bring about desirable changes in the patient. The reader can now appreciate that the changes create greater congruency between inner and outer selves.

THE MIND

Psychological adjustment is carried out in the mind. This entity, the mind, is discussed by all, but visualized and understood by none. Sigmund Freud, a brilliant neuroanatomist who began his work in Vienna in the latter half of the nineteenth century, studied the human mind and recorded his observations in numerous papers. Freud, who is often called "the father of psychiatry," recognized that human beings sometimes act upon thoughts and emotions of which they are not consciously aware. He demonstrated that these unconscious thoughts and emotions exert a strong influence upon mental functioning and ensuing behavior. This material is often spoken of as being "out of awareness," and can be thought of as existing at the deepest level of the mind, which we call *the unconscious.*

Freud studied the unconscious and developed techniques for helping his patients to bring into awareness the thoughts and feelings buried there. His principal technique is called psychoanalysis. This is a form of long-term psychiatric treatment in which the patient works with the analyst to understand his own behavior, and ultimately the person he is, by bringing into his awareness as much as possible of the unconscious content which influences his behavior.

The object of Freud's studies, the unconscious, possesses qualities which are specific to it. They are as follows:

1. The content of the unconscious consists of primitive instincts and concrete ideas.[10] Primitive instincts are those needs which demand satisfaction and the drives which channel energy into finding satisfaction. They evolve during infancy when the human organism *must* have certain needs met in order to survive. Examples of primitive instincts are the drives for food and comfort.

Concrete ideas are formed through memories of perceptions and sensations which originally entered the central nervous system by stimulation of sensory organs, thoughts and bodily sensation. A concrete idea is that mother is good. In the unconscious the individual does not justify the goodness of mother, but he experiences the thought of her as inherently positive.

2. The method of functioning in the unconscious is called primary process. The word "primary" indicates the first developmental stages of infancy. The language of thought in this phase, primary process, is characterized by displacement and condensation. Displacement means the ability to relate to another object instead of the one originally encountered. Condensation is the tendency to perceive a scene or object, with many implications or characteristics, through the medium of only a select number of those characteristics. Thus, the baby who sees the breast thinks of mother and food and feels comfort and security. He has condensed the being of "mother" into the sight of the breast. Primary process is disorderly. It is observed in the dreams of healthy individuals when such people report their inability to understand the meaning of their dreams. Dreams are usually not understandable because they are made from primary process. The dreamer cannot easily find the perceptions which have been condensed, nor can he identify the sources of his displaced feelings.

3. The unconscious does not recognize contradictions. Again, the dream, which reflects the unconscious, demonstrates how opposites can exist together.

4. The unconscious has no concept of time. There is no past or future; only present exists in the unconscious. Again, the reader is asked to consider dreams. In them the dreamer always experiences *now*. Delights or horrors of many years past are re-experienced in the present.

5. External reality is replaced by internal reality. In the unconscious, reality is based on what is felt, not what is known.

Consciousness is focused toward the external world. It is awareness based in reality. Thoughts that are readily identified by the thinker are called conscious.

Preconsciousness is between unconsciousness and consciousness. It contains content of both the unconscious and the stored impressions from the external world. The individual can usually bring into consciousness that which is preconscious by focusing his attention on the material to be "remembered." On the other hand, preconscious material can also be moved into unconsciousness.

AGENCIES OF THE MIND

When a neurosurgeon cuts into the brain, he finds a conglomerate of soft tissue that is gray in some areas and white in others. The tissue is divided into sections by fissures and convolutions. Its gross appearance does not indicate functional areas. Yet students of the mind have given names to imagined parts, based on functions of the mind which have been observed. Some, like Freud and his student Jung, chose names taken from the Latin. The translations of the Latin words give some indication of the work done by the parts so named. Others like Sullivan, who also developed schools of thought in psychiatry, have used names for the functional designates which are derived from the English language but still indicate the functions attributed to them. In most of the terminology, the mind is separated into three or four areas, or agencies. Though the names differ, depending on the school to which one adheres, the identified functions tend to be divided into:

1. An area of awareness that interacts with the external world and also communicates with the intrapsychic world.
2. An area that is purely intrapsychic; that is, one which does not cope with the limitations of reality but considers primarily the survival of the organism.
3. An area that deals with the influences from the external world which will ultimately shape the development of the organism.

Though the areas of the mind are spoken of separately, they converge in conscious process sometimes, and in unconsciousness most of the time.[3]

To understand the Freudian frame of reference, it may be helpful to envision the mind as a three-layer cake. The bottom layer will be called the *Id.* The middle layer is the *Ego,* and the uppermost layer, the *Superego.* Actually, one might more accurately envision the cake as a marbleized one in order to understand the interlocking of the three areas, for part of the middle layer, or Ego, extends into the top layer and part of it reaches into the bottom, or *Id.**

Id

The id, or "it" in Latin, is mainly unconscious. This means that we cannot recognize communications from this area of our minds without special psychiatric treatment, usually psychoanalysis. The id is the

---

* Sullivan's theory, called "interpersonal theory," identifies a "self system" which is roughly analogous to ego; a "dissociated self" which roughly parallels id; and a "central paranoia" which shares some common characteristics with the superego.

most primitive part of the mind. It develops first in the infant and is partially responsible for the individual's survival. It is the id which demands to be satisfied. Thus, the young infant who is hungry cries to signal his condition. Mother recognizes the need and places the bottle on the stove to heat it. The infant screams more loudly. It is unlikely that the infant's internal signals of hunger have become more intense, but it is likely that the id is demanding satisfaction *NOW*. This is a characteristic of id behavior—"I want what I want now." Freud coined the phrase "pleasure principle" to describe the demands of the id. In addition to being the repository for all needs and basic drives, it is also the storage facility for the early experiences of each individual. Thus, it contains many important memories. The id dictates all mental behavior of the infant until the ego begins to develop.

Ego

That part of the human mind which will be most evident to the nurse is called the ego. In Latin, *ego* means "I." It is the part of the human mind that is, in the main, accessible to awareness; this is to say, the ego is partially conscious. When an individual thinks, "I am Karen. I am breathing and seeing. I am alive," the person is using data which is in her awareness or conscious experience.

When people discuss "personality, character, intellect, aspects of self," they are usually referring to the ego, which is that part of the mind that is evident to others. Thus Sue, who has such a sparkling personality, or Earl, who is a "real brain," or even Dick, whose "character is blameless," are people who are known to others by the activities of their egos.

Ego is present when one observes the delightful phase of infancy in which the child begins to be aware of himself. Those who have had younger siblings or have raised children will recall with pleasure when the baby began to study his own body. He may have lifted his hand and studied it, or gazed with apparent interest at a raised foot before placing the bare toe in his mouth and sucking it. Another sign of the infant's beginning awareness of self is when he smiles in delight when mother enters the room. These behaviors and others similar to them represent the early development of ego, that is, of awareness of self as a unit separate from the mother. The ego meets demands from the other two agencies of the mind. It acts as a sensory end-organ to the mind, for it perceives reality—the external world, and the ego makes possible whatever actions an individual takes, based on the limitations of the external world and the demands of the id and the superego. The ego is a tireless worker. It is always bringing messages into the individual which tell of the outside, real world. It is equally busy sending out messages from the internal world. The id and superego need not wrestle with the outer world, and so their needs and demands go to the ego undiluted by recognition of external world prohibitions.

The tireless ego must constantly referee between demands of the id and the superego and the expectations of the outside world. This is more than a full-time job. By the end of a full day of thinking, perceiving, and feeling one needs to relax and sleep. It is important for mental health that the individual has sufficient sleep. The unending work of the ego is partially responsible for this health requirement.

Superego

The uppermost layer of the marbleized cake represents the last agency of the mind to develop—the superego. This is the conscience. It is that part of the mind that says, "No, that is wrong; don't do it." In other words, it is the censor of behavior. It is also the core of integrity. When one is eulogized as "an honest man, a person who lived by his ideals, a moral citizen who upheld the greatest ethic to which men aspire," it is known that a highly developed superego has been influential in the eulogized individual's life.

Superego arises from three sources: The first is the child's *image* of his parent's ideals and prohibitions; the second is the parent's *real* attitudes and, later, those of his teachers. Finally, superego arises from the culture in which the child is raised.

ADJUSTMENT AND DEFENSE MECHANISMS

The reader has now had an opportunity to consider mental health and mental illness as fluid states which are constantly altered through the need to maintain equilibrium. Like other biological entities, human beings are subject to the vagaries of internal and external environments over which they have only partial control. One means of regaining and maintaining psychological equilibrium is through the utilization of defense mechanisms. The effective use of these measures determines the individual's state of mental illness or health. In the following section, the reader will see *what* the mechanisms are and *how* they are used to create and to maintain equilibrium.

> Alan W. is a 35 year old dentist. He has a good practice and enjoys his work. Alan lives with his 70 year old mother and claims to enjoy this living arrangement. Alan W. occasionally dates women his own age; however, he is most often seen in public with his mother.
> Allan W.'s intrapsychic life is far different from his observable external life. He is kept quite busy (and entertained) by his fantasies. While at work he daydreams of a succession of beautiful young

women with whom he enjoys various sexual encounters. Occasionally and inexplicably Alan has a fantasy about the death of his mother.

In the case of Alan W. one can observe the use of defense mechanisms. He has done well professionally, but socially his life has not developed. Instead, he fills his days with dreams of a companionship he has never known. Though he cannot, consciously, express his feelings concerning his mother, who is responsible for his lack of social-sexual fulfillment, he does deal with her in his fantasy life. Here he expresses his anger toward her by fantasizing her death. Alan W. has made a partial adjustment to life. He is successful in his chosen work and enjoys it. In the sexual-social aspects of his life, however, this man has not developed. In order to tolerate this situation, Alan has turned to an intrapsychic life which is rich in fantasy. This is his substitute for the life he cannot attain as long as he acquiesces to mother's wishes.

All people use some defense mechanisms from time to time in order to adjust. Both the kinds of mechanisms utilized and the frequency of their use indicate the degree of individual adjustment/maladjustment. They are utilized in order to bend reality into such form that the individual's perceptions of himself and the world around him are acceptable. Without this, the mind would be overrun by anxiety.

Defense mechanisms can be divided into groups of those which are successful in maintaining the security of the individual by decreasing his anxiety, and those which are unsuccessful because they do not prevent the anxiety from recurring.[5] According to Freudian hypothesis, the cause of the basic anxiety is impulses from the Id which threaten to break through the restraints of the Ego and the Superego. In the case of the neurotic, the defense mechanisms used to ward off the intolerable impulses are not entirely successful, and there is a continuous battle to maintain control.[5] In the case of the psychotic, the battle is clearly lost and the impulses emerge into consciousness.

SUCCESSFUL DEFENSES

The following defenses are termed "successful" because they tend to diminish anxiety that threatens to become conscious and because their use permits the individual to become more like others in his society.

Sublimation

The infant exhibits overwhelming urges, or drives. They can be inferred through observation of the child when he is hungry and screams without end until the bottle or breast is presented. From this behavior one can see that the urge to eat—or looked at another way, the need to change the character of hunger pains—is urgent. The toddler continues to show highly energized behavior toward that which he desires, as does the young child prior to school age. At about this time, however (two and a half to four years), the child becomes able to control his drives to the point that he does not exhibit the desperation of need fulfillment that he showed at earlier stages of his development. He does this partially through the utilization of the mechanism, sublimation. The process represents the individual's unconsciously turning away from that which he cannot have and, instead, focusing on another object that is attainable. The mechanism is useful in the socialization of the child, for it assists him in becoming more like the people to whom he must ultimately conform. Sublimation is evident when the toddler gives up stooling in his diaper so that he may have mother's approval. In this instance, he relinquishes one kind of pleasure, i.e., the feeling of the warm, moist bowel movement and the pleasure he feels in controlling its expulsion, for the love of his parent, who demands that the stool be expelled when she wishes and where she indicates.

This mechanism is successful because it enables the individual to conform to society by becoming toilet trained. It is defensive in nature because it permits the child to become aware of the great price he has paid for mother's love, i.e., giving up his pleasurable behavior. When the child is fully trained, he no longer finds pleasure in his stool, but instead has pleasurable feelings from the control he exerts over his bowel habits.

Substitution

This behavior is related to sublimation; however, it involves a more superficial effort. In sublimation, the individual's entire drive, his effort, and his enthusiasms are turned from one type of object to another. In substitution there is merely a replacement of one object by a similar one. Using the example of the child again, a broken or undesirable toy might be replaced by another one like it. Through substitution the individual is able to give up his possession of one object for another which is like it. Substitution is usually a conscious behavior, i.e., the individual chooses to give up one object for another. The mechanism differs from sublimation because it is conscious and also because the *substituted* object has properties which are similar to the original object. In the example of sublimation provided, the reader will note that the characteristics of the stool and mother's love are vastly different. The characteristics of the broken toy, in the example of substitution, and the new toy are similar.

Substitution is considered a successful mechanism because, again, it permits the individual to become more like the members of the group in which he lives. It permits him greater control of his feelings and drives because they continue to have an object. Without the latter, they would provoke anxiety.

Compensation

When, because of a basic inadequacy or disability, a person is unable to accomplish some task that he has identified for himself he can sometimes derive satisfaction from achieving in a related but different area. Such is the case of the manager of the high school football team who cannot actually play because of a congenital hip dislocation.

> The case of Beth A., an adolescent girl who hoped to become a Broadway dancer, demonstrates the usefulness of compensation. This girl studied eagerly and practiced her art enthusiastically until a fateful Wednesday afternoon when she broke her hip and her leg in several places. One of the x-rayed areas showed the bone to be shattered. Beth's dreams were shattered as well. She found herself with no hopes, no aspirations, no goals. Beth's convalescence was not easy, nor was it pleasant. The girl struggled to regain some sense of herself as an individual, for without her goal of dancing on Broadway, Beth felt that she was without identity. In the months that this young girl spent recuperating, she went regularly to a community hospital for physical therapy. There, Beth was encouraged to explore ideas about alternative careers as she exercised her healing limb. By the anniversary of Beth's accident, she had decided to become a choreographer.

This happily ended vignette demonstrates the successful use of defense mechanisms in adjustment to a physical problem. The girl could not realistically pursue the goal she envisioned. Over a period of time she accepted this situation by identifying alternative objectives and was able to reformulate her goals in a realistic manner.

Identification, Introjection and Imitation

Social roles are learned, in part, through imitation and identification. The child observes his family and peers in order to find models. By imitation, which is a conscious behavior, the child copies others. Another means of development is through identification, which is an unconscious defense mechanism. The child becomes socialized by identifying with parental behavior, attitudes, and expectancies. Through these he evolves internal standards and images of what he wishes to be or to achieve. Identification is defensive in nature because it relieves the feelings of helplessness and anxiety that the individual has when he cannot adequately handle a situation. Through identification, such a person borrows the means of a significant model to handle his problem. Psychiatric patients sometimes find themselves in difficulty because they have unconsciously identified with a poor model, i.e., one that is ineffective, or one that does not permit the individual to attain his goal. Because the process is an unconscious one, the individual is unable to give up the behavior, attitude, or expectation until he is helped to recognize its origin and meaning to him.

Repression

This defense mechanism must be viewed as both successful and unsuccessful. It can either be used in a healthful way or its use may promote mental illness. Repression is the most basic mechanism. It is present in all defenses. Through the use of repression, that which is perceived as dangerous to the self (and provokes anxiety) is rendered out of awareness. When an impulse is repressed it becomes inaccessible to the person. Thus, he cannot identify its nature and modify it so it does not present danger. Such a solution would be useful except that some repressed content is not completely handled, so that it keeps reappearing in disguised form or in incomplete form in consciousness. As such, it continues to bother the individual who cannot cope with it because he cannot recognize it.

Examples of healthy repressed content are the feelings of omnipotence experienced by the infant, as well as the pain, the frustration and the anger of that same period of life. It is only under tremendous stress, such that the individual becomes mentally ill, that any of these primitive feelings are re-experienced, i.e., become unrepressed. Thus, an operational description of severe mental illness might be stated as the experiencing of events which have erupted from the well of the unconscious and have swarmed up into the preconscious and even bubbled out over that barrier into awareness.

Sometimes young children have school phobias. They feel terror about leaving home to attend classes. When such children are given psychiatric treatment, it usually is revealed that they have unconscious fears that their mothers will die or disappear in some way while they are in school. The children experience anxiety regarding their departure for classes; they do not recognize the underlying theme of abandonment by mother because this theme is repressed. In this instance the mechanism is pathological because the child is unable to cope with a fear (abandonment) that he cannot even recognize. Secondarily, the repression influences a behavior (not attending school) which is dysfunctional.

UNSUCCESSFUL DEFENSE MECHANISMS

Suppression

Repression differs from suppression because in the latter, the individual consciously decides to be inattentive to needs, affects and thoughts. Thus, the person is aware of restricting his self. Handling of anxiety-provoking impulses in this way, such as curiosity and anger, is common. Suppression is evident in the person who says, "I am just not going to think about it," and is able to put whatever the undesirable content is out of his mind. Material that is suppressed is rather easily refocused in awareness by the simple effort of remembering. Such is not the case when repression is demonstrated.

Rationalization

Rationalization is discussed after suppression because it too can be used consciously as well as unconsciously. It is a mechanism that serves to justify a thought or action. It relieves anxiety by helping the individual to maintain his self-image. The student who flunks an examination and explains his failure by the inadequacy of the teacher is likely to be rationalizing. (If the teacher really is poor, such reasoning does not demonstrate the use of defense mechanisms, but is evidence of normal ego functioning, i.e., reality testing.) Rationalization is not useful to the individual because it removes the anxiety that might otherwise motivate growth. The individual who flunks an exam and blames it on an ineffective teacher is unable to see, or to admit, that he himself is inadequate. Thus, the studying that might result from such an observation, and the growth of the individual that would result from studying, do not occur. It is likely that the ill repressed notion of the person's inadequacy will continue to foster anxiety, and he will be chronically uncomfortable but unable to modify his condition because he cannot identify its source.

Isolation

Isolation is another mechanism that is used to defend against anxiety. It is related to the more pathological mechanism, repression. In isolation, events and feelings that occurred together are separated in the individual's memory. The painful aspects of an event are repressed and the person recalls only partially what occurred. This mechanism is operant in compulsive behavior in which the individual feels driven to complete a prescribed ritual, but he cannot indicate the reason for his action.

In situations like the labor room, isolation is useful. The mother recalls her labor vaguely, but she cannot re-experience her pain; however, she remembers very vividly the arrival of the baby.

Isolation, like the majority of defense mechanisms, becomes a precursor of pathology because it prevents the individual from being able to cope with that which influences his anxiety. When the individual is unable to identify what it is that has caused his discomfort, he cannot modify it. A patient who had recurring nightmares told the therapist, "Yes, I do have terrifying dreams each night, but they don't cause me any problems." This person had isolated his feelings about the dreams from his awareness that the dreams occurred. He could not begin to analyze the content of the dreams in order to gain control over them until he could become aware of his strong feelings in reaction to them.

Reaction Formation

This mechanism involves the replacement of an original attitude with another one which is opposite to the first. The mechanism is defensive, for it permits the individual utilizing it to deny or to repress some impulse. The secondary, opposite attitudes are notable for their cramped and unbending character. Common themes in reaction formation are anger, hatred and the need for disorder. Since the ego cannot tolerate these feelings for reasons peculiar to the individual, he defends against them by assuming an opposite attitude. The toilet trained child illustrates a constructive use of reaction formation. In this case, the child begins with a desire—an actual appreciation for his body wastes— and ultimately assumes the attitudes of his parents, who express their distaste for the child's urine and feces.

Undoing

Undoing and reaction formation are related. In reaction formation a new attitude is assumed that contradicts the original one. In undoing, the manipulation of *actions* rather than of thoughts occurs. The behaviors or actions observed in undoing serve to annul previous acts. Undoing is an expression of belief in magical acts. It demonstrates that, by performing a given act, the individual unconsciously feels that another act, already completed, can be undone. This mechanism is evident in the child who speaks an untruth and crosses his fingers behind his back to negate it.

Displacement

Displacement is an important mechanism for those in the health fields to understand. It is commonly used by patients as they attempt to cope with the stress of hospitalization. Displacement involves the transfer of feelings from one situation, where their expression would be inappropriate, to another, where the feelings can be safely demonstrated. Thus, a patient who feels anger and resentment toward the doctor might not openly react to him. This is because patients often, unconsciously, perceive the doctor as the omnipotent, sometimes punitive father they perceived in childhood. Fearing retaliation, again unconsciously, the patient does not permit the doctor to know of this anger. Instead, he expresses these feelings toward the nurse. She is perceived, unconsciously, in the light of the accepting, warm, security-providing mother of bygone days. Feelings are also vented on inanimate objects. Slammed doors, kicked over wastebaskets, and drawers hastily pulled out often reflect displaced anger.

Denial

Unconscious denial is a mechanism that distorts reality. Through its use, the threats of reality are negated. Denial is utilized to hide the existence of defects, dangers and illness. According to Waelder, it is the foremost defense in psychosis.[15] The staff nurse working in a general hospital sees evidence of denial when she deals with a terminally ill patient who has been told his prognosis, but who reports to the nurse that he will recover.* Denial is exhibited by the psychotic patient who reports his state of excellent health and claims no problems.

Projection

At an early age the child wishes to separate that part of himself which is pleasurable from those elements which are offensive. This can be done as long as the line of demarcation between the ego and the world outside the ego is not sharp. Such is the case in early childhood and in psychosis. Projection is easily observed in the child of two and a half to four years (the Oedipal child) who feels rivalry toward his parent of the same sex; these feelings often become focused in a wish to be rid of the parent. Another strong sensation the child feels is the smoldering resentment which explodes into anger at the rival parent. These feelings are unacceptable to the small child. They are dangerous to him because he fears his own lack of control as well as the power of the parent to retaliate. Defensively the child projects his own feelings onto the rival parent and experiences that individual as a frightening, dangerous person. He perceives the parent as a person who is likely to harm him. In this situation the child unconsciously attributes to his parent those feelings which really originated in himself.

This mechanism can be used extensively only if the ego's function of reality testing is severely impaired. Thus, an adult who utilizes it is quite ill. The psychosis in which projection is most often observed is called paranoia. In this disorder the patient has delusions of persecution which actually represent his own internal reactions. In order to remove the odious feelings from the ego, they are attributed to another

---

* So common is the use of denial in the early phase of the dying patient's response to his fate, that Kubler-Ross, authority on death and dying, has called the phase Denial, after the mechanism used.

person. Neurotics use projection also, but to a lesser degree. They misunderstand the actual situation in terms of their own unconscious needs.[5]

Regression

Regression is a defense mechanism which is also unconscious. It means that the individual involuntarily feels and responds as he did at an earlier age. Regression is a symptom of the person in stress. When regression occurs, it signifies that the individual is so uncomfortable psychologically that he has automatically sought the security of earlier phases of development. Thus, the youngster who suddenly finds that mother has a new baby is often observed to return to crawling, pants wetting, and thumb sucking. Regression, in some situations, causes reduction of anxiety, but at the same time results in such inappropriate behavior that the individual cannot be tolerated by the community and is excluded by it and termed "sick." The mother of seven children who, having been overwhelmed by stress, ceases to speak or eat and curls up in the fetal position has regressed. She may have temporarily decreased some of her anxiety by returning to infantile modes of behavior, but this very mechanism renders her incapable of continuing her life style effectively. Thus, use of the mechanism is ineffective as an adjustment mechanism and the woman is seen as ill.

There are other defense mechanisms which are used in an effort to control anxiety; generally, mechanisms are used in combination. It is rare to see one type utilized alone. All people buffer themselves against stress by using defense mechanisms. Very sick people, i.e., those whose egos are unable to tolerate the stress of living because of the demands of the external world and those of the intrapsychic world, use more mechanisms more often than better adjusted people. The more realistic a picture one has of himself as a feeling, reacting person, the more realistic one's assessment is of his talents and skills, the more congruent his inner resources are with his external social role, the less an individual has to use defense mechanisms to adjust to the stresses of his life.

Hopefully when the psychiatric nurse observes these mechanisms in use, she will have a greater appreciation of them because she is able to recognize them in a behavioral framework. It should be kept in mind that *all* defense mechanisms serve the purpose of alleviating anxiety, or of holding it in check. It is an academic exercise to recognize defense mechanisms. If one goes no further than observing their use, then one can only say: (1) the patient is utilizing a mechanism, and (2) his perception of reality is not accurate because of the use of the mechanism. Of basic importance when the psychiatric nurse observes defense mechanisms in play is her awareness that *the patient is anxious.* It is not the goal of the nurse to recognize the use of defense mechanisms; her task is to discover *why* the patient is anxious and *how* to make him more comfortable.

REFERENCES

1. Alexander, F., and Selesnick, S.: *The History of Psychiatry.* New York, Harper and Row, 1966.
2. Bexton, W., Herron, W., and Scott, T.: Effects of Decreased Variation in the Sensory Environment. *Canad. J. Psychol.* 8:70, 1954.
3. Brenner, C.: *An Elementary Textbook of Psychoanalysis.* New York, Doubleday Anchor, 1957, p. 2.
4. Eysenck, H., and Prell, D.: The Inheritance of Neuroticism. *J. Ment. Sci.* 97:441, 1951.
5. Fenichel, O.: *The Psychoanalytic Theory of Neurosis.* New York, W. W. Norton and Company, Inc., 1945.
6. Frankl, V.: *Man's Search for Meaning: An Introduction to Logo-therapy.* New York, Washington Square Press, 1963, p. 172.
7. Joylon, L., Janszen, H., Lester, B., and Cornelison, F.: The Psychosis of Sleep Deprivation. *Ann. New York Acad. Sci.,* 96:66, 1962.
8. Kallman, F.: Psychogenetic Studies of Twins. *In* Koch, S. (ed.) : *Psychology: A Study of a Science.* Vol. 3. New York, McGraw-Hill Book Co., Inc., 1959.
9. Kallman, F.: The Genetics of Mental Illness. *In* Arieti, S. (ed.) : *American Handbook of Psychiatry.* Vol. 1. New York, Basic Books, Inc., 1959.
10. Nunberg, H.: *Principles of Psychoanalysis.* New York, International Universities Press, 1955, Chapter 3.
11. Redlich, F., and Freedman, D.: *The Theory and Practice of Psychiatry.* New York, Basic Books, Inc., 1966.
12. Rosenthal, D. (ed.) : *Genain Quadruplets.* New York, Basic Books, Inc., 1963.
13. Sabshin, M., and Offer, D.: Concepts of Normality in Psychiatry. *In* Freedman, A., and Kaplan, H. (eds.) : *Comprehensive Textbook of Psychiatry.* Baltimore, The Williams & Wilkins Company, 1967, p. 256.
14. Slater, E.: Psychotic and Neurotic Illness in Twins. *Medical Research Council Special Report Series,* No. 278. London, H. M. Stationery Office, 1953.
15. Waelder, R.: *Basic Theory of Psychoanalysis.* New York, International Universities Press, 1960.)
16. Weiner, H.: Schizophrenia III: Etiology. *In* Freedman, A., and Kaplan, H. (eds.) : *Comprehensive Textbook of Psychiatry.* Baltimore, The Williams & Wilkins Company, 1967.

chapter 5

THEORIES OF GROWTH AND DEVELOPMENT

To understand the mature individual as he makes use of self in adjusting to life and achieving those goals he has identified, it is necessary to understand how the adult develops. One can witness physical growth, but it is more difficult to observe and comprehend the complex development of the mind.

Many theorists have offered explanations of human growth and development. The better theories explain growth in a way that is meaningful because it can be related to those events which are observable; they correlate biological and psychological growth. The differences between the theories are chiefly in their frame of reference.

Freud proposed a theory of development which focused on a concept called libidinal energy. To understand the concept of libido, one must first be familiar with Freud's concept of instincts and drives. The latter are complicated phenomena. They result from tension within the individual pressing for release.[1] Instincts consist of responses to stimuli which make the individual aware of alteration in his inner state of equilibrium. This alteration and his awareness of it cause coordinated, purposeful behavior to bring about a renewed state of equilibrium.[1] The feelings that press for re-establishment of equilibrium are what Freud called "libido." Libido in Freudian theory is pleasurable feeling. It is the energy of the instincts.[9] In the Freudian formulation, libidinal energy focuses in various zones of the body. The particular focal area at a given time is dependent on the physiological level of maturation. For instance, the infant is known to experience much of his life through his mouth; he sucks his thumb, takes in food, cries, coos, and explores objects about him by taking them into the mouth. In Freudian theory this phase of development is known as the "oral" phase. Libido, or the energy to satisfy the instinct, is concentrated in the area of the mouth. At later stages of development the excretory organs and the genital organs become the foci of libido.

Another theorist of great repute was Harry Stack Sullivan, whose theory differed from Freud's in philosophy and terminology. Sullivan utilized the concept of conscious and unconscious agencies of the mind as did Freud; however, Sullivan proposed a different vocabulary to identify the mental apparatus. His basic frame of reference was not instincts but anxiety—how it evolves and is handled within the interpersonal relationship. In the Sullivanian framework the ongoing interaction between the human organism and the people in the organism's environment is the main focus of study. Sullivan attempts to explain growth and development in terms of the maturing capacities of the individual. (This roughly parallels Freud's focus on the biological factor.) He focuses also on the influence of the environment in terms of the significant people influencing the developing child. The latter focus is not seen distinctly in the Freudian framework.

Sullivan does not utilize the idea of instincts as did Freud. Instead, he proposes a new concept called the dynamism. In the Sullivanian framework, a dynamism is "a relatively enduring configuration of energy which manifests itself in characterizable process in interpersonal relations."[11] Dynamisms arise out of interaction between the individual and the interpersonal situation.* They are patterns that are not only readily observable, but whose development can be traced. For some students of human behavior this fact is more acceptable than the theory of instincts which Freudian thinkers acknowledge, because the Sullivanian theorists can actually trace the formation of the dynamism and utilize systematic evidence to demonstrate the concepts they identify. Basically the individual pursues satisfactions, both physical and psychological, in order to feel secure. As situations which threaten his security develop between the individual and his interpersonal environment, anxiety appears. It is built upon heightened bodily tension. In the Sullivanian framework it is the inevitable consequence of the child's relationship with the mother. Anxiety is the fear of disapproval, which brings loss of security. The Sullivanian theorists perceive human growth

---

* Dynamisms and instincts demonstrate a fundamental difference between Sullivan and Freud. Sullivan focuses three dynamisms on the individual's maturation via external influences, i.e., interpersonal exchanges. Freud views maturation through instinct development which is basically internal. Freud did not acknowledge the importance of influences external to the individual as being of fundamental significance in the individual's development.

and development as the individual's orderly maturation of his capacities (influenced by his genetic potential and his resulting physiology) and the influence of those in his environment who bring security to him or bring about anxiety in him. The study of the individual's mode of interaction is a major focus of the interpersonal theory.

A third and more contemporary theory is that formulated by Erik Erikson.[3] He proposes that the human being is endowed by those agencies of the mind described by Freud; however, Erikson envisions the development of the individual to be influenced not only by hereditary or biological factors, but by social factors as evidenced in the exchanges with the family and the peer group and, in addition, by cultural dictates. Thus, Erikson has formulated a theory of growth and development that includes the influences of Freud (biological, instinctual drives, libido), the influences of Sullivan (social experiences with significant persons who mold identity), and also includes a rationale for the cultural influences which we recognize today as influencing the way an individual experiences himself as a living entity.

The discussion to follow will be eclectic; this is to say, it will attempt to draw upon the best of several theorists in trying to explain how the individual grows and matures. It is important for the reader to remember that concepts are being utilized; thus, one cannot hope to see or touch a "libido" or a "self." These are only terms used to explain those events occurring in the process of development. The terms, the concepts and the theories discussed are presented in order to provide the psychiatric nurse with a theoretical base upon which to build nursing intervention.

INFANCY

Infancy is the period of development from birth to approximately one year of age. It is a time when the individual is most helpless physically. Infancy is a time of rapid development; in fact, aside from prenatal development, this will be the period of most rapid growth in the entire life of the human being. The infant enters the world with a relatively "clean slate." He comes equipped with a biological heritage which will influence, to a degree, who and what the mature individual will be. Aside from this biological heritage, however, which is embodied in the genetic code, the newborn arrives in the world ready and equipped to absorb the experiences of interacting with his environment.

In the first several weeks of life the infant appears to be governed by the basic needs for survival. Thus, sleeping is the major activity of life. The infant awakens, presumably because of hunger which is signaled by discomfort. Once this stimulus is reduced, the infant sleeps again. Wetness and perhaps coldness are also experienced as noxious stimuli to which the infant reacts by crying and kicking. Again, when the discomfort they cause (which will be labeled tension) is reduced, the infant returns to his resting state, sleep.

It is thought by most theorists that the infant is unaware of forces outside of himself in the early weeks. Thus, comfort and discomfort come in waves. Warmth, comfort and dryness simply occur. It is likely that the infant experiences feelings of great power, since he seems able to change the badness to the good. This is called omnipotence. It is a normal feeling for the infant. When it is experienced in later life, this feeling is considered inappropriate and is a symptom of severe mental illness. The infant is an organism that is physically helpless, yet one that experiences himself as being all-powerful because his discomforts become comforts, seemingly through his communication that they exist. For instance, the hungry infant screams, and warm, filling fluid is placed in his mouth. It is usually three to four weeks after birth before the infant recognizes that the breast or bottle belongs to another. It is at this time that he discovers a very important fact; there is a separate being who responds to him, who comforts, who gives to him; he alone is not responsible for his comfort. It will be the prime task of the infant to learn to trust this all-important mothering one. He will learn trust if the mothering one is responsive. He will learn trust through the regular provision of his needs and comforts. He will learn through mother's touch, her voice, and the tension he feels from her body. If the conditions for a warm, satisfying mother-child relationship are not present, the infant will learn to mistrust others, and as he continues to grow and mature, his "set"—that is, his basic assumption—will be that others cannot be trusted to care and to provide. He will not experience others as dependable and trustworthy. If his basic needs are met by an uncomfortable, anxious mothering one, the infant will feel her tension empathically and experience anxiety himself.

ONE TO TWO AND A HALF YEARS

The toddler of one year is normally an enchanting child. He has discovered, if he is lucky, that the world as it is represented by mother is a warm, comfortable place where he can feel loved and secure. If such a base has been established, the toddler is prepared to move on to a new series of discoveries and accomplishments. If the infant has been unfortunate and has not had sufficient good and rewarding experiences with the world, as he perceived it primarily through his mouth, he may continue into his next phase of development with lingering needs from the earlier period. Such a situation is called *fixation*. It means that personality development becomes caught, or fixed, at a given point. One can witness the results of fixation at the oral level (newborn—one year) in adults who must eat or smoke or drink without end. This is reflective of the infant who tries out new experiences and is gratified and communicates—all through his mouth. More mature integrations of behavior have not been possible because the infantile experience was not adequate.

The toddler is in an enviable position for learning on a physical level. He has developed remarkably. His muscles and nervous system are sufficiently mature that he can stand and walk. Bladder and bowel control are now possible. Mother and father are highly esteemed by the toddler, and he learns much by mimicking them. His efforts at walking and talking reflect the will to be like his trusted, loving companions, his parents. All is not well, however, for mother and father feel very differently about the toddler's products of excretion. The child enjoys his urine and feces. They are part of him—warm and comfortable. His parents do not seem to appreciate these waste products as he does; in fact, they show disgust and lack of love for these possessions of his. The showdown occurs when mother communicates openly to the child that she wants him to control the time and place of his evacuations. This is very uncomfortable for the toddler because, in essence, he loves mother, but he loves his excretions too! What is he to do? The toddler finds himself loving mother because she loves and comforts him. At the same time he feels resentment toward her for not allowing him to continue to evacuate when and where he pleases. The feeling of love, on the one hand, and anger, on the other hand, when experienced at the same time is called *ambivalence.* It is an emotional quandary that will occur over and over again. If the toddler has developed sufficient love for the mother and he wishes to please her enough to sacrifice his own pleasure, he will attempt to take responsibility for his excretory functions. This is a giant step forward. It is one of the first moves toward independence and socialization.

The first step in the bowel and bladder training will be a change in the toddler's attitudes toward his body's waste products. Where he once felt at home, warm, and accepting toward his feces, he will take on the attitudes of his parents. This process demonstrates the use of *identification,* introjection, and reaction formation. It demonstrates the taking on of certain qualities of another. Thus, the toddler becomes more like his parents by becoming like them in attitudes. At a deeper, more profound level, the child will later assume other facets of the parental personalities, such as values and morals.

Reaction formation must be used as a defense because it permits the toddler to sacrifice what has been dear to him. He gives up part of his self-esteem in order to please his parents. Such a move would be terribly harmful for such a young mind, but the toddler, in assuming the parental attitude, is no longer aware of his earlier learnings. Now he is only conscious of being like his parents and wishing to become more like them and to please them. Thus, the toddler strives to control his impulses to urinate and defecate. As he succeeds, he feels greater self-esteem and self-confidence. When he fails, he feels guilt, shame and dirtiness. This is a period fraught with danger because it is the first instance in which the child is not totally accepted. It is a time when he may feel uncherished if mother cannot communicate her fundamental love during those times when she is unable to accept the toddler's behavior. Because of this, the mother-child bond is in jeopardy, and that bond is the basic building block for all the child's attempts at exploration and growth.

If the relationship is badly disturbed, the child may develop the need to be stubborn and withholding. These traits are directly related to holding back feces, despite mother's requests. If mother has been overly demanding and controlling, the adult personality may be one of meticulousness, cleanliness, tightness and obstinacy.

Provided this period has not been too coercive and the rewards of responsibility have been freely experienced, the toddler, toilet trained and self-confident, will move into the next phase of development. Interest in feces will be replaced by delight in play with mud, clay and other soft, moldable materials. For some, these pursuits will continue into adult life, where they will be reflected in the creativity of sculpture. This process utilizes the mechanism of sublimation. The toddler who completes the tasks of this period, often called the "anal phase," is for the first time able to experience a sense of autonomy. The unsuccessful child feels shame and doubt. The toddler has now enlarged his social horizons. Father, though not so important as mother, is recognized and accorded love. Siblings (brothers and sisters) are also accepted by the toddler as part of his world. All these people are now "significant others" in the child's environment who may influence his development through interpersonal relations with him.

TWO AND A HALF TO FIVE YEARS

The child of two and a half years is still, essentially, a baby. He has learned to control his voluntary muscles; he talks; and he experiences himself as a member of the family. It is at this time that the child begins to show signs of interest in his sexual self. The two and a half year old obviously does not label, or even sense, his interest as sexual or genital. He only knows that it feels good to touch and stimulate his penis or, in the case of the girl, her clitoris. Masturbation becomes a daily occurrence, and through it the child comes to appreciate more of his body and his capacity for sensation and responsiveness.

At this stage of development the child also takes a greater interest in the bodies of others. He is very curious about mother's and father's anatomy and what they do behind the closed bedroom door. It is at this time that the little boy's activities become more intrusive. He seems to put himself in a position of being more exploring, more daring. He goes after what he wants. The little girl acts more receptively. She is more passive than her masculine counterpart and seems to be softer, more willing to accept. Children of both sexes, however, are actively seeking to explore their own bodies and to compare them with the bodies of their siblings and parents.

Up until this time both boys and girls have felt that mother was their first love. Father was loved also, but there has always been a special kind of relationship with mother. Now, that relationship is to be tested and strained. The little boy, who has become pleasurably aware of his penis, begins to resent father's attention to his mother. He cannot identify his feelings and the strivings he experiences; however, they are there, driving him, making the little boy uncomfortable in the home situation with mother and father. The little boy, aware that mother feels differently toward father than toward him, attempts to be more like his father. He mimics father. He attempts to protect his mother, to take her away from father. The little boy's behavior, however, is not consistent, for he is afraid. He wants mother for himself, but he is afraid of father's retaliation. This is not a pleasant phase of the child's development. It is one in which fear and desire intermingle. This phase, often referred to as the *genital* or *phallic,* is characterized by swings toward sweetness and lovable behavior, with shifts to resentfulness and irritability. The phallic or "oedipal" child* often suffers from grotesque nightmares as he attempts in his dreams to escape from lions, tigers and monsters, which represent the angry father (for the boy) or mother (for the girl). The boy wants only one other object as much as the mother, and that is his penis. While he is acting intrusively and aggressively, that is, as he attempts to compete with father for mother's affection, he fears that father might cut off his penis as a means of punishment. (The penis is focused upon because it is a prized possession.) Finally, the exquisite torture of these embroilments diminishes when the little boy resolves to leave his mother to father. He compromises by regarding her with affection, but controls his infantile sexual desires for her. This is a long, painful process for the boy, but it is only when this phase has been resolved that the child is ready to mature further, to become more like father in order to gain mother's love, and to continue his growth, no longer afraid of father's wrath.

For the little girl the "oedipal phase" is more complicated. She must renounce the original love object, that is, mother, and turn her

---

* According to Greek legend, Oedipus was the central figure in a saga in which he was separated at a young age from his parents, the King and Queen of Thebes. According to Homer, Oedipus unwittingly killed his father and married his own mother. (Odyssey XI, 271.) The term "oedipal" is derived from the main character of this unfortunate saga and it has come to refer to the child of two and a half to four years who experiences sometimes ungovernable longings to replace the parent of the same sex in a relationship with the parent of the opposite sex.

interest to father. The little girl begins this phase just as the boy does. In exploring her body the girl eventually finds her vagina and clitoris. She stimulates the latter and soon finds her body capable of delightful feeling. At this time the little girl, too, is interested in the bodies of others. It is inevitable that she find her own body sadly lacking. Father has a penis; she does not. In families in which there are other children, the little girl usually compares her body with those of her brothers and sisters. It is a source of frustration to the little girl that she cannot urinate from a standing position. She may feel her inadequacy keenly because she does not have an appendage that is visible between her legs.

It is sometimes difficult for mature adults (and almost-mature students of psychiatric nursing) to understand the role of the penis in the life of the oedipal child. This is partially due to the mechanism of repression. Our minds have efficiently hidden from our quest for information our own painful experiences in the period. In order to regain some of this experience, however, we can observe the two and a half to four year old child at play. We see the little boy urinating in the communal toilet at nursery school. Sometimes there are two or three little ones in the room at the same time. Notice how they handle their penises, compare them, and use them as objects of fun. They aim them in the toilet to urinate, but if one watches closely, it may be seen that the penis becomes an object with which to make configurations as voiding continues. (Have you ever seen two little boys surreptitiously urinating outside in the snow? It appears to be great fun for the two as they giggle and observe the yellow stains they can make on the snow bank.) Another typical game of prowess is to see who can urinate the farthest. The little girl may observe these games, but lacking the basic object, the penis, she cannot participate in the sport. Unlike other toys that are desired, this one can *never* be acquired. It is difficult for any child to be deprived of something that is desirable. One can observe her longings when the little girl is seen playing "horsey" with a broomstick between her legs. Sometimes the girl child will even show her envy more openly by walking about quite exhibitionistically with a banana, ruler, or other long object at her pubic area.

The little girl begins to disengage her affections from the mother when she becomes aware of her body's inadequacies. She resents the mother, whom she holds responsible for her lack of a penis. During this period, the little girl begins to flirt with father. She attempts to imitate mother's feminine wiles in an effort to capture father's interest. The little girl is often perceived as "cute" or "just a little lady" during this stage of her· development. She is much more than these things, however. The little girl is engaged in a developmental struggle, the outcome of which is essential to her continued growth and development. Just as the boy does, so the little girl vacillates between the more infantile position of loving and accepting mother totally, and resenting and hating her for being the main object of father's affections, and also for taking away her penis.

It comes as a further shock to the little girl that mother has no penis either! At this phase of her development, the little girl now becomes more actively concerned with becoming like mother. She no longer holds mother in the position she held her prior to this phase, nor will she ever do so again. Mother will now provide a model for the little girl to imitate so she too might someday be cherished as mother is by father.

The unconscious maneuverings of this period are many, and they are highly significant in the later sexual development of the individual. It must be understood that the basic concerns are not consciously identified; they are experienced through bodily discomfort, i.e., tension and frustration. The child has strong, physical feelings for the parent of the opposite sex but cannot identify these feelings for he has not had prior experiences with them, nor does he have the opportunity to "compare notes" with others who might identify these feelings for him. Thus, the child experiences unnamed bodily sensations and he feels tension.

The child does not consciously want to kill the rival parent, but he does wish to get rid of that parent. The "getting rid of" is equivalent to killing, to putting to death. Another strong sensation the child feels is the smoldering resentment which explodes into anger at the rival parent. These feelings are unacceptable to the small, vulnerable child who is in a position not unlike that of David with Goliath. And so, another defense mechanism is demonstrated. It is *projection;* this occurs when the child experiences the rival parent as a frightening, dangerous person who is likely to harm him. In this situation the child unconsciously attributes to his parent those feelings which really originate in him. This mechanism is observed often in persons who are mentally ill. It originates in the oedipal child.

Why is it that the reader cannot remember these painful struggles of the early years? If the complex happenings of the phallic phase occurred and they were so highly charged, so fraught with feelings of love, hate and murderous death wishes, why are they not recalled instantly, with pain and embarrassment? The answer is that repression is operating. The oedipal phase is marked at its end by *repression.* It is relegated, along with most earlier experiences, to the unconscious and is not brought to awareness again, except in special instances of psychoanalysis or psychosis. The successful termination of the oedipal, phallic or genital phase marks the beginning of the child's more mature attempts to cope with the world. The child now has a sexual identity. The boy, proud of his penis, moves forward, imitating his father— aggressive, intrusive, protective and affectionate toward mother. The girl, resigned to her anatomy, looks to the mother for a model to copy.

She behaves somewhat passively and is more accepting and receptive than the boy. Though not actively engaged in seductive efforts toward father, she regards him with deep affection. Thus, the basic behavioral differences between the sexes are established. This has been a long, difficult journey, and at its end the child will put aside these genital concerns and seem totally unaware of them for approximately six years. The child who has successfully completed the oedipal phase will feel capable of taking the initiative. The child who has not been patiently loved will feel guilt.

SIX TO 12 YEARS

By the beginning of the period that extends roughly from six through 12 years, which is often called "latency," the personality has formed in the rough. The id, which was present at birth and reflects the basic instincts and needs of the individual, has been joined by the ego. This agency of the mind which reflects the thoughts that are in awareness has been well developed, starting in the first year of life. With the advent of the oedipal phase, the child has introjected much of the conscience of his parents and so the rudimentary superego joins the id and the ego. The child of six is ready to go into an enlarged world for the first time. He is prepared to leave the confines of his home and the safety and predictability of parents and siblings whom he has come to know intimately.

The "latency child" is a calmer, less troubled child than the youngster in the oedipal phase. He has repressed the need to possess one parent and to do away with the other. He does not remember the pain of physical inadequacy. In short, latency is a respite from sexual drives and the friction produced from intimate strivings toward and against parents. Latent drives are hidden drives. Life is essentially good for the latency child.

For many children school attendance begins at the age of six. This is a very wise choice, because the child has much available psychic energy which can be used to ponder the mysteries of "reading, writing, and arithmetic." The six year old is ready to become absorbed in the business of peer group involvement. This is the age that has been immortalized by such famous characters as Charlie Brown and Christopher Robin.

The child in the latency period turns his attention from home and parents to school and peer group. He learns to use tools, to play with others, and to behave in ways which are acceptable to his cultural group. The child continues to identify with the parent of the same sex. In addition, he admires a variety of people who attract his attention via television, movies, books, and the stage. Such people provide *ego ideals,* which offer role models for the child to copy. This is a time of broadening and solidifying bases of behavior. The basic personality is formed. Additional means of coping will be tried, but the direction of growth has been established. The child in latency becomes industrious, and he is gratified by his efforts. Should he feel incapable of drawing upon his innate resources in work and play, he will approach puberty feeling inferior.

This is a "betwixt and between" phase of development. The child seems to grow, to flourish. Then he regresses and is unhappy. Things go well for a while, and then they decline. The years of elementary schooling go quickly. It is necessary for parents to support the healthy personality that demands freedom to experiment and to expand. Wise parents also allow for the swings back to immaturity. Of most importance, the superego is strengthened as the child has more experiences which permit him to choose between right and wrong. While in the oedipal phase, the child felt constrained to behave in a given manner because mother or father desired it. As he develops through latency, the child chooses a course that is right because it is *his* wish. Thus, the child has come from an infantile position of behavior prompted by needs and a desire for gratification and parental approval to a position of awareness that some of his needs and desires are not always of primary importance to others. The child had begun during the anal phase to be aware of the mother's prohibitions. Eventually, through reaction formation, he experiences mother's attitudes and values as his own and, finally, during latency he incorporates enough of parental and societal values that he acts upon these and performs out of personal choice, rather than because of the coerciveness of the earliest years or the rigidity imposed by reaction formation in the late anal and early oedipal phase.

Neither Freud nor Sullivan lived to see the conglomerate of stimuli and demands focused upon the latency child of today. Had they observed the rapid social change which has led to new cultural values, but also to confusion of values and uncertainty on the part of parents, the deluge of technological data confronting the latency child, and the electronically produced stimuli which bombard the child, they might have concluded that the luxury of latency no longer exists. In many children of the sixties and seventies, we observe a continuous heightened sexuality in dress, dance and other social behavior which indicates that the concerns of the genital phase are not being "turned off" temporarily. There is evidence in the increased rate of venereal disease, the number of illegitimate births and the use of drugs to indicate that the developing individual is not capable of handling all that confronts him at the age when these stimuli appear.

12 TO 15 YEARS—EARLY ADOLESCENCE

The relative quiet of latency is interrupted violently by the onset of adolescence. This period is heralded by puberty, the physical basis of adolescence. This is a catastrophic phase of development for the youth. He is overwhelmed with physical sensations up to now unknown. Bodily changes—that is, the secondary sex characteristics—cause the individual to feel that even his body is strange to him. Thus the youth, no longer a child, begins a journey that he has not voluntarily chosen. It will be frightening and at times harrowing. It will be, at times, a lonely period, and he will not be able to communicate with anyone about the pain associated with it.

The youth in early adolescence must become reacquainted with his body. For the girl, *menarche* brings with it questions, doubts or pleasure, depending on the earlier laid foundations for sexual identity. For the boy, *nocturnal emission* heralds the same. If the oedipal child has turned without undue trauma to the business of becoming like the parent of the same sex, early adolescence will bring with it the opportunity to solidify sexual identity and to develop a social role. If the oedipal years have been unsuccessfully traversed, early adolescence can bring Hell.

The early adolescent grows with a rapidity not seen since infancy. In addition to the secondary sex characteristics, his body suddenly grows larger, and clumsiness and an inability to control finer movements do not add to the young person's self-confidence. Problems in control of his outer body are compounded by problems in control of his inner self. At this time there is an upsurge of the sexual drives which racked the oedipal child. The young adolescent must now master once and for all his overwhelming sexual and aggressive feelings toward his parents. He does this, in part, by turning away from them. It is at this time that intense friendships are formed with individuals of the same sex. These are unconscious homosexual relationships, and they stem from a need to relate to one who substitutes for the parent of the same sex. The youth is, in effect, protecting *himself* unconsciously from the feelings he experiences toward the parent. He is protecting the *parent* from these same uncontrollable strivings. The pairing off in intense friendships will continue until the adolescent begins to explore the world of heterosexual relationships. The boy-girl relationship is not to be realized, however, until the adolescent is comfortable with his sexual identity.

The primary business of this period is to realize, finally, sexual identity and, partially out of this set or group of related attitudes, to find a comfortable role in the social world. To solidify sexual identity, the adolescent builds on the base he established during the oedipal phase when he renounced his sexual longings for the parent of the opposite sex and began the work of identifying with the parent of the same sex. In addition, the early adolescent compares his perceptions regarding himself and his sexual identity with his friends. He tries to be as much like his friends as possible because he is in the throes of role confusion and it is safer to be, at least externally, like his peer group. Thus, teen-agers are observed to be very clannish. They seem driven to dress alike, talk alike and think alike. Those who deviate are excluded from the group and treated cruelly. Such behavior is prompted by the teen-ager's insecurity. It is terribly threatening to see a contemporary who is different, for the question arises, "Who is right? Who is real?" These are frightening kinds of questions, so they are not allowed to arise. Differences are not permitted to exist.

Teen-agers are known for their mood swings and their lightning-like switches in objects of affection. These signs are, again, symptoms of the struggle that is being waged to find identity. Adolescents swing from moods of maturity and self-confidence to periods of more infantile behavior in which the teen-ager feels less capable and demands the type of guidance and protection bestowed upon him at an earlier period. It is not easy to be consistent and supportive toward the young adolescent.

The "crushes" and hero worship that are observed are an attempt to reach out, to find identity by copying the admired person and to interact with that person in order to find some stable identity for oneself. To say the least, this is a hectic time. It has been said that youth is wasted on the young; however, it is only youth that has the energy to *be* youth! Early adolescence is a time of frantic searching. It is in these years that serious mental illness is often first encountered. Those who cannot tolerate the loneliness, the insecurity and the frightening lack of control of feelings often begin to exhibit behavioral symptoms of a serious nature at this time.

16 TO 21 YEARS

At the time when the teen-ager begins to live comfortably with himself as a sexual being, he then turns to the task of relating to those of the opposite sex. Secondarily, his quest turns to finding a role for himself in the social world. This role grows out of his cognizance of himself as a sexual person, his awareness of his talents and skills, and the opportunities provided by the social world. The successful conclusion of this search requires the youth's ability to comfortably integrate his perception of his *inner* self with his perception of his outer person as observed by others.

The main work of this phase, however, is to gain heterosexual experience and to begin the business of finding a mate. This is the time of dating and of beginning to experiment sexually. One's level of experience is very much dictated by opportunity, peer group standards and the degree of permissiveness of the cultural group. The early "love," which reflected a need to receive, gives way to more mature feelings, signified by the wish to give. The healthy individual experiences himself comfortably and can extend himself to another. An analogy can be made by comparing a child and a 17 year old, both of whom desire to reach out from a standing-still position to some object. The child is likely to fall because he will be off balance; the 17 year old can stretch and reach and obtain because his base is secure. He can maintain balance as he extends himself. It is the goal of this phase of development to extend oneself repeatedly until one finds a partner with whom it is pleasurable to be intimate. If this does not occur, the penalty is a life of isolation.

ADULTHOOD

It would be desirable to break down the next decade into phases because, in truth, there are still distinct tasks to be accomplished; however, as a result of socioeconomic factors, individuals continue the growth process at widely varying ages. Some are ready to marry and begin a family at the age of 17 years. If the individual has finished as much schooling as he can obtain or absorb, if he has a job which makes him financially and psychologically independent of his parents, then he can give vent to his desires to be sexually intimate and to procreate. In our society today, when many youths continue in graduate education far into the third decade, they cannot be financially independent of their families, and social mores influence parents and offspring to maintain the psychological bonds of dependency. For this group, adulthood and generativity must be postponed. Thus, we cannot divide into years the remaining developmental tasks.

Generativity, which grows out of the successful quest for intimacy, implies not only the creation and guidance of the next generation, but also the freedom and the desire to create such inanimate objects as reflect the innate nature of the individual. For instance, a talented person composes lyrics which reflect his artistry, or another gives expression of her inner self through the colors and groupings of flowers she plants or raises in a garden.

This is not to say that for those who cannot raise children, life is a failure. If the desire to create is present, these people *compensate* by becoming involved with other productive endeavors.

For those who do not achieve the ability to lose themselves in the minds and bodies of others and to gain the benefits of expanded interests and investments, stagnation and personal impoverishment occur. For these individuals life becomes stale and loses meaning. These are the people who mark each day as another sign of drudgery on the way to death. Finally, in the development of maturity the individual must come to the pinnacle of life and look back. If his existence has been rich and full, if he has realized himself as a lovable and loving person, if he has created out of a need for self-expression, he will look back on his lifetime with joy. Contentment will be the gift of the declining years. If he has not had, or availed himself of, these opportunities, his final years will be marked by despair.

RELEVANCE OF THEORETICAL BASES
TO NURSING INTERVENTION

So, one may ask, what is the meaning of all these words? For what reason has a whole chapter been devoted to intangible, unprovable theories of personality development? Hopefully some of the reasons were evident as the thoughtful reader noted the tasks that each human being must accomplish in order to continue the business of development. Without these accomplishments, which are like building blocks, the individual cannot stand unsupported. The lack of accomplishment, the incomplete development of the individual, is equivalent to mental illness. This is why one must understand and appreciate developmental concepts. The psychiatric nurse will actually observe the structural weaknesses she has read about. Her work will involve an understanding of the "missing ingredients," so that she can assist the patient in compensating for the weakened area, or in seeking the type of therapy that tears away the defect and rebuilds with stronger materials.

PATHOLOGICAL BEHAVIORAL PATTERNS REFLECT
ADAPTIVE BEHAVIOR PATTERNS FROM
EARLIER DEVELOPMENTAL PHASES

The reader now understands the behavior and developmental tasks associated with each phase of growth. Also, there is an awareness of defense mechanisms which arise during the various phases of development. It will be of use to the reader to understand some of the behavior patterns she will observe in patients in terms of the developmental phases from which they arise. This knowledge makes theoretical bases of development relevant to nursing intervention. Though some behavior will be unacceptable to the psychiatric nurse, and this reaction should be communicated to the patient, the nurse will be more comfortable in helping the patient to modify inappropriate and ineffective behavioral patterns if she understands their meaning. It must be constantly kept in mind that *all behavior is meaningful.*

The nurse will encounter ill persons who withdraw and seem unwilling or unable to relate to others. Such people are extremely ill. The most severe form of withdrawal is called the *catatonic reaction.**

---

* See Chapter 9 for a more complete discussion of this syndrome.

Patients exhibiting this behavior pattern are usually found in hospitals where their basic need for survival can be met. Individuals who withdraw, who are unable or unwilling to speak and interact, are utilizing behavior that was appropriate in the first two years of life. Thus, the nurse seeing such adults knows that these individuals have regressed markedly.

Other behavior that reflects the earliest years of life includes withholding patterns, such as are seen in those who will not cooperate in their medical regimen, patients who are stubborn and procrastinating, and those who seem unduly argumentative. To be traced to these early years, also, are those patterns of behavior that reflect the individual's inability to make decisions concerning his daily life. Individuals who have not experienced the pleasure of "being their own boss" may be afraid to assert themselves. Their early experiences with this behavior may have met with such strong disapproval that they have learned it is safer not to "stick their necks out."

Such behavior patterns as these can be most annoying and frustrating for the psychiatric nurse in her attempts to help patients. This is the job of the nurse, however, who deals with psychiatric patients. This is the challenge—to identify the behavior which is inappropriate or ineffective, to understand its meaning, and to help the patient to find better modes of expression. It is often said in psychiatric circles that one "begins where the patient is." This is a valuable maxim, and one to be heeded. If the patient's behavior reflects regression to infantile levels, then it is necessary to approach the patient at these levels. This is not difficult if the patient is grossly regressed; however, most sick individuals demonstrate some healthy aspects of personality, and when both sick and well aspects are present, the nurse must try to address herself to the healthiest parts of the patient's personality. It is part of the job to motivate the patient to perform at his best possible level of behavior.

Thus, if the severely ill patient smears his feces and does not speak, the nurse may have to communicate with him on a very primitive level. The best a nurse and patient can do together may be, for a while, sitting in the same room, perhaps sharing some candy. However, it is well for the nurse to keep in mind that the time may be near when she and her patient can share experiences with modeling clay or plasticine, or paint with finger paints. In other words, if smearing is the best level of behavior that the patient is capable of—fine; the nurse must intrude herself into his world at that point. If, however, she can offer him an incentive to sublimate his smearing needs by using clay substitutes, then it is a waste of time to indulge the patient in more regressive pursuits.

It is a fine art to be able to sense when a severely ill patient is ready to respond to "pushes" from the nurse. This awareness comes with much exposure to patients. It is really a sense of timing. The psychiatric nurse observes her patient's behavior in order to understand when more mature behavior can be expected or demanded. She obtains cues of patient "readiness" from the patient whose behavior is no longer consistent. She may notice, for instance, that the severely withdrawn, silent patient is beginning to follow the nurse's movements with his eyes. The patient who is always smearing may show signs of collecting his feces in one spot only or of saving them for one special person. The chronically stubborn, argumentative patient may become gradually amenable to suggestion. The patient who could not decide to get out of bed in the morning and get dressed might now show signs of "awaiting" the nurse who gets him up and started. Such signs of change in an otherwise stable behavior pattern are the cues that tell the psychiatric nurse that the patient is ready to be pushed.

Thus, an understanding of developmental theory offers a frame of reference for the nurse's observations. She can generally recognize the level at which an individual operates and can begin to infer, tentatively, some meaning to the behaviors she sees. This step is never complete, however, until the nurse is able to confirm her impressions through the patient's explanations. Such a sharing of thoughts may be months in the offing, but it should occur. The patient is most unlikely to say, "I reacted as a six month old infant because the stress was overpowering and I had to regress"; however, it is quite likely that a patient will, at some time in the therapeutic endeavor, tell of his feelings of fright and his overwhelming inability to cope with the events that threatened his very being. It is worth the nurse's time and effort to arrive at this point of reflection with her patient when he is well enough to put the total picture in perspective and to look at it. This is like preparing old treasures to be wrapped and packed for storage in the attic. One understands the illnesses that have been incorporated in whatever form that understanding is possible. The last step is "mothballing" the memories, tying them up in red ribbon and putting them away.

In the psychiatric sense, understanding equals the mothballing and wrapping; repression is equivalent to putting away in the far reaches of the attic. The repression represents a healthy process, in this situation, because the former patient understands the meaning of his illness; he uses his understanding for effective living but the torment of illness is left behind. It is satisfying as a psychiatric nurse to be part of this process.

REFERENCES

1. Arieti, S.: *The Intrapsychic Self*. New York, Basic Books, Inc., 1967.
2. Brenner, C.: *An Elementary Textbook of Psychoanalysis*. Garden City, New York, Anchor Books, Doubleday & Company, Inc., 1955.

3. Erikson, E.: *Childhood and Society*. New York, W. W. Norton and Company, Inc., 1950.
4. Erikson, E.: *Identity: Youth and Crisis*. New York, W. W. Norton and Company, Inc., 1968.
5. Freud, A.: *The Ego and the Mechanisms of Defense*. London, Hogarth Press, Ltd., 1937.
6. Freud, S.: *A General Introduction to Psycho-analysis*. New York, Washington Square Press, Inc., 1952.
7. Friedenburg, E. Z.: *The Vanishing Adolescent*. Boston, Beacon Press, 1959.
8. Munroe, R.: *Schools of Psychoanalytic Thought*. New York, Holt, Rinehart, and Winston, 1955, p. 357.
9. Nunberg, H.: *Principles of Psychoanalysis*. New York, International Universities Press, 1955, p. 62.
10. Pearce, J., and Newton, S.: *Conditions of Human Growth*. New York, Citadel Press, 1963.
11. Sullivan, H. S.: *Conceptions of Modern Psychiatry*. New York, W. W. Norton and Company, Inc., 1940.
12. Sullivan, H. S.: *The Interpersonal Theory of Psychiatry*. New York, W. W. Norton and Company, Inc., 1953.

chapter 6

ANXIETY AS A FUNCTION OF THE MAINTENANCE OF SELF

Anxiety is a term that is central to all discussions of dynamic psychiatry. It is an abstract concept describing a feeling state that may range from the minuscule to the most immense proportions. Anxiety is a household word. In this highly technical, swiftly changing century, which has been called the "Age of Anxiety," everyone has experienced at one time or another "having the jitters," "being nervous," "having a bad case of nerves," or "climbing the walls." Anxiety undoubtedly has been part of the human condition since before recorded history, but life in the twentieth century seems to be leading to its wider prevalence.

The child born into this era may expect to live fast. As a by-product of his pace, he will probably live intimately with anxiety. He will be primed on energizing, growth-producing foods; he will be encouraged to develop sooner. He will be bombarded by exciting stimuli via television, movies, books and parents who wish him to absorb all that is presented. Though the child may not be psychologically ready to cope with the wide range of feelings generated by the stimuli around him, he will, nonetheless, be exposed. If he cannot handle the resultant feelings, anxiety will erupt.

Attendance at school will be accompanied by strivings to achieve. For the financially secure child, there will likely be incentives to compete. The successful competitor will be recognized; he may receive material rewards from proud parents. After toys are outgrown, there will be monetary gifts, bicycles, motorcycles and cars; later there will be admission to sought-after schools, colleges and jobs. The child is likely to learn that seeking and acquisition are accomplished by aggression, competition and winning. To win, however, one must compete. Woven into the competition will be the threads of anxiety, for whenever one must pit himself against opposing forces, anxiety arises.

Perhaps the reader can recall feelings of anxiety when she measured her accomplishments against a standard in the form of a testing situation. Can the reader remember the sudden awareness of excessive warmth, a sensation of rapid movement in the abdomen? Now the feet get cold; the hands are cool also, and they are moist. One is aware of a feeling of faintness; in the back of the head is a pulsing throb.

Is this the feeling of anxiety? Could it be fear? It is a response to threat. But what is the threat? What is the very worst possible outcome in this testing situation? The student may fail the quiz. Such a failure could not bring physical harm; bodily injury is not a possible outcome in this situation. Thus, the individual experiencing such a reaction is feeling *anxiety* in response to an internal, or intrapsychic, threat. Were the student facing a runaway tiger instead of an instructor in the test situation, one might describe the subsequent physical sensations in terms of *fear*. Such a reaction is a response to an interpersonal, or external, threat.

It is important that the student of psychiatric nursing develop an appreciation of the concept of anxiety. As has been said, this concept is the key to all psychiatric work, whether done by doctor, nurse, psychologist, occupational therapist or allied workers. All personnel work to decrease anxiety, to bring it into awareness, sometimes to increase it, or to harness it into constructive work. Anxiety is generated by all human beings who have a stake in maintaining their identities. It may be felt through a variety of symptoms, ranging from a slight "nudging" undercurrent to the vast oceanic panic that is observed in very ill people who scream, run and try to escape when there is no observable danger.

Basically, anxiety is tension.[1] It arises from threats to the individual's sense of self, that is, his identity. The threats to identity usually result from conflict. If one can imagine the engines of two trains (which are analogous to conflicting impulses) colliding, with sparks fanning out at the accident site, this is similar to the production of anxiety. Were either engine permitted passage without obstruction, its motor, which provides the energy for movement, would propel it down the track; however, the engines meet head on. The energy from them (which is analogous to psychic tension) is unable to discharge smoothly because their movements are impeded; it is transformed into sparks, spitting from the site of the collision. This is like the conflict that is created when opposing impulses meet: decision and action are impossible; generated energy escapes, unchecked, undirected, in the form of anxiety.

Another useful analogy is that of the steam pressure cooker. One might envision the bubbling of boiling water as the seething conflict in one's mind. If the temperature is not lowered, the water boils harder and faster, causing steam (anxiety-energy) to form. For many, a pressure valve is available which regulates the flow of steam (anxiety). Mental illness occurs when one's regulating mechanism is stuck or altogether absent and anxiety simply pours out without pause.

SYMPTOMS OF ANXIETY

When reading lists of symptoms, it is a temptation to simply memorize the words. (This is, in a sense, using the defense mechanism, isolation.) To really understand the concept, however, the reader is requested to remember his own personal experiences with anxiety. No words, no looks nor any lecturer can be so vivid as personal experience. All people feel some of the following symptoms; few experience them all.

Vital signs demonstrate the presence of anxiety through rapid and shallow respirations and increased pulse and blood pressure. The nurse may also observe that anxiety is reflected in changes of skin color, nausea and vomiting, changes in appetite, diarrhea, perspiration, restlessness or immobilization, and insomnia. Other subjective symptoms of anxiety are "butterflies in the stomach," cramps, tense muscles (which often result in tension headaches), dryness of the mouth and feelings of fatigue. The nurse is cautioned to remember that there are numerous reasons for the signs and symptoms just described. It is folly to ascribe them to anxiety when other causes are equally plausible; however, when physical conditions do not warrant the symptoms observed, it is reasonable for the nurse to consider anxiety. She must then try to identify the *cause* of the anxiety and perhaps *why* the patient experiences anxiety in the face of the stimulus.

Of most importance is the nurse's memory of her own anxious moments. From these very personal experiences she will appreciate the exquisite agony that her fellow human beings feel.

ANXIETY AS A MOBILIZING FORCE

Anxiety is not necessarily bad. When it is experienced in small, controllable amounts, anxiety is a motivating force. It is the energy which motivates the individual to change.

Patients receiving psychiatric treatment sometimes complain of anxiety. They are puzzled because their therapist, who formerly attempted to control their discomfort with drugs or other measures, now insists that the patients live with their anxieties. Patients sometimes feel hurt and angry with their therapist; they may find it difficult to understand that the therapist considers patient anxiety a motivating force which, when the patients' egos are strong enough, can make them just uncomfortable enough to work steadily in psychotherapy, searching for "gut level" answers to alleviate their illnesses.

Laura W., a 37 year old mother of four children came to the psychiatric clinic after she experienced difficulty in sleeping over a four-month period. Mrs. W. explained to the psychiatrist who saw her that she felt constantly irritable and tired. For several months the doctor prescribed tranquilizers. During this period, Mrs. W. kept her appointments. She was always punctual and worked hard to understand her feelings of anger at her husband and children. She slept well at night and assumed this to be the result of taking the prescribed tranquilizers and the psychotherapeutic work. During the seventh visit Mrs. W. asked the psychiatrist for more pills, explaining that her supply was exhausted. The therapist said, "Mrs. W., I think we have done enough work now so that you will not need drugs anymore."

"But doctor," she exclaimed in distress, "I can't sleep without them. My nerves get all jittery. The kids, my husband . . . come on. You don't understand."

"No, Mrs. W. I'm going to help you over this thing, but not with drugs any more." He smiled and touched her arm. "You're doing pretty well and this is the time to try living without that crutch."

Mrs. W. looked doubtful, but she trusted her therapist and was willing to follow his advice. He, in turn, increased her appointments to twice a week and told Mrs. W. to call him if she became particularly anxious.

At her next appointment Mrs. W. reported an inability to sleep during the previous two nights. Her therapist asked Mrs. W. to join him in searching for answers to the insomnia. He reminded the patient that they had discovered in previous appointments that Mrs. W. felt anger towards her family when she was tired and they clamored for various favors without noticing her inability to give more. The therapist recalled how Mrs. W. felt unable to express her anger and that she would instead keep it bottled up until everyone had gone to bed. Mrs. W. listened carefully and she began to smile. During the remainder of the visit she recalled incidents of the days preceding her insomnia which had angered her, and together doctor and patient identified the factors that kept Mrs. W. from expressing her feelings at the time to the appropriate person.

This patient had been given tranquilizers to make her more comfortable when she began psychotherapy. When the doctor thought Mrs. W. had established a pattern of trusting him and of working effectively in psychotherapy, and when she had once again regained her normal sleep pattern, he felt she had the "ego strength" to continue without drug therapy. At this point, Mrs. W. might feel more anxiety than she had experienced since coming into psychotherapy, but she had learned to recognize her anger. Also, she had an ally in her therapist, who encouraged her to identify and to express her feelings. In addition, Mrs. W. had had the opportunity to mend physically, for the drugs she had taken had enabled her to feel less anxious and to sleep at night. Now the therapeutic task was to look directly at her anxiety, to recognize it, to understand *why* it arose, and to use it as a signal of problems in the future. In this case the symptom, anxiety, was utilized constructively by the patient in coming to understand her problem— expressing anger.

When anxiety is present in small, controllable amounts it enables the individual to be more alert, to be more quickly aware of danger to his integral self. In this way, anxiety is constructive. It can be viewed as a safety feature built into each human being. Unfortunately, this "safety feature" sometimes multiplies out of proportion. It grows like a cancer, crowding out rational, constructive thought and the ability to make decisions. The person experiencing this phenomenon is aware that he is "losing control." His feelings are frightening and can run the gamut from mild discomfort to outright panic. The degree of mental illness that an individual experiences can be evaluated in terms of the amount of incapacity he suffers as a result of his anxiety. Thus, individual A may be very anxious. He may express much fear and foreboding, though he manages to earn a living and follow a complex schedule. Individual B, on the other hand, may feel less overt anxiety; however, he is compelled to wash his hands after each episode of touching wooden objects. On the surface one might judge individual A to be more ill than individual B; however, when it is considered that individual B is strongly hampered in his daily movements, it can be seen that individual A has more resources to work with and he is not made an invalid by his anxiety. Individual B must spend a considerable portion of each day washing because he cannot readily avoid contact with wooden objects. The washing is time-consuming, and unless individual B is self-employed, he must account to others for his behavior, which results in less efficiency on the job. Thus, it is evident that individual B is in rather dire straits. He needs psychotherapeutic aid in order to return to a semblance of his normal day's routine. Individual A has been able to maintain this much organization without help; thus, he is evaluated as being better integrated.

ANXIETY AND THE NEUROTIC PERSONALITY

The reader will recall the discussion of mental illness (Chapter 4) in which psychopathology is described in terms of the defense mechanisms needed to maintain equilibrium. The mechanisms utilized are employed to fend off anxiety which threatens to erupt as the individual meets those stresses which are part of living. Neurotics are described as individuals who utilize multiple mechanisms in an effort to maintain adjustment. They are people who are constantly anxious, tense and on guard. They are uncomfortable and unable to identify the source of their feelings without help.

The neurotic person is not entirely in touch with his real self. This is not to say that he experiences frank delusions as does the psychotic, but rather that his impressions of self and others are not entirely valid. The neurotic must constantly struggle to maintain his self-image which is not a valid reflection of the personality resources which actually make up the individual. Thus, the neurotic's fantasies, or daydreams, are concocted. These, in turn, influence his perceptions and actions. The neurotic individual is one who has not made strong, healthy adaptations to the problems (or developmental tasks) of childhood. He uses a set of repetitive responses (behavior patterns) to maintain his pseudo-image. Subjectively, these maneuvers keep the individual's anxiety at manageable limits; in reality, they keep the individual from evolving an identity consistent with his resources, from which he might experience real security and a sense of worth.

As a result, the neurotic individual has continued to mature, but his basic personality is not strong. His ego needs the assistance of numerous defense mechanisms to maintain equilibrium. He feels unsafe because he has not had the growth experiences which would promote a sense of adequacy and autonomy. The end product of the assumptions that the neurotic makes about his life, and the unproductive activities that he engages in, result in a basically unhappy, chronically dissatisfied individual who cannot hope to come to a realistic awareness and appreciation of his real self. Such individuals may live long, physically sound lives. They love, work and procreate. Their inner agonies are often unrecognized by others. Why, the reader might ask, should these persons be identified as "mentally sick"? The answer is, basically, because they themselves can never approach an awareness and understanding of their own significance. Such people are under constant pressure, which results in a type of behavior influenced by fear, the predominance of negative over positive motivation and the predominance of fantasy over direct experience. They are a vulnerable group, for their egos are always working harder than those of people termed "well adjusted." The following example illustrates the kinds of behavior shown by such an individual and her feelings concerning these involuntary behavior traits.

> Some of the nursing students in Muriel's physiology class did not like her. She was always the one to volunteer for extra reports or odd jobs that the instructor wanted done. At first, it was a relief

when Muriel raised her hand and settled the question of who would do these jobs, but after a while the other students began to find her an "apple polisher" and rather "pushy." It was observed that Muriel was bright and received very good grades.

She was very intense when talking with small groups of her peers. The girls noticed that she bit her nails down to the quick and, when she was with them, she had a disconcerting tic in her left eye. Muriel was one of the least popular students in the class. It was not until the second year in the nursing program when a small group of students were receiving their psychiatric training with Muriel that they were able to find out more about this basically unhappy girl.

One day when the group was having a discussion of neurotic behavior, Muriel began to sob. She said, "It's never enough for me. I feel like the ballet dancer in 'Red Shoes.' I must dance on and on. I do all my work. Most of the time I do at least half of my friends' work as well. I get all A's, but it only helps for a few minutes. I'm so tired from proving myself. My instructors write 'good,' 'excellent work,' or some other gibberish on my paper, but I just can't believe it. I have to push all the time to feel okay about myself. . . . I wonder if I shall ever be able to rest?"

People like Muriel exhibit the more usual type of neurosis, often called *psychoneurosis*. They have basically maladjusted personalities. In this group are individuals for whom a mild or moderately stressful incident is enough to precipitate anxiety of such proportions that defense mechanisms must be used to keep it in check, and these maneuvers result in unproductive behavior. The various types of psychoneuroses can be classified into categories such as anxiety reaction, phobic reaction, and several others. These individual types will be discussed later.

TRAUMATIC NEUROSIS

Sometimes an individual who has previously demonstrated an adequate adjustment, when exposed to overwhelming stress, may develop neurotic behavior temporarily in response to this stress. Such a disturbance is termed a *traumatic neurosis*.

A 19 year old college coed was seen for evaluation in the Emergency Room. Her roommate brought her to the hospital eight hours after she was involved in a car accident in which a friend was killed. The patient had been interviewed at length by the police at the scene of the accident. After it had been established that she was not responsible, the patient had been brought back to the dormitory by the police. The roommate reported that she was asleep at the time and did not see the patient until the following morning. At that time the patient was observed to be sitting on the edge of a wooden, straight chair. She sat bolt upright, both feet on the floor, hands folded in her lap. She was expressionless and her eyes stared ahead of her. The roommate reported that the patient did not respond when she was called by name and she did not seem to hear any attempts at conversation with her.

The roommate was alarmed and brought the patient to the hospital. The admitting physician found the patient to be in excellent physical health. Questioning of the roommate by the physician revealed that the patient was a good student who did well in college. She was well liked and dated frequently.

Because of her behavior subsequent to the accident, the patient was admitted to the psychiatric unit. She was willing to walk and to follow simple directions, but she could not or would not speak. For several days the patient sat on the ward in the dayroom. She ate her meals, but did not respond to the approaches of other patients or staff members. A psychiatrist saw the patient every day. In their work together the patient and therapist slowly began to reconstruct the events leading to this young woman's mutism. On the ward the patient began to converse haltingly with others. She was observed to flinch noticeably whenever sirens were heard. On the fifth day of hospitalization, a nurse on the unit entered the patient's room and found her looking out the window at a car being towed behind a truck. When the nurse called the patient's name softly and placed a hand on her shoulder, the patient turned, put her arms around the nurse and began sobbing. She cried without pause for quite a while. The patient sobbed that she had loved her friend and she felt that she, and not her friend, should have died in the accident.

This critical incident was the turning point in the patient's hospitalization. Several weeks were needed to work through the patient's feelings of guilt and grief. During this period the members of the nursing staff were central in supporting the patient by their constant presence and their willingness to sit and listen. In addition, the nurses identified times of the day that were particularly difficult for this young woman—early morning and bedtime. A nurse was assigned to be with the patient at these times, to support the young woman by listening to her, by telling her that these were difficult hours because of her painful thoughts, but that she would not be left alone. By the end of a month, the patient was speaking freely. She was able to hear sirens and observe wrecked cars without undue pain. The psychiatrist permitted her to leave the hospital in order to resume her studies.

The traumatic neurosis is not observed frequently. During periods of war it becomes common among soldiers who have seen or been part of overwhelming events such as attacks, capture by the enemy or the death of buddies. In civilian life such catastrophic events as floods, earthquakes, severe accidents or the witnessing of unexpected death may also result in traumatic neuroses.

TYPES OF PSYCHONEUROSES

Some types of neurotic behavior are seen so often in the acutely anxious individual that they can be identified as specific patterns of defensive behavior; some of these patterns will be described. It should be remembered that though the behavior patterns differ in specific observable ways, their goal is the same; that is, to control the anxiety which threatens to reach overwhelming proportions.

ANXIETY REACTIONS

A person who is uneasy, irritable, "tense" and unable to sleep may be suffering from an anxiety reaction. If the anxiety is not too overwhelming, the individual may demonstrate no symptoms other than chronic tenseness, an inability to "unwind," timidity, apprehension, indecisiveness, sensitivity to the opinions of others, or the chronic fear of making mistakes. As anxiety builds, symptoms become more intense. Highly anxious people may release their feelings through crying, restlessness, irritability leading to aggressive acts, and paralyzing indecision. Fantasies involving neurotic individuals' feelings of inadequacy and their vulnerability to injury from the environment can become so rampant that they begin to suspect that people are *purposely* trying to impinge on them, or that events which occur in the environment are meant specifically to cause them frustration.

People suffering acute anxiety reactions are often found in emergency rooms. Here, they complain of tightness of the chest, dyspnea or bandlike pain around the head, accompanied by elevated blood pressure and pulse and profuse perspiration. They are often examined for physical illnesses before the diagnosis of anxiety reaction is made.

Generally, the individual has been faced with a situation that symbolizes such stress for him that his resulting anxiety cannot be handled. Feelings of unbearable discomfort overwhelm him. Immediate management requires identification of the stressful situation (if the individual has been in therapy and has sufficient insight) or support through drug therapy and the presence of a trusted, helping person.

> A 22 year old graduate student was seen in the Emergency Room because of a series of symptoms which had begun two hours prior to admission. He had been in the library studying for a test. Suddenly, without warning, he became very anxious. He trembled all over and was unable to stop. His mouth became dry, he could feel his heart pounding, and his legs felt rubbery and weak. The young man could not imagine what was wrong, but he feared that he was dying. Friends took him to the Emergency Room of the University Hospital where a medical examination failed to disclose any organic irregularity and he was diagnosed as having an acute anxiety attack.

CONVERSION REACTION

Conversion reactions and dissociative reactions (see p. 85) are often grouped together under the heading of hysteria. These are particularly interesting illnesses to observe clinically because there actually *is something to observe*. One does not have to infer the process that is occurring; the observer can actually *see* symptoms. In the conversion reaction, the observable symptom is the dysfunction of an organ of special sense or movement. In this case there is no physical lesion causing the dysfunction. The underlying process involves anxiety, resulting from an emotional conflict which is expressed on a symbolic level. The mental mechanisms of repression, displacement and conversion are used in creating the symptom, which has unconscious meaning and motivation for the patient.

The classic conversion symptoms involve deafness, blindness, anesthesias, involuntary muscular movements such as tics or tremors, and problems with speech. As would be expected, the patient with such a symptom is intensely concerned about his "illness," that is, the physical illness that he believes he has. His *real* illness, of which he is unaware, allows him to focus his anxiety in the *conversion* symptom, rather than the emotional conflict which is hidden from awareness.

The primary, unconscious purpose of the conversion reaction is to decrease the anxiety aroused by the emotional conflict. All behavior is learned, and neurotic behavior is not an exception. The individual with a conversion reaction soon learns that his symptom prompts behavior from those around him that is *gratifying,* or pleasing to him. His symptom, as it is responded to by those around him, may permit the patient to control others through attention getting or by frightening those around him into submission to his wishes. Such gratification is termed *secondary gain.* Thus, the symptom fosters the primary gain, which is the alleviation of anxiety; also it promotes the secondary gain, which is control of the environment. From the latter, an individual may gain some measure of security.

> R. L., a 17 year old high school student, went out with her boyfriend on Saturday night. She was unprepared for his announcement that he no longer wanted to go steady. When he said haltingly and with decided anxiety, "I want to split," R. L. experienced a sharp pain in her head. She put her hands over both ears. The pain disappeared, but when she lowered her hands R. L. could no longer hear her boyfriend's words. She watched his lips move, but heard no sound.
>
> R. L.'s "deafness" continued throughout the evening. The next day, still unable to hear, she reported the problem to her parents. They took her to a doctor. The girl had a thorough neurological workup, but the examination revealed no physical cause for her deafness. R. L. was eventually referred to a psychiatrist. The girl was able, in psychotherapy, to develop insight into her problems and her symptom gradually disappeared.

The conversion symptom in R. L.'s case, that is, her deafness, had *meaning.* The message it pantomimed was "I do not want to hear this." R. L.'s psychotherapy consisted, in large part, of making her psychologically strong enough that she could tolerate hearing the interpretation of the meaning of her symptom. This therapy takes a long time. As in nursing intervention, patient and the therapist must devote whatever time is necessary in order to become acquainted with one another and to establish a trusting relationship. If this goal is reached, the patient is ready to share with the therapist the kinds of information necessary to understand the patient's conflict. The patient is better prepared to risk the pain of facing his anxiety and the underlying conflict.

In the nursing of individuals with conversion reactions it is very important to understand the patient's *need* for his symptom. No "happy, well-adjusted" person really wishes to be blind, deaf or paralyzed. Such a problem is handicapping, and the victim's life must be altered in many inconveniencing ways to accommodate his problem. Keeping this in mind, it is easy to feel empathic toward such a person and not to scorn his situation. The nurse must attempt to steer a "middle of the road" course in which necessary adjustments are made for the patient's welfare, but special arrangements are not created which would provide secondary gain. Such nursing care is not easily planned and implemented. It requires a thorough evaluation of the neurotic individual to learn what he really can accomplish independently and when he needs assistance in order to achieve. Such an assessment should be the result of thoughtful observation during which assumptions are recognized as such and replaced by data collected through observation. This type of planning for prevention of secondary gain is not unkind. It is based on the fact that this type of gratification may delay the patient's recovery by interfering with his wish to be well.

It is well to identify the differences between the neurotic individual and the malingerer. The former demonstrates a symptom over which he has no control; the meaning of the symptom is not in the person's awareness. The malingerer, on the other hand, describes a symptom when, actually, he has none. Such a person's motivation is quite conscious and his *primary* gain is similar to the conversion patient's secondary gain.

DISSOCIATIVE REACTION

The dissociative reaction is often grouped with the conversion reaction under the heading of hysteria. Like a conversion symptom, the dissociative reaction is a symptom of conflict and anxiety. It is interesting clinically because it is so dramatic, sometimes even bizarre.

The dissociative reactions are defensive patterns of behavior offering flight from crisis and danger. In emotional dissociation there is "an isolation or splitting away from the total personality of some element, which can then be separately conceived, observed and studied. Through the process of dissociation there is unconsciously secured the separation of an idea, wish, function, greater or lesser segment of attention, behavior, or awareness from the mainstream of consciousness."[1] Unlike the conversion symptom, it cannot be seen in the physical make-up of the person, but it is obvious to one who *listens* to this individual that he is missing a large segment of his consciousness. Such an observation is really quite awesome! Dissociative reactions are sometimes broken down into more definite categories, including *twilight states, amnesia* and *fugues*. Each of these categories involves the individual's repression of his identity and the situation that has generated his overwhelming anxiety. The dissociative reaction usually occurs suddenly, following a situation which is catastrophic to the individual. Such a situation might be externally catastrophic, such as a fire, hurricane or war, or it might be intrapsychically so.

One occasionally reads in the newspaper about a person having a dissociative reaction. It is reported that an unidentified person has been found wandering aimlessly about a train station, airport or bus depot. The account usually reports that the person seemed dazed and was unable to identify himself. It is most common to find persons manifesting dissociative reactions in places of travel because they are usually unconsciously trying to escape situations that have proved too overwhelming for them. Their escapes often begin as physical withdrawal and then proceed to psychic escape through repression.

Try to imagine how it would feel to wake up dressed and in a strange place where no one was recognizable and no one seemed aware or interested in your plight. Think how lonely and frightening such a situation would be. Compound the fright until it becomes terror because you do not even know your *own* identity. There is no recourse to "I'll-call-home-for-help" or "I-can-ask-anybody-to-help-me"; when one is not certain of his *own* identity, it is not easy to approach a stranger for aid.

This terrifying situation is often made worse because well meaning people alert the police, who then take responsibility for the individual. It is good that there are police, who are willing to take responsibility for the fate of the amnesiac; however, not knowing one's identity, not recognizing one's surroundings, and on top of this, being taken to a strange hospital by police, whom most people associate with criminals or lawbreakers, is indeed a terrifying situation.

It is often the Emergency Room nurse who first encounters the individual with a dissociative reaction. The patient is frequently accompanied by one or more policemen. He usually looks frightened, and his expression should tell the perceptive nurse much about the treatment he needs. The nurse must try hard to communicate her awareness that the patient is not a criminal. She needs to let the patient know that she, as a representative of the hospital, and the police, as representatives of another agency interested in his welfare, are going to help him to find the answers to his identity. The nurse needs to take time to comfort this patient. He is afraid and alone. On a busy Saturday night in "the pit," as many Emergency Rooms are affectionately dubbed by their staff, it is sometimes hard to find time, energy and sympathy for a patient who isn't hemorrhaging to death, or suffocating. However, the patient who does not know his identity is frightened to death; he, too, requires nursing care. It is true that the ultimate therapy of this patient will rest with a psychiatrist, and the law-enforcement officers may be instrumental in establishing the patient's identity, but the creation of an environment in which the patient feels safe, welcome and, hopefully, *nurtured* is the task of the nurse.

PHOBIC REACTION

It is not unusual to hear someone described as being "phobic" about something. The term "phobic" has gotten to be almost a layman's label. Just what does it mean? Is the reader afraid to touch a worm or a harmless black snake? These are common feelings, especially among females. But consider the rationality of the intense fear of worms. Can an earthworm injure or kill a human being? Of course not. Yet there are many people who would not touch the simple earthworm or black snake unless the situation were dire. Such strong feelings are phobic.

Phobic reactions are intense, irrational fear responses to external objects and situations. As with the other neurotic disorders, the individual's behavioral symptom, i.e., the phobia, begins with overwhelming anxiety which must be controlled by the ego. In this type of reaction the anxiety is transformed into fear through the use of projection. This is to say, the fear that has its unconsciously focused object within the person is *refocused* outside of him; an object outside the person becomes that which is feared. Such a process utilizes displacement. This rather complex unconscious operation helps the individual to control his anxiety because he now has a specific object to which he can attach his feelings. He can then control the intensity of his discomfort by avoiding the object to which his anxiety has become attached.

There are numerous types of phobias. Several of the more common ones are claustrophobia (fear of closed places), acrophobia (fear of heights), and zoophobia (fear of animals). People who fear closed places go out of their way to avoid such situations. An elevator, for the claustrophobic individual, may generate disorganizing fear. For such a person it is a worthy investment of his time and energy to use the stairs—even if it is four flights of steps to his destination.

When a phobic person is forced to confront the feared object, he may become extremely fearful or even panicked. The mere possibility of contact can cause sweating, faintness, nausea and other symptoms of anxiety reaction. Thus, it is well to cooperate with the need of a phobic individual to be protected from that object or situation that generates strong discomfort in him.

Intensive psychotherapy, sometimes in the form of analysis, is necessary to get at the deeply unconscious (repressed) events and feelings which are symbolized by the object of the phobia. This type of psychotherapy is prolonged and difficult. The nurse's role in such an individual's recovery will vary considerably, depending on whether the individual is hospitalized or is living in the community and whether there is a psychiatrist available.

No matter what the setting in which nurse and patient meet, it is appropriate that the nurse *not force the patient into contact with the feared object(s)*. The patient is well aware of the irrationality of his fears; his real problems begin when he must cope with the agony of the onslaught of anxiety that would inundate him were he forced into contact with the symbolic object of his feelings.

The intelligent nursing of neurotic patients is somewhat like exploratory surgery. Consider, for example, the stab victim who is brought into the Emergency Room. The astute surgeon would not simply pull the knife out of a vital area; rather, he would explore the region to ascertain the depth and width of the injury. So it is with the psychiatric nurse; she does not simply confront the patient with the feared object but, instead, she becomes familiar with the patient's feelings and thoughts about significant factors in his life. She does not precipitate a crisis; rather, she works from the outside in, coming to know the patient well, and at such time as the patient shows readiness, or the psychiatrist indicates the patient's readiness, the meaning of the phobia is examined more minutely. If interpretations are made prematurely, that is, before the patient is prepared for them, he will simply not accept them or, worse, will be thrown into an acute anxiety attack.

The following cases illustrate phobic reactions. The first two are not particularly handicapping; the last patient became so disorganized that intense nursing measures had to be instituted.

> A. L., a 70 year old pianist and grandmother, had remained active throughout her life, both in her social activities and her musical career. She was well liked by others, especially her family, who found her ever willing to help others and always concerned for the welfare of those she loved. Her concern was normally expressed verbally, except in one instance—her piano. Whenever her grandchildren, grandnieces or nephews came to her home and they showed interest in playing her piano, A. L. felt it necessary to clean the keyboard with Lysol. When asked about this strange habit, she claimed that the keyboard harbored cold germs which she did not wish the children to contact.

> N. R., a 35 year old doctor, was secure in the majority of his undertakings. He had succeeded in educating himself and embarking alone on a practice that was developing well. N. R. was known to others as a self-confident, occasionally brash young man who was independent and conscientious. Those who knew this young man might have been surprised had they seen him on the Empire State

Building observation deck, ashen colored and clinging to the inner wall of the building.

There are many people like A. L. and N. R. That is to say, many individuals are able to lead successful, productive lives in spite of symptoms of neurosis. Those who are able to live effectively in spite of their problem can do so because their symptoms are not grossly handicapping. Most individuals exhibit some signs of neurotic behavior, and mild phobic reactions are a common manifestation of it.

In the next example we meet "Frank Jones" who, because of his phobia, became progressively handicapped until, finally, he was unable to leave his apartment. Frank did not identify a particular object that he feared; rather, he suffered from a pervasive discomfort when he was out of doors. As his illness progressed, his phobic symptom indicated that Frank feared danger in any place outside the safety of his own apartment; he feared open spaces. The technical name for this particular phobia is *agoraphobia*.

Mrs. Wise, a public health nurse, was making a monthly visit to a family living in a housing development. The identified patient was being treated for tuberculosis. The patient's mother asked the nurse if she could possibly stop at the flat below to see a neighbor who was in need of help. The nurse promised to stop by.

Mrs. Wise knocked at the door of the apartment. She heard movements within, but it was several moments before the door was opened. An elderly woman with thin white hair framing a chestnut colored face lined with age stood in the doorway. She was slightly bent over and the hand that held the door knob was gnarled and swollen from arthritis. She looked up at the nurse questioningly.

"Hello, I'm Mrs. Wise, the public health nurse. I understand you wanted me to visit."

The stooped over woman seemed to stand taller. "Oh, yes. Thank you for coming. I'm Letty Jones. It's my son, Frank. He don't want to leave here. He lay 'round the bed all day long and I can't get 'im out." The elderly woman beckoned Mrs. Wise into the apartment and led the way to a small, cluttered living room. The window in the room was surrounded by potted African violets. The overstuffed chairs and sofa were old. The sofa had a tear in it which could not quite be hidden by a throw cushion.

The two women sat on the sofa while Letty Jones related the story of her 40 year old son who had begun acting "queer three months ago." It seemed that Frank was in the habit of looking for work on construction gangs. When the weather was good, he had no trouble finding jobs. As the cold weather came heralding winter, work became scarce, and when it was available, it was at distant points to which there was no public transportation. Frank had been forced to spend more and more of his time on the street corner or in the local bar with his friends.

Frank's mother first noticed his strange behavior when he stopped going to the bar. He reported to her that he simply was "tired" of his friends. Then, several weeks later, Frank stopped going to his favorite corner. At this point, his mother was aware of difficulties because her son wanted his friends near him, but he would see them only if the men came up to his apartment.

The next problem occurred when Frank refused to go out to get groceries for his mother. She was elderly and unable to get around unassisted. Frank's help, both financial and physical, had been counted on for many years. It was at this point that the mother asked Frank just what *was* happening. He told her, with a small embarrassed smile, that he really was ashamed; however, he was frightened to go out. The problem had begun the last time he was laid off a job.

Frank described to his mother how he became aware of an unexplainable fear of the bar where he and his friends gathered. Soon after that, Frank felt equally uncomfortable as he stood on the street corner with his friends and watched others. It was at this point that he began staying in the apartment and inviting his friends up to visit. This arrangement was satisfactory; however, Frank's friends could not be persuaded to stay in the apartment and Frank could not bring himself to go out on the street. He was lonely, but worse, he was afraid.

Letty Jones asked her son just *what* he was afraid of, but he could not say. She tried to force her son to go out, but she could tell from his tear-stained face and trembling body that he was truly terrified, and so Frank became a prisoner of his fears. He had now been in the house for three months. Thanks to the kindness of neighbors, food was procured and other necessities found.

Mrs. Wise listened to the story. She wondered where Frank was now. What had happened to him three months ago? Did he have a physical problem such as a brain tumor that could be responsible for his seeming aberrations of thought? Mrs. Wise wondered also if she should request consultation with one of the black supervisors, for she recognized her typical white concerns about Frank Jones' "laziness" or his desire to malinger. She tried to push these thoughts from her mind but could not, and she knew that this was good, for she recognized her need of sociological consultation in order to better understand the role of a culture that was alien to her and its influence, if any, on Frank Jones' illness.

Mrs. Wise asked the elderly woman if she might talk to Frank. The mother nodded and called, "Frank, come on in here. The nurse come to see you." Mr. Jones entered the room minutes later. He was dressed in slacks and a pullover. Mrs. Wise saw that he was good looking and alert, and his face reflected kindness. She wondered how to begin.

"I'm Charlotte Wise, Mr. Jones. I'm a public health nurse."

"Glad to meet you," he nodded. "We're gettin' pretty low 'round here. I got some kind of thing 'bout bein' outside."

Mrs. Wise listened and nodded. She asked the man if he could tell her about it. Frank's mother and the nurse listened as he repeated essentially what the mother had described. Mr. Jones said repeatedly that he knew it was silly, but he just could not bring himself to leave the apartment.

At the end of the recitation the nurse said, "I can imagine how uncomfortable it must be for you to think of going outside. I'm not sure I can help you, Mr. Jones, but I am going to try. I shall come back as soon as I know what I shall be able to do. Have you had any illnesses or accidents in the last six months?" The public health nurse put her coat on as Mr. Jones thought about her question and answered, "No."

The two occupants of the apartment walked her to the door, thanking her for coming. Mrs. Wise promised to return as soon as she found out what would be available in the way of help for the Jones family.

Mrs. Wise kept her promise. She spoke to her supervisor, who directed her to the nearest Community Mental Health Clinic. There she made a referral by describing Frank Jones and his problem to the intake nurse. When a patient conference was scheduled Mrs. Wise was invited to come and to present Mr. Jones to the other nurses, psychiatrist, social worker, psychologist, and mental health workers. It was decided that Mrs. Wise and one of the psychiatric nurses would go to the Jones' apartment the following day to further evaluate the problem.

During their visit the next afternoon, the two nurses outlined a plan to Mr. Jones involving a time, twice a week, when the nurse from the Mental Health Clinic and Mr. Jones could talk. In the plan it was anticipated that, when he felt able to, he and the nurse would travel together to the clinic for an appointment with the psychiatrist. In the interim a social worker would also make a home visit to speak with Mr. Jones and his mother. The plan was agreed to and the nurses left. Back at the Mental Health Clinic a conference was held with the staff, outlining what had transpired.

The psychiatric nurse began her regular visits to Mr. Jones. It was necessary to spend many weeks identifying each person's expectations from the collaborative work. Then Mr. Jones began to describe his feelings. It did not surprise the nurse that her patient had very strong, ambivalent feelings about his mother. The nurse did not comment specifically about Mr. Jones' feelings, but she did acknowledge that she heard and that she could imagine that it was difficult to live with these kinds of feelings. The nurse felt certain that the emotions Mr. Jones described played a part in his phobic reaction. She did not interpret this to the patient but made a note to report these observations to her psychiatrist consultant.

At the end of the fifth month Mr. Jones felt that he could risk a trip to the Mental Health Clinic, if *his* nurse went with him. The expedition was arranged and it took place uneventfully (though Mr. Jones would probably not agree). The nurse, who touched his arm often as he spoke, noted that her patient looked fearful, but he managed the trip. The psychiatrist talked with Mr. Jones and he seemed satisfied with the progress being made. It was decided that the nurse would continue seeing her patient biweekly and the psychiatrist would see them together at the center every six weeks. The doctor noted on the record that the patient suffered from a phobic reaction.

The interviews continued for several months. Mr. Jones spoke more and more of his dread, *not* of the outside, *but of leaving his mother.* As he unloaded these feelings, Mr. Jones felt freer to venture outside. At first he would not go without his nurse. Later, he did go out unaccompanied, though he was not at ease. Finally, after nine months, Mr. Jones was able to resume his former way of life. The Mental Health Clinic was instrumental in locating regular work for this client. The public health nurse was sent a report of the work that was now completed. At the patient conference in which Mr. Jones was discussed after the closing of the case, the psychiatric nurse presented a resumé of her work with the patient. The psychiatrist remarked that, though Mr. Jones did not fully understand the relationship of his feelings toward his mother, his feelings about the gang boss who laid him off the job, and his primitive feelings toward a long forgotten father, nonetheless he had made a good symptomatic recovery, and his prognosis was fair, provided he did not encounter a similar "triangle" of problem-feelings.

OBSESSIVE-COMPULSIVE REACTIONS

Obsessive-compulsive reactions in their severest forms can result in almost total incapacitation. In milder cases, however, they are regarded as constructive by various segments of the population. One cannot generalize about *all* such persons; however, the reader should try to recall when a clinical instructor was encountered who seemed harsh and rigid concerning various activities related to asepsis. Or, again, think of the nursing instructor who checked the students out on the administration of medications. Were there "bull sessions" in the dormitory where someone mentioned how compulsive these nurses were? Yet no one described them as "sick." In fact, the women in question perform a function that is basically advantageous to the community.

Obsessive-compulsive behavior is seen normally in the anal phase of development as the child masters muscle training. Again, in early adolescence it is not unusual to observe post-pubertal individuals managing their anxieties with compulsive activity. The obsessive component of obsessive-compulsive behavior is the involuntary thought, recognized by the individual as irrational, if it is so, that keeps recurring despite the person's wish to avoid or ignore it. The compulsive part of the behavior is an act that is performed by the individual, either to avoid anxiety or to make an obsession disappear. Like the obsession (and the phobia), the individual recognizes his compulsive behavior to be "silly, stupid or illogical." The problem is, he *cannot stop it.*

If the reader has caught herself listening to the accounts of symptoms and patient's plights from a distance, if she has fallen into the trap of observing with a "cold, clinical eye" and it is difficult to imagine these symptoms attached to *real, feeling,* live persons like herself, let us consider a closer example. Is it possible to dredge up the memories of the elementary school years? Who remembers walking home from school saying "step on a crack, break my mother's back"? How many young children were comfortable enough to put a foot on the divisions in the sidewalk? Is it possible to remember discomfort if a crack was stepped on by mistake? Such memories are not always vivid, and an inability to recall these early years may be a good solid example of repression at work.

Obsessive-compulsive reactions are, like the other neurotic behaviors noted, an attempt to control anxiety arising from unconscious conflict. In Freudian terms, this reaction involves the unconscious id impulses which tend to be hostile and aggressive. The id is in conflict with the ego, which attempts to modify these unacceptable impulses. The behavior that is labeled obsessive-compulsive represents an attempt by the ego to control the actual, unacceptable id impulses.

Persons who suffer from overwhelming anxiety often displace these feelings on unrelated objects, as in the process that creates phobias. The individual then negates the "harm" done by the feared object, which may be just a thought in this case, by completing some compulsive act.

> L. G., a 16 year old high school boy with acne, was admitted to the psychiatric service because he could no longer function at home or in school. The boy spent literally hours each day thinking of the nonsensical rhyme "snips and snails, and puppy dog's tails."
>
> When he wished to control the obsession, he had to complete a complicated ritual for washing his genitals. The boy suffered greatly because he recognized the absurdity of his symptom, but he became uncontrollably anxious whenever he tried to break the cycle.

The nursing students were particularly interested in L. G., who was close to their own age and obviously distressed. They approached the resident who explained that, as in each case of this kind, the patient's symptom utilized four mechanisms. The first was *regression*. In effect, the patient's thoughts, his attitudes and his emotions were from an earlier period of development. The second mechanism was *isolation*. This was evidenced by the boy's inability to identify any emotions that accompanied his obsession. *Reaction-formation,* the third mechanism, makes the individual able to act opposite to the unconscious feelings that actually threaten and batter the person who displays the symptom. Thus, it is usually observed that patients with obsessive-compulsive reactions are sweet and cooperative, sometimes to the point of seeming obsequiousness. Staff members often feel uncomfortable in the presence of such individuals. When members of the staff can discuss their own feelings, it is generally found that their discomfort is related to the *rage* they perceive in these patients who are experiencing difficulty in "keeping the lid" on their unconscious emotions.

The fourth mechanism utilized is *undoing*. This mechanism enables the individual to negate the unacceptable (though unconscious) feeling. In this particular case, the emotional component attached to the thought was undone by washing the genitals.

Nursing Care

The nursing care of individuals who use compulsive or ritualistic modes of behavior can be particularly taxing for the nurse. This type of patient is usually encountered in an institutional setting, for if his problem is severe enough to come to the attention of the health professions, it is usually too incapacitating for the individual to continue living outside a hospital.

Patients who utilize compulsive acts to allay their anxiety should not be prevented from carrying out their rituals. To do so would be cruel, for the anxiety which might emerge could precipitate overwhelming panic. In order to accept the necessity for the ritual, staffing patterns must be established which leave nurses free to use limitless amounts of time in being with the patient and getting the things done that need to be accomplished such as eating, toileting and drug administration. In the case of any one of these objectives, it should be recognized that many hours might be consumed completing the compulsive acts in order to get to the goal of the nurse. To say the least, patience is not only a virtue but a decided necessity in the attending nurse.

As with all patients who are in acute distress, a nurse or other psychiatric worker should be in constant attendance as long as the patient displays the need for constant compulsive behavior. The underlying assumption is that compulsive behavior is utilized to control anxiety and, for the psychiatric patient, overwhelming anxiety represents a condition of acute distress.

It is expected that a combination of chemotherapy and psychotherapy will alleviate the patient's anxiety; however, before these two elements have been able to "take hold," that is, to become effective, the nurse must provide first aid measures. These consist of:

1. Remaining with the patient. This does not require that the same person be in constant attendance. In fact, it is absolutely necessary that staff members be relieved often, for it is terribly taxing, in terms of frustration, anxiety and anger, to remain with compulsive patients.

2. Providing satisfying channels for substitution. If the patient washes his hands, perhaps he will be equally comfortable washing other things, such as his dirty clothes or medicine glasses. Also, helping to keep his own belongings or things on the ward straightened may be satisfying because he is performing a needed task for which he can accrue recognition and praise. (This kind of "substitution" may not be possible for the patient and should not be pushed.)

3. Protecting the patient's right to his ritual and protecting him from the scorn of other patients.

4. Maintenance of physical well being. Often the rituals of compulsive patients endanger their health. For instance, the handwasher is likely to develop dermatitis. His hands should be protected by rubber gloves (if the patient permits them), and lotions should be applied that offer some protection against constant exposure to soap and water.

Another likely problem is the need for rest when the patient's ritual does not leave time for this. Drugs may be necessary in order to free the patient for sleep. It may be necessary to administer medication parenterally, and every effort should be made to explain the necessity to the patient.

5. Above all, a nursing care plan must be initiated that offers limitless time for the nurses attending the patient to accomplish necessary tasks. This protects the patient. The staff must be rotated frequently in order to protect the nurses.

HYPOCHONDRIASIS

This disease is described by many texts as the most serious of the neuroses. In its severest forms, the symptoms border on psychosis; this is to say, the sick individual has poor reality testing ability which is manifested by his rigid belief that a physical illness is present.

The hypochondriac represents an example of severe regression. His position is similar to that of the infant; that is, he is extremely concerned with himself and his body. (The psychiatric term for this concern is narcissistic*). Much of his energy (libido) has been withdrawn from the world around him and is refocused on his own body. He spends countless hours considering the possibility of having one disease or another. Such a person is often encountered in the general hospital where he is hospitalized for extensive work-up. The test results are always negative; no physical lesions are found. Such patients tend to be badly received by staff members who are geared to the curing of demonstrable disease.

Individuals who manifest hypochondriasis have difficulty establishing meaningful relationships with others. This, the reader may recall, is a developmental task of infancy. Thus, it is interesting to see the dynamics of the neurotic behavior. It reflects an early phase of development which is characterized by the infant's consuming interest in his body; relationships with others have revolved about the mutual concern of mother and child for the infant's physical welfare. In adulthood the hypochondriac can only interact with others, in an effective way, if all parties are concerned with his now adult body.

Hypochondriasis involves a transposition of behavior which was appropriate for an infant to a later period of life when it is not appropriate. The neurotic individual unconsciously wants and demands to be treated in such a way that infantile needs are met. What makes this situation pathological is that the adult is not an infant. Thus, the

---

* Narcissism, a term implying a morbid interest in one's own body, is a word that is derived from the Greek myth about Narcissus, son of the river god Cephissus and the nymph Leiriope. Narcissus loved his own reflection in the water, and he either pined away while gazing at himself or perhaps drowned one day as he leaned too far over the spring.

adult's conscious behavior, which seeks gratification of his unconscious needs, is doomed to failure. Other adults, from whom he expects gratification of his needs, do not respond to him as he unconsciously desires. Anxiety and frustration are generated in the neurotic person because he is ineffective in the communication of his needs.

The caretaking staff in the hospital unconsciously represent parents. Their ministrations symbolize the loving care that the infant demanded and received. For the hypochondriacal patient, problems arise when the tests are negative and the hospital staff tacitly demands that the patient mature and become independent again. The hypochondriacal patient *simply cannot do this.* Staff members become anxious; the patient becomes more symptomatic.

The hypochondriac presents a challenge to the nurse. As a rule, this type of neurosis does not respond well to psychotherapy, and the nurse's concern must be as much for her own attitude and behaviors as for those of her patient. Interaction with a severely regressed individual can be quite irritating because it is anxiety-provoking. The psychiatric nurse or the nurse who encounters hypochondriacs in other settings must be willing to recognize her own feelings if she is to be able to cope with the strain that the hypochondriacal patient can potentially impose. The nurse must be aware that the patient's demands cannot be met through literal response to his requests, because the actual needs are unconscious and cannot be expressed by the patient. Thus, most nursing intervention represents stop-gap measures because it is a response to the patient's conscious request for gratification only; the unconscious needs remain unmet. The patient is chronically anxious and demanding. If not insightful, the staff becomes frustrated, then angry and sometimes, finally, retaliatory.

The discussion of hypochondriasis clearly illustrates the functions of regression and fixation in all neuroses. As has been previously discussed, the personality develops much as a foundation and wall are constructed. Structural weaknesses in the wall make it vulnerable to stress; when stress occurs, it is the area of structural weakness that crumbles. That area is represented by the neurotic individual's unconscious yearning to have the needs of the earlier chronological period met. The regressive needs are inappropriate in later periods of life. *This is the disorder.* Mothers, fathers and siblings cannot be magically recalled. The family of origin cannot be reconstructed so that the sick individual may live through the phase of development that he needs to re-experience. In order to surmount this problem it is sometimes necessary to provide substitute parents. In the case of hypochondriacs, hospitalization often represents gratification through secondary gain for the patient because he is placed in a setting in which regression is actually encouraged. The same circumstances account for some of the attitudes and behaviors exhibited by hospitalized patients in general toward their doctors and nurses, whom they unconsciously treat like the parents who formerly cared for them.

ANXIETY AS A PROBLEM TO THE NURSE

As the reader has seen, anxiety plays a major role in all the psychoneurotic disorders mentioned. At their base is unresolved conflict. The product of the conflict is anxiety, which is observed within the behavior patterns organized to control it. Individuals who experience moderate to severe amounts of anxiety are very uncomfortable. One of the main goals of the psychiatric nurse is either to decrease the anxiety of her patient if the cause can be identified in the environment and the environmental factor can then be manipulated, or to actually assist the patient to withstand the ravages of anxiety if the cause cannot be manipulated. Techniques will be discussed in depth to provide the nurse with a variety of means to achieve these goals.

A notorious occupational hazard of nursing that is not always discussed is the nurse's own anxiety and the means at her disposal for caring for herself. By now the observant reader has not only learned the symptoms of anxiety but, hopefully, she has looked into her own past experiences and recalled situations in which she, too, felt the symptoms described in these pages. This is a very important learning experience, and if the student has failed to do this "exercise," she should close the text, sit back and consider quite honestly what her experiences have been.

The majority of human beings have had both good and bad growth experiences. Usually the good outweigh the bad, and the individual matures and produces effectively. Occasionally a situation arises that calls forth the unconscious areas that represent the "bad" experiences. At these times the individual may not recognize and identify what is happening, but there is usually awareness that all does not feel "right." Nurses who work in high-risk areas are vulnerable to this kind of mishap because they deal with sick people all the time, both in psychiatric settings, in general hospitals and in the community.

Sick people tend to regress, and their behavior reflects this movement. For patients in a general hospital setting who are severely ill, regression is a normal occurrence and it is useful insofar as it permits the patient to accept his care with less psychic discomfort. For those nurses who also have need to regress, the behavior of these patients is severely taxing. The recognition by the nurse of the patient's demands is not conscious, and her response is influenced by her own needs. Thus, the nurse who responds to the regressed patient may find herself irritable, tense or tired. These feelings, while they come in part from true physical fatigue, are also the result of mental strain. The strain is from anxiety generated by contact with patients whose unconscious demands are similar to the unconscious needs of the nurse. This, then, can become a vexing problem. The nurse is uncomfortable and dissatisfied with herself in the job situation. The patient is anxious and his feelings influence behavior which generates discomfort in the nurse. One can see that this is a circular situation, and if it is not interrupted, it can continue without end.

There are several techniques of interruption that may operate in the general hospital setting. The nurse may have sufficient curiosity about herself to research her own feelings; perhaps her experiences have led her to develop insight; or if she is fortunate she works with an observant supervisor who channels the nurse's perceptive powers into efforts directed at analyzing the nurse-patient situation to find answers to the mutual discomfort of both parties. Either alone, or with objective help, the nurse can and most surely will benefit from examination of her feelings, her actions, and the patient's apparent feelings and his actions.

The end product of such an investigation will be the nurse's recognition of her own discomfort. She will label it appropriately as anger or anxiety. This is a good and an important beginning, because the nurse can then explore further the causes of her feelings in regard to this patient. It is *not* recommended that the nurse attempt to uncover her unconscious motivations without psychiatric consultation; however, it is of use for the nurse to explore those feelings and thoughts that are available to her. Through such an investigation she can modify her behavior, which is likely to cause alteration in the patient's behavior, which, in turn, will bring about modification of both the patient's and the nurse's feelings.

Anxiety is an ever-present problem in dealing with psychiatric patients. The reader now knows that anxiety is basic to all psychiatric illnesses, so that it is present whenever the nurse encounters a sick patient. Anxiety is also contagious. This means to the psychiatric nurse that she will be affected by it; she may either recognize its presence in herself and work with it appropriately, or she will not identify it and either be uncomfortable for unknown reasons or she will control it through involuntary (that is, not consciously determined) acts. The latter is definitely an undesirable situation, for this is just the problem that the nurse is trying to alter in her patient!

Causes of the nurse's anxiety in the care of psychiatric patients tend to stem from several sources; sometimes the nurse's basic anxiety is aroused when she encounters a patient whose presenting problem represents a conflict that the nurse also has been unable to resolve. It is important to remember that this process is unconscious and the nurse may not be able to identify the problem fully. She will do quite well if she can simply identify her feelings of discomfort so that measures can be instituted to alter the process that is occurring between nurse and patient.

Sometimes the nurse will become anxious because she feels the need to control her patient. She may not realize the problem immediately, but her discomfort will be lessened when she is able to identify the situation, for it is readily understandable to logical, conscious thought that one human being cannot hope to control another. In the case of neurotic patients who demonstrate specific behavior patterns to control their anxiety, this problem is very prevalent between nurse and patient. Sometimes the nurse, in her unconscious need to change the patient, becomes highly anxious when the patient continues to exhibit behaviors that the nurse hopes to modify. As she feels greater discomfort she either withdraws from her patient or presses more for behavior modification, or she expresses annoyance with the patient. None of these behaviors is of use in the therapeutic process. The patient, unaware of the nurse's underlying feelings of caring, is likely to feel hurt, rejected or misunderstood. Such reactions are obviously untoward, considering that the psychiatric nurse has spent untold hours trying to develop a trusting relationship with the patient in which he can feel comfortable presenting himself as he really experiences self. He will feel free to do this, in part, because the trust in the relationship is based on his awareness of the nurse and his assumption that he knows enough about her to predict her responses to him. If the nurse then responds in a new, negative and inexplicable manner, some of the trust that has been developed between the two parties will be destroyed.

It is highly important for the nurse to identify her own feelings in regard to her patient. If she cannot do this and then go on to handling them, the feelings are likely to spill over into the relationship with the patient, and the latter will then be forced to handle them. It is much more likely that the healthier party in the relationship, the nurse, can deal with her feelings than that the handicapped party, the patient, can identify correctly what is occurring and act appropriately.

> M. G., an elderly widowed patient, was admitted to the psychiatric unit because of his compulsive activity. He washed his hands continually and mumbled to himself. The gentleman had been living with his married son and family ever since the death of his wife. M. G., it was reported, had adjusted well to his new home and the family had seemed to accept him comfortably. About one month prior to admission the patient was noted to have become more critical of his young grandchildren. Specifically, he could not tolerate their use of his belongings, such as his towel or napkin or glass. When another family member touched these items, the elderly man would

become quite upset and demand that they be washed and sterilized. Then he began mumbling unintelligibly. Shortly after this the man began washing his hands repeatedly, as often as every 20 minutes.

The other patients on the unit seemed to notice this patient almost immediately. They did not bother to introduce themselves or to make M. G. feel welcome. Staff members were also aware of their own lack of motivation to make him feel comfortable and wanted. At an admission conference on M. G. where the nursing care plan was to be formulated, the staff voiced their lack of enthusiasm. The ward resident interpreted the staff's lack of enthusiasm, not as such, but as a sign of their withdrawal because of their own discomfort in the situation. The interpretation was accepted and the staff tried to deal with their underlying feelings about the patient. Several persons explained that they dreaded going into the patient's room. They said they felt isolated from the other staff and they felt inexplicably blue. One of the nurses described her feeling of annoyance when she took medication to M. G. and then had to devote one to two hours to getting the medicine into him. Interestingly enough, there was an attendant on the unit who was, himself, getting older; he moved more slowly than the rest of the staff and completed his assigned tasks in a leisurely fashion. This particular man did not feel uncomfortable with M. G. He was able to sit in the patient's room and observe his ritualistic behavior without discomfort. He talked with M. G. about various topics when the patient was able to stop mumbling.

The staff considered everyone's contribution to the discussion. They decided that their anxiety level was very high in the presence of this patient for two reasons: The first was that the patient was elderly. He seemed quite frail, and the staff were made uncomfortable by the realization that youth and vigor do decline as people age. The patient was an unconscious reminder to each of them that they, too, would become less competent over the years. Such an awareness brought anxiety, as well as a sense of loss, which was represented by the "blue" feelings expressed by some. The anxiety was compounded by the staff's inability to make M. G. stop washing his hands. It is true that they had not tried overtly to influence his activities, but their underlying assumption was that the patient was in the hospital to get well. Staff were the purveyors of that which would heal the patient, but he was not healing! The staff found themselves responding to the patient's continued ritualism by anxiety and unconscious attempts to be out of the situation.

The resident said that these feelings would not simply disappear because the staff recognized them, but that the patient would benefit because the staff members could protect M. G. by consciously *not* withdrawing, and that they could protect themselves by assigning staff personnel to the patient in such a way that no one had to be extensively exposed to the patient while he was highly anxious and ritualistic.

Staff members were then assigned on a rotating basis to Mr. G. Each person spent no more than a half hour with him when he was observed to be highly anxious. The attendant who was not affected by his exposure to Mr. G. was given freedom from some of his other duties so that he could devote more time to this patient. The two of them could converse or engage in some activity together.

It was decided that while one nurse was assigned to medications for the entire unit, a second assignment would be made for administration of medication to Mr. G., who often required as much time as the entire patient group for administering the medicine. Thus, every attempt was made to cover those situations in which anxiety might be engendered in working with this patient who was so ritualistic. The staff tried to identify each instance in which anxiety began to crop up and cause behavioral responses in them. The behaviors were interpreted and altered.

As Mr. G. began to feel less anxious, his compulsive activity decreased, and the staff's anxiety level also decreased. It was noted and jokingly reported by an aide that by the time Mr. G. was well enough to be discharged, the staff would be well enough to give up their therapy hours (ward conferences) and return to work.

In summary, anxiety is a pervasive problem to nurses in their work with patients, both in the general hospital, the psychiatric hospital and the community. The symptoms of anxiety are as applicable to the nurse as they are to her patient, and the discomfort experienced because of anxiety is similar in all people, be they nurses, doctors, patients or relatives. Anxiety can be used constructively if the individual who feels it is able to identify the true nature of his discomfort and then is able to alter the source of his anxiety, that is, the conflict. Anxiety is destructive when the individual who experiences it does not realize its true nature and acts involuntarily to alleviate his discomfort. Thus, the nurse who paces the floor rather than finishing her charting and going into a patient's room to spend a few minutes with him is depriving that patient of a beneficial experience. If the nurse were able to identify her feelings of discomfort and then to come to terms with the basic problem, she would not have to pace in order to become comfortable, she would finish her required work more effectively, and she could then devote a few extra moments to a patient who needs the attention of an insightful, compassionate nurse.

Anxiety can be used by the perceptive nurse in the same way she utilizes the mercury column in a thermometer. If the nurse knows herself to be well and can rely on her own insight, she can then observe herself with interest as she becomes anxious in a clinical stuation. If other causes are not evident, the psychiatric nurse is then justified in questioning the process occurring between herself and the patient. It is likely that the patient is more anxious, or is struggling to express something that is difficult for him or, conversely, is trying *not* to express some consciously felt situation. Thus, if there is an overload of anxiety that is experienced by the nurse in her encounter with the patient, and if the nurse is confident that the anxiety does not stem from a personal problem of her own, she can then safely look to the patient for the cause of the feelings between the two parties. In this case, anxiety has been used as an indication of a problem; it has acted as a signal light flashing green to the nurse, telling her to go ahead with her investigation.

NURSING INTERVENTION TO ALLEVIATE ANXIETY IN THE HOSPITALIZED PATIENT

Anxiety is an often observed phenomenon in the patient hospitalized for a physical illness. Some of the causes of anxiety stem from the patient's lack of control over his test outcomes or the choice of procedures done to him and his inability to find a psychological position that enables him to assume the "patient" role comfortably.

Assumption of patient status is sometimes difficult when the sick individual is basically a person who must control his life situation in order to feel comfortable. This is not a person who can regress "gracefully," and the nurse is obliged to arrange the patient's care in such a way that he feels that he really does have some say in the procedures pertaining to himself. This is the patient whom we question regarding his preference in matters of routine care. This is the patient for whom a special effort is made by staff not to "overpower." In talking with such a patient, it is well to remember that his room is his property while he uses it and, as such, we are visitors in it. Thus, it is appropriate to ask the patient if he would like company for a few minutes. If the answer is "no," then the nurse must be prepared to leave without feeling rejected. She should be aware that the patient may be tired; he may want some privacy, which is difficult to find in the fish bowl called "hospital"; or he may need to keep distance between himself and the nurse. It may be that the patient simply needs to know that he controls the situation; that is to say, he may really want company, but perhaps he needs to see first that through his words he can cause the nurse to leave. The nurse who leaves, saying that she will return at another time, offers the patient the chance of further contact.

Let us return, however, to the patient who *does* invite the nurse to enter. She should, if at all possible, be seated in the patient's presence. Not only is this more comfortable for her, but it allows the patient in bed to be physically higher up than she is and, therefore, symbolically, in a more powerful position. This may seem like a contrived maneuver, but it does allow the patient a greater sense of control, which is certainly hard to achieve while hospitalized.

With the patient who seems anxious, it is important, basically, to be with him. Next it is urgent that the nurse listen in order that she might actually hear. This is easy to suggest, but the skill takes time to acquire. It is unusual to hear a patient say, "I am afraid. I cannot tolerate the thought of another eight hours in this place." It is more likely that the nurse will hear a patient say, "It's kind of dull around here. Don't you ever feel like getting your coat on and departing the place for a while? How did you ever get into nursing anyhow?" The actual question is directed to the nurse's feelings but, between the lines, the patient is saying something about his own feelings. (For the nursing student who wonders about the plausibility of such an interpretation, it should be pointed out that the patient is making a statement about the nurse's feelings, but his assumptions about her come from within his own awareness, unless he has seen her behave in a manner that he interprets as her wishing to leave. Thus, he really projects his sense of longing to leave on to the nurse.)

In response to this kind of statement the nurse needs to indicate that she has heard and that she wants the patient to continue. She does this by saying, "It is hard to be around here sometimes" or "What are some of the things about hospital life that you think would make it difficult to stick around?" or some other statement that gives the patient the opportunity to say out loud what it is that is bothering him. For a while it may seem that the discussion is about the nurse, but sooner or later, depending on the patient's ability to trust the nurse and his willingness to recognize his own feelings, he will begin to speak in terms, not of her feelings, but of his own. This is progress and will be helpful for the patient because he can take a look at what is bothering him; perhaps the nurse can modify his environment in some way to decrease the anxiety-provoking elements in it.

> A patient confided to the nurse that he dreaded the mornings because the laboratory technician left his cart outside the patient's door. The patient, listening to the technician's footfalls approach and depart many times, never knew which time the technician was going to open his own door and enter. The patient had blood drawn each day. He explained that it was really not painful, but he had come to dread the simple stick of the needle because he relived the moment each time he heard the rubber wheels of the cart and the many footfalls of the technician.

In this situation, the nurse was able to ask the technician to leave his cart elsewhere. It was a simple manipulation of the patient's environment. Doubtless there were other anxiety-provoking factors, but this identified one was easily altered.

In the case of procedures to be done to the patient, especially of a diagnostic nature, the nurse must assess her patients carefully. For the anxious individual who needs to know in order to control, it is necessary that the patient have complete information about procedures. For such a patient, real problems might be precipitated in the form of panic if something is done that was not anticipated by him. On the other hand, there is another type of anxious patient who should have a minimum of details presented to him because his anxieties grow with each detail and offer him more with which to be concerned. This is a difficult nursing assessment to make, and it is well to check with the patient's doctor for guidelines.

Generally (and it must be kept in mind that it is dangerous and unrealistic to generalize), patients who seem aloof and "tight," the ones who seem unwilling to share or to be friendly, are the patients who need more information. Patients who are quite outgoing, dependent to the point of seeming rather infantile (typically, the patients who are emotionally explosive), do better with less information about their tests. For this group it is well to present the broad outlines of tests to be done. For instance, consider a gastric lavage. For a patient who needs detailed information one might prepare the individual by explaining: "It is a simple procedure. The resident [or whoever does the test in that hospital] will probably come early in the morning so you don't have your breakfast delayed too long. He will take a rubber tube that has been iced and slip it up through your nose into the back of your throat and down into your stomach. The whole procedure takes only a few minutes and it is painless, though slightly unpleasant. You may feel like gagging, but the doctor will instruct you to breathe deeply or to swallow at intervals. This will help in the passage of the tube. When it is in your stomach (and you will have no sensation of this), the doctor will then take a syringe attached to the tube and withdraw some of the fluid in your stomach. This is painless, and after he gets the sample, he will pull the tube out." For the patient whose anxieties multiply with numerous details, the following kind of presentation might be more appropriate. The reader will notice that the broad outline is given, but the details are omitted. "As your doctor told you, he has ordered an analysis of the contents of your stomach. The doctor will come in the morning before breakfast to do the test. He will get the sample by placing a tube in your stomach, through your nose. The whole procedure does not take more than five minutes and then we can bring you some hot coffee and breakfast."

Note in the example that the nurse finished her description with mention of food. This is not an idle selection of words. Food is important to all of us, and for the more regressed patient, it is important and usually satisfying. The nurse has completed her discussion of the unpleasant and hopes to focus the patient's thoughts on that which is pleasant and will follow the procedure.

In summary, the patient hospitalized for a physical illness is vulnerable to anxiety. It is most helpful if the nurse can recognize her patient's anxiety. She will observe its presence through the same kinds of symptoms described earlier in the chapter. In addition, she may note an increased stream of conversation initiated by the patient that is used to hold the listener in the room; she may observe an increase in the patient's restlessness, a decrease in the patient's interpersonal communications, or the emergence of specific behavior patterns which indicate that the patient is attempting to keep his feelings under control. Such behaviors include excessive use of the bell cord followed by numerous demands, pacing in the hall, or rigidity in respect to room arrangement and daily scheduling of events. (To be honest, one could not hope to describe all the manifestations of anxiety in the patient hospitalized for physical illness. It is realistic to point out that, aside from the symptoms described earlier, anxiety might be suspected when any behavior is observed that is different from that known to be part of a particular patient's life style.)

The nurse who will ultimately be of help to a patient in controlling his anxiety is one who can take the time to sit down and listen. She is the nurse who is willing to sacrifice that time for a cigarette and a chat in the nurses' lounge for a talk with a patient. She is the nurse who listens carefully to her patient's stream of conversation and hears *themes*. Though the patient may not come right out and say what is bothering him, the nurse may detect hints in the patient's choice of conversational topics.

NURSING INTERVENTION TO ALLEVIATE ANXIETY IN PATIENTS WHOSE PRIMARY DIAGNOSIS INVOLVES A PSYCHIATRIC ILLNESS

It is of utmost importance to be available to the anxious patient. The psychiatric patient who displays specific behavioral patterns identified as measures to control anxiety is in a state of emergency. The overwhelming anxiety is the factor that represents the emergency and the job of the nurse is to be there to provide first aid and then maintenance care. This objective is met by the nurse's provision of physical support; she is there. If the patient washes, the nurse remains with him; if the patient paces, the nurse is beside him; should the patient become destructive, the nurse (and whomever she deems necessary) restrains him. The nurse, in effect, lends her strength to the patient when he is weakened and unable to control the emotional storms within himself.

In order to be perceived as real and helpful, it is absolutely necessary that the nurse *be* real. She must listen to the patient and respond. The content of her remarks is not so important as the fact that she listens and acknowledges that she has heard. When gross distortions are evidenced, it is the nurse's task to clarify reality. Conversational content should be related to the topics initiated by the patient. It is reassuring and therefore supportive of patients to experience the closeness of another understanding and accepting human being when a situation is particularly difficult.

When the press of an acute episode is past, the anxious patient will often try to piece together or to integrate the experience. His efforts might be directed to identifying the events that have caused his anxiety. In this case, the nurse can be of help to the patient if she can help him to sort out the loose threads. This involves, once again, listening carefully and pointing out where there is an area that is not clear, or one that seems distorted.

In a setting in which the patient is in a therapeutic relationship with a psychiatrist, it is helpful to direct the patient's thinking to that which the doctor has discussed with him. It is necessary, however, to try to contain the patient's anxiety so that he continues to work productively in therapy. To do this the nurse must be careful not to allow the patient to funnel off his anxiety by discussing with her the material that should be saved for the therapeutic conference. It is not always easy to recognize this content. As the student becomes more proficient in its recognition, she should feel free to say to her patient, "I think you should discuss this with your doctor."

A related problem is that of privileged communication. The patient sometimes wishes to confide in the nurse. Usually the content of the proposed confidence is material that belongs in the therapeutic hour. For various reasons, both conscious and unconscious, the patient wishes not to confide in his therapist. It is important to communicate to the patient that it is necessary to his well-being and progress for his therapist to be aware of the patient's thoughts and feelings; thus, the nurse cannot commit herself to hearing a confidence. After this statement, if the patient chooses to pursue the discussion, the nurse must evaluate its contents. If it seems central to the patient's psychotherapy, the doctor should be informed.

A good psychiatric nurse will record factually for the doctor what she has observed. This means placing on the chart an account of what was actually *seen* and *heard*—not an interpretation. Thus, the record would read, "Mary met her mother at the door of her room. She took the older woman in her room where they conversed during visiting hours. After her mother left, Mary began pacing the hall." It will be of less assistance to the doctor and the patient if the record reads, "Mary got very upset after her mother's visit."

For patients who are hospitalized, the nurse has an added responsibility for their physical health. There is often a temptation to overlook this component unless the patient is physiologically ill. Also the assumption is sometimes made that reported physical symptoms are actually signs of psychiatric illness. Patients admitted with physical symptoms who are not known to the staff should be examined for demonstrable organic problems before a psychiatric diagnosis is made.

A patient was admitted to the quiet room on Saturday night. He smelled of liquor and he was combative. The Emergency Room staff was particularly busy and transferred the patient before a careful work-up was done. During the night the nurses checked this patient's vital signs often. They became concerned because his blood pressure and pulse were rising. The nurses called the resident several times, but it was almost six hours before he was able to get to the unit. At this time it was determined that the patient was not intoxicated at all, but had suffered a subarachnoid hemorrhage.

Such a situation is rare, but the psychiatric nurse should always keep in mind that the patient with psychiatric symptoms can be physically ill!

Patients who are extremely anxious are often not hungry. The nurse needs to observe whether such patients are getting proper nourishment. If the patient cannot stop to eat because of his anxiety-alleviating activities, it is helpful to provide nourishing snacks that can be "eaten on the run." Food from home may be tempting, and if the institution's regulations permit, this is another means of nourishing the patient and also a useful means of helping the family to feel a part of the patient's care. It is necessary to see that the patient maintains personal hygiene. But with many anxious patients the focus will be reversed, and the nurse will have to protect the patient's skin from too much cleanliness.

Activities that use up the "other 23 hours" are very important. Planning for the patient's day is a necessary part of his care. The psychiatric nurse has an opportunity to exercise her creative talents in this area, for activities can be devised which will provide the patient with the kinds of experiences he needs to meet his particular needs, be they recognition and approval, security, self-esteem, closeness with another human being or whatever. In addition, as was mentioned in the section on compulsive behavior, activity can sometimes be devised which permits the patient to sublimate his impulses into a behavior which is socially acceptable and productive. For instance, the patient who must clean and organize can be invited to help with the ward cleaning activities. The patient who gets jittery and then paces might be sought out by an athletic staff member and challenged to a friendly game of 21 in the gym if a basketball and basket are available. For the patient who seems paralyzed by apprehension, the experience of finger painting with the nurse close by (this means sitting beside him and encouraging him) can be very useful. The nurse can then offer praise and approval for the effort made, and if the product is pleasing to her, she can be lavish in her evaluation of it.

Group activities need to be planned for patients who can interact and support one another. The activities should be planned in such a way that competitive activities are kept to a minimum; in this way patients will not be exposed to loss of self-esteem. It is also well to plan opportunities for the patient group to organize segments of their own time. In so doing the patients are encouraged to focus on ideas outside themselves. They are able to witness events occurring as a result of their planning, and this is satisfying as well as productive.

Last, it is necessary for the nurse to protect the patient who displays particularly aberrant behavior. Such a patient sometimes arouses such anxiety in others that the patient group acts in a way to ostracize the deviant member. Thus, the psychiatric nurse must either interpret to the other patients something of the deviant member's need for his behavior, or she must segregate the severely anxious patient while the crisis is occurring. In some hospitals the therapeutic community model is utilized. In such a unit, the patient is not protected from the others but is encouraged to join them and to hear what they think of his behavior. Usually some members of the group support the patient who is "attacked"; if this does not occur, the nurse, being part of the community herself, can speak of the patient's motivation as she sees it. She should also try to sit near the patient during the meeting.

REFERENCE

1. Laughlin, H.: *The Neuroses*. London, Butterworth & Co., Ltd., 1967, p. 726.

SUGGESTED READING

Berliner, B. S.: Nursing a Patient in Crisis. *Am. J. Nursing*, 70:2154-2157, October, 1970.

This article gives a clear and concise account of care given to a woman who was about to have a baby. The author speaks from the viewpoint of a worker in the community mental health field, but her handling of the patient's anxiety demonstrates techniques that will be useful to all workers in all settings.

Knowles, L.: How Can We Reassure Patients? *Am. J. Nursing*, 59 (No. 6):834-835, June, 1959.

This is a readable presentation about the nurse's handling of patient's anxiety through the interview. It is pleasant to read and at the same time, factual.

Levine, M.: The Intransigent Patient. *Am. J. Nursing*, 70:2106-21111, October, 1970.

This rational yet amusing treatise focuses on the reality of the nurse's position vis-à-vis her patient. The author demonstrates the illogical position of the nurse who becomes "morally indignant" when her patient does not perform as expected. The article presents a fine discussion of the nurse's anxiety and it is well worth reading.

Norris, C.: The Nurse and the Crying Patient. *Am. J. Nursing*, 57:323-327, 1957.

The material in this paper gives helpful insights concerning the care of the crying patient. It is a sensitive though practical article.

BOOKS

Fromm-Reichmann, F.: On Loneliness. *In* Bullard, D. (ed.) : *Psychoanalysis and Psychotherapy*. Chicago, University of Chicago Press, 1959.

It is a bias of this writer that Frieda Fromm-Reichmann is one of the outstanding contributors to psychiatry in the 20th century. Her short paper on loneliness reflects the profound thinking of its author and should be read by all serious students.

Rhodes, L., and Freedman, L.: *Chastise Me with Scorpions*. New York, G. P. Putnam's Sons, Inc., 1964.

This very interesting account of Mrs. Rhodes' illness and hospitalization affords the nursing student an opportunity to see anxiety at the "gut level." The patient permits the reader to see how it feels and influences behavior. The book is extremely readable and does not bog down in terminology. The commentary at the end of each chapter by Dr. Robbins, a psychiatrist, permits the student to see how the patient's thoughts and behavior might be interpreted. This book, written as a novel, gives a good look at the world of the neurotic.

Stone, I.: *The Passions of the Mind*. New York, Doubleday, 1970.

This long novel confers on the reader a deepened understanding of neuroses, their treatment and, most importantly, the author of our understanding of neurosis, Sigmund Freud.

Tao-Kim-Hoi, A.: Orientals Are Stoic. *In* Skipper, J. K., and Leonard, R. C. (eds.) : *Social Interaction and Patient Care*. Philadelphia, J. B. Lippincott Company, 1965.

The writer published this account originally in the New Yorker. It is not organized as a text-like presentation. It is short and witty, pungent and true. The nursing student reading this article might develop a new appreciation of the patient who comes into a general hospital with all his normal faculties, evaluates his situation realistically, and reacts. This article gets star billing.

Toffler, A.: *Future Shock*. New York, Random House, 1970.

This best seller of the seventies does not focus on psychiatry. It does, however, explain very graphically the kinds of stresses induced by this Age of Anxiety and the ways in which citizens of today and tomorrow must ready themselves in order to survive.

chapter 7

THE INDIVIDUAL WHO IS DEPRESSED

Depression, grieving, sadness and "blue spells" are all feeling states that are related in quality; the subjective differences among them are in degree, not kind. Most people have experienced these feelings which influence mood, or *affect,* as the term is known psychiatrically. Feelings of sadness or depression are not uncommonly felt on Monday morning as the carefree weekend gives way to work, school or the responsibilities of providing sustenance. For some these feelings come at the end of the week and they reflect the discomfort that accompanies the realization that the organization and predictability of the work week are coming to a close. For others the weekend means a loss of structure, perhaps the loss of human contact until Monday morning. No matter the cause, the feeling is unpleasant. It is a dullness, a hopelessness mixed with pessimism. It weighs heavily on the individual experiencing it.

There are many life situations that bring unhappiness and psychic pain. Death is the most obvious. Those who suffer a loss through the death of a loved one go through a type of depression that is considered normal and necessary; this is called grief. The individual who cannot accept the death of a significant person is not psychologically well, and he will not be so until he has gone through the grieving process in which he becomes aware of, accepts and works through his feelings toward the dead person. Only then can he effectively resume his life's work.

Death, however, is but one situation that causes unhappiness and psychic pain. What of lesser life problems? What of the tricks of fate that bring bankruptcy, hunger, sensory deprivation, failure? What of the life situations that most people would not even notice, i.e., a watched mailbox that does not yield the desired letter, the school grade that does not rise despite hard work, the fantasied invitation that is not extended? All these situations from the catastrophic to the seemingly inconsequential can evoke equally intense feelings in the individuals involved.

DEPRESSION

The oppressive quality of depression, the lack of limitations on its duration, make it quantitatively different from either "blues" or the grieving process. Depression is a response that can be precipitated by disappointment, shame, guilt or feelings of loss. The particular kind of loss is known in psychiatric terminology as "object loss"; the object may be a person, thing or ideology. Depression can be fleeting and easily altered, or it can be intense, of long duration and distinctly handicapping. Differences in the basic personality of the person and the meaning of the precipitating events will influence its profundity. Depression is manifested by feelings of sadness, worthlessness, hopelessness and emptiness. The person who experiences this constellation of feelings is sensing that he *is* nothing, he can *become* nothing, and the world around him contains little or nothing for him. Such an individual lacks interest in the outside world; all activities seem dull, flat and meaningless.

Daily routine is experienced like the tastelessness of food eaten when one has a cold. Getting up in the morning, dressing and planning one's activities for the day have the same relevance for a person lost in depression that they would have for someone in prison. Facing the morning is often agonizing; to wake up means to open one's eyes, to acknowledge that the dreams just past were only that. Reality remains —cold, bleak and cheerless. To appreciate severe depression is beyond the capacity of most readers; it is too hopeless, too flat and too despairing for most to imagine.

SIGNS OF DEPRESSION

In the acutely ill, drooping facial musculature is present, making the patient appear far older than his chronological age; sometimes the eyeballs are sunken from loss of weight. Such a person assumes a slumped position when seated; when he is walking, the gait is slow and dragging. The depressed patient cries frequently, and sleep disturbances are common. He is uninterested in personal hygiene, and if those around him do not tend to this problem, the patient is apt to become dirty and perhaps physically ill from the growth of pathogens in and around him. Subtly his condition reinforces his evaluation of himself as a worthless person.

> A young woman, recalling a childhood when she was chronically depressed, described herself as dirty and unkempt. Again and again in her analysis she recalled that she was different from her classmates because they always looked clean and well groomed. She wore soiled dresses, had messy hair and her nails were dirty and bitten off. She lamented that neither she nor the adults responsible for her seemed interested in cleaning her up and sending her off to school to compete on equal footing with her peers. The young woman cherished the fantasy that she could be "dipped in Lysol" and would then be cleansed physically and psychologically.

PHYSIOLOGICAL ASPECTS OF DEPRESSION

In the severely depressed patient there are numerous physiological changes which result in alterations of body function. Generally there is retardation of action; for instance, respirations are slower and alimentary tract motility is retarded. The latter causes delayed emptying of the stomach and intestines. The patient feels the effects of this problem through loss of appetite, feelings of fullness in the stomach, belching and constipation. It is not difficult to lose track of the living patient as one reviews the long list of signs and symptoms that represent the effects of depression. It may be meaningful to sit back and consider how having such a multitude of problems might really feel. Recall the last time a very heavy meal was eaten when afterward there was no opportunity to lie down and rest. Perhaps the reader had a date for the movies, the theater or a concert. Recall the miserable feeling of sitting in a cramped, uncomfortable chair, almost gasping for breath, trying unsuccessfully to stretch out one's middle section so the food could "go down." Most people have occasionally had this very uncomfortable experience. The depressed patient with decreased gastric motility has it often, perhaps constantly. Thus, depression is not only a painful state of mind, but it also has a physical component which is uncomfortable. Just as there are nursing interventions to alleviate the psychic condition, so there are approaches to decrease the physical discomfort. They will be discussed in the section on nursing care.

ETIOLOGY OF DEPRESSION

What of the underlying causes of depression? They are basically similar for the reactive depression (neurotic illness) and the psychotic depressions. The precipitating factors, as have been described, are usually loss of a person, an object, self-esteem, security, part of one's body or a health function. The loss may be actual, anticipated or imagined; however, it is always real and meaningful to the person involved. It is theorized that the loss evokes hostile, aggressive impulses which arise from the unconscious. These feelings conflict with Ego responses, which are more positive. Thus, the patient is beset by ambivalent feelings. During this struggle, the punitive superego enters the picture in response to the erstwhile repressed Id impulses. While the psychic battle rages between Id and Superego, the patient experiences guilt, and self-deprecation. Hostile, aggressive feelings are turned inward and vented on the self.

The psychotic depression may be precipitated by severe environmental blows to security and self-esteem or by the mobilization of extreme guilt feelings. The severity of the illness is determined by the basic personality of the individual who is afflicted and by the meaning of the precipitating event. Heredity and physiological predisposition are factors that are also being scrutinized by investigators. The latter two elements are implicated, but are as yet unproved etiological factors.

TYPES OF DEPRESSION

There are three basic types of depression: the neurotic, sometimes termed reactive or exogenous; the psychotic, or endogenous; and the cyclic psychotic disorder called the manic-depressive psychosis, depressive phase. It is sometimes difficult to make a clear-cut distinction between neurotic and psychotic depressions unless the patient verbalizes delusional themes about his worth.

Depressed patients, whether neurotic or psychotic, feel that they are worthless. The psychotic patient demonstrates more severe symptoms, however. He usually exhibits delusional ideation. The delusional themes of the psychotic patient often involve body image, sinful acts and punishment. This ideation may cause the nurse endless frustration in her attempts to maintain the patient's physical health because he clings stubbornly to the delusion that he is without stomach, that his bowels have turned to worms, or that some other visceral organ has rotted. The patient may be convinced that he cannot eat. Breaking into such a delusional pattern is very difficult. Also the depressed psychotic has severe psychomotor retardation that leads to physiological symptoms. The stupor of severe retardation sometimes gives way to agitation which is reflected in constant, aimless activity. Insomnia may be intractable.

Both neurotic and psychotic patients who are depressed may ruminate about self-destruction, though such ideation is more persistent in the psychotic. Both have mood alterations, though they tend to be reversed as influenced by the time of day; the neurotic patient usually feels his best early in the day. His somber mood increases as evening approaches. The psychotic patient has difficulty in the early morning when he feels at his lowest. As the evening approaches, this patient begins to feel better.

Finally, there is a difference in the way the patients view their conditions. The neurotic usually fights his problem. He may not do so effectively, but he is in pain and he is dissatisfied. The psychotic patient *lives* in his illness. He seems to make it a part of himself, not questioning it and not fighting the terrifying pain that engulfs him.

The Manic-Depressive Cycle

The manic-depressive reaction is similar in symptomatology to other psychotic depressions; however, it is different because of its cyclic pattern. The following case illustrates the behavior of a manic-depressive individual in whom wide mood swings are predominant.

> Anthony C. is a 55 year old professional who has been hospitalized six times in the 30 years since his cum laude graduation from college. He was committed each time by his wife, who observed the symptoms of his psychotic illness emerging. Mr. C. is normally an outgoing, energetic person who works hard. He is unstinting in his willingness to give of self, and his enthusiasm is acknowledged by all who work with him. Mr. C. has short periods of depression, but his co-workers are usually not aware of them; only his wife and family know about Mr. C.'s dejection, anorexia and insomnia. These occur at home. The office and laboratory staff see only the vivaciousness, warmth and enthusiasm that are Mr. C.'s external self.
>
> Each time Mr. C. becomes severely ill, the psychosis is heralded by this increasing activity. He sleeps shorter periods, goes to work in the early hours of the day, and is unable to accomplish much because concentration is not possible. During this phase of his illness, Mr. C. experiences overwhelming urges to give. Unable to concentrate, he will turn from his work in annoyance and go to the department stores to buy excessive quantities of gifts for his family and co-workers.
>
> As his feelings of well-being increase, periods of work and sleep decrease. Mr. C. may be found dancing, singing and joking. He has no appetite and feels he does not have time to eat. During these periods he talks loudly, sometimes shouting. He elaborates grandiose ideas, and his wife feels it necessary to monitor his telephone conversations in order that her husband not consummate business involvements that they cannot afford.
>
> When Mr. C.'s manic illness reaches these proportions, his wife always recognizes the need to hospitalize him. Attempts to discuss it with him are futile for he always thinks himself to be at the zenith of his development. He feels his wife's demands for hospitalization and treatment are an attempt on her part to discredit and ruin him. Thus, the family doctor is called in order to sedate Mr. C. sufficiently so that an ambulance crew can transport him to the hospital.

Mr. C.'s courses of hospitalization follow a pattern. Initially he is extremely overactive and requires sedation to protect him from exhaustion. Gradually the frenetic behavior gives way to periods of depression which are characterized by inactivity and verbalizations of worthlessness. The depressive phase of Mr. C.'s psychosis tends towards alleviation after a three- to four-week period. The patient is usually hospitalized for two to three months and discharged to outpatient status where he remains in psychotherapy for approximately one year. Mr. C. always leaves therapy when his symptoms have abated and he no longer experiences psychic discomfort. He will not consider long-term psychotherapy with its potential for basic personality reconstruction.

The cycles of the manic-depressive psychosis are repetitive. Sometimes the manic phase is seen only briefly before the depressive symptoms appear. It is felt by some that the manic phase represents an unconscious attempt by the patient to protect himself against the ravages of the depression which is to follow. The depressive phase is thought to represent an expression of hatred for self; the manic phase, an appeal for love.

Some theorists feel that the manic-depressive is the product of a home in which there was an abundance of affection and care during the first year or so of the child's life. Then another child came along, and the mother had to turn her attention to the new baby. At this point her care of the older child became perfunctory. She did what she could for him out of a sense of responsibility rather than because of her love and orientation of nurturing for the older child.[1] Rado feels that the meaning of the depressive illness is a despairing cry for love. He writes that it is probable that the patient's unconscious feeling is, "If I punish myself, I shall be accepted again."[1] Thus, the depression is punishment which is self-inflicted by the patient in order to regain mother's love. The nurse can make her own judgment on this theoretic issue as she observes people with manic-depressive disorders. The cycles of their illnesses are well differentiated, and from observation one can see obvious alterations in mood. The depressive illness seems to reflect a negative orientation; the manic phase communicates more positive tones.

It has been noted that the incidence of manic-depressive psychosis is greater in women.[1] Suicidal attempts by the manic-depressive patient are seen as an attempt to kill that which has been incorporated into his personality from another person. This psychotic individual is a person who has taken into himself much that he has accepted without question. His situation is similar to that of the trusting puppy that swallows whatever is given and even such contraband as grass, buttons and rags. Sooner or later the pup begins to feel rather ill from the effects of his highly unselected diet. It is at this point that the puppy's stomach rebels and the hapless little dog begins to regurgitate, relieving his stomach of its odious contents. The puppy is a far cry from the manic-depressive patient, but the analogy may help the reader to focus on the process of taking in (introjection) and later extruding (destroying by suicide). The theory is an interesting one not only in itself, but as a comparative frame of reference for another psychotic illness, schizophrenia. It is felt that in the latter illness the individual does not take in as a basic process, but sends out, or projects.

It is theorized that as the manic-depressive patient experiences repetitions of his illness, the prognosis grows worse. The patient who is hospitalized in a true manic illness is in a precarious life-threatening state. Activity is constant and death may ensue from fatigue or coronary insufficiency. Nursing intervention must be directed to providing opportunities for sleep.

TREATMENT OF DEPRESSION

Depressive reactions are treated by both psychological and physiological intervention. Primary is psychotherapy, in which an effort is made to understand the etiology of the patient's illness. In this endeavor the therapist studies historical data, i.e., the patient's childhood and his background, as well as the patient's current life style and his patterns of communication in order to understand the psychologic trauma that has given rise to the depression. The therapist tries to facilitate the patient's expression of the feelings that determine his affect. When the patient has learned to communicate them and his depression begins to lift, the therapist then focuses on an exploration of the meaning of the patient's depression. In this segment of the therapy the patient experiences less support from the therapist, but he is helped to gain insight into his problems.

For some patients psychotherapy alone will not be effective because the level of depression is so profound. In such patients, chemotherapy is also instituted. Drugs which cause mood elevation are prescribed in order to make the patient more amenable to psychotherapy. (See Chapter 11.) Because of the availability of these drugs, some practitioners prescribe them for minor depressions, *substituting* them for psychotherapy. This is not a wise practice, for the depressed patient does not have an opportunity to gain insight into his problem. Unfortunately, too, the trend toward "popping pills to make the world right" is thus subtly and unwittingly encouraged by those who are perceived as leaders in the community.

When a patient is deeply depressed and cannot be reached through verbal and nonverbal communication, or when he is in danger of suicide and seems to have taken an intractable position, electroconvulsive therapy is sometimes utilized. This treatment has an immediate effect on the patient, whereas chemotherapeutic agents require two to three weeks before their effects are felt. With a prompt regression of symptoms, the patient becomes more amenable to psychotherapy.

ASPECTS OF PHYSICAL CARE FOR THE HOSPITALIZED PATIENT WHO IS DEPRESSED

PROVIDING A SAFE ENVIRONMENT

Nursing care in all cases of depression, whether neurotic, psychotic or cyclic, is similar. Attention to the physical well-being of the depressed patient is the first concern. This is to say, it has priority over other problems because a dead person is not one whose psychological condition can be modified! One should not lose track of the possibility that death may result from a depressive illness. Threat of death comes from two possible dangers: starvation and suicide; the more common is suicide.

It is basic to one's understanding of depression and the nursing care of depressed people to keep in mind that aggression, hostility, hate and bottled-up anger are key concepts. Depressive symptoms reflect these feelings, which, if not expressed, are there under the surface, unable to be spoken and understood by the sick person. Instead, the feelings are packed into the unconscious, acting as a tightly coiled spring, ready to catapult the individual into acts of aggression directed at himself. Sometimes the patient is too immobilized to act on these impulses—he may be so stuporous that he is described as showing "vegetative signs" of depression. At other times, however, his energies may be sufficient to allow for that momentary act which would result in death. It is rather ironic that our therapeutic efforts often result in a phase of the patient's recovery in which he has sufficient energy and motivation to destroy himself. The treatment we prescribe for the convalescing depressed individual is not without danger.

Depression is often signaled by the individual's sudden increase in irritation and anger. He is propelled downhill by the unconscious forces that dictate his journey into the morass that we label as depression. As the ravages of self-doubt and sadness turn into the abyss of worthlessness and bleakness, the individual who has embarked on this fated journey relinquishes fantasies of the relief of death because he is now imprisoned by his mood and a consequent inability to act. It is this stage that is physically least dangerous to the depressed patient, but which is most injurious to him psychologically. Now he is completely without self-direction and ability to lessen his pain. The depressed person, in this stage of his illness, must have help from others if he is to begin the long, arduous climb to mental health. Though it is felt that most depressions are self-limiting, the severely retarded patient might well die from starvation if he were left to his own devices while his illness moved to its natural termination.

In the prodromal phase of depression, the patient has the potential for suicide; as he progresses into the depths of despair, he loses this potential. Not until the patient begins to mobilize his physical and psychic energies does the threat of suicide reappear. The desperate need is to protect the patient from turning his hatred and aggression inward and taking his own life. This is a simpler task in the hospital than that undertaken by any individual who tries to protect a suicidal person who is not in such a controlled, regulated environment. Happily this situation does not occur frequently, for when a person is diagnosed as suicidal he is generally committed to an institution or he voluntarily admits himself. Once he has been hospitalized, it is the task of the nurse to provide a safe environment for the suicidal patient.

Suicidal threats and rumination should be taken seriously. It is an unfounded fable that the person who talks about suicide will not take his own life.

Of rather academic interest are the themes that run through the content of patients' suicidal fantasies. Often the listener will hear preoccupation with the fantasized feelings of guilt that surviving relatives will feel. The observer can detect in the neurotic patient's ruminations an urge to destroy himself in order to make the family sorry. There is little regard for the fact that such a move is a fatal form of cutting one's nose off to spite one's face! In contrast, the fantasies of the psychotically ill suicidal patient tend to involve thoughts of self-punishment, remorse and sin. This patient is not so interested in the reactions of those around him; his thoughts are centered on himself and his projected suicide is more a punishment of himself for his supposed worthlessness and sinning than an instrument for the evocation of remorse in surviving relatives.

The neurotic individual can usually develop insight concerning his anger at others and his use of suicidal plans as a threat against them. He can eventually be brought to a dialogue concerning the effectiveness of venting his feelings outwardly at the appropriate targets, rather than chancing the loss of his own life.

For the psychotic patient, emphasis will be on support of his weak ego. The patient will be brought to an understanding that his life has not been sinful and that his guilt is ill-founded. For this patient, insight may be more difficult or even impossible to achieve; however, the nurse can provide effective protection as long as the patient seems delusional and actively suicidal.

Provision of a safe environment is interesting, but sometimes difficult, requiring ingenuity. It is silly for the student to try to memorize long lists of things to be confiscated. Rather, she should relax and think logically of those objects that could be used in a lethal manner. Obviously, anything sharp is dangerous; this includes such things as razors, knives and scissors. Metal nail files and sharp-edged pieces of miscellaneous metals might also be used to sever arteries.

Belts, ties and shoelaces might be utilized for strangulation. Also, surplus materials used in O.T., such as the strands from which lanyards are made, might be used. These kinds of articles need not necessarily be taken from the patient during the day when they are needed, but at night their whereabouts should be known. Even such things as light bulbs are occasionally used by the resourceful patient who puts all his energies to work to find ways of injuring himself. Panes of glass might be shattered in the windows and the broken edges used to sever blood vessels.

Finally, medications can be stored up and taken when a lethal dose is accumulated. In order to protect against calamity it is wise to make sure individual doses of medicine are taken at the proper time. Inventive patients roll pills under their tongues and into the sides of their mouths. The careful nurse will, if necessary, use a tongue blade and flashlight to examine the patient's mouth to see that this has not occurred.

The nurse feels awkward doing these things to another adult, but she must keep in mind that she is constantly trying to protect his life. If the patient expresses irritation or anger toward her, this is not a personal derogation; it merely indicates that patient and nurse do not have the same goal. It is reasonable, and even indicated, that the nurse explain as many times as it is necessary that she means to protect the patient while he feels so bad about himself that he wishes to take his own life. Admittedly, however, the final responsibility is his. Such a statement indicates that the nurse's purpose is not to punish the patient, which is an elaboration of his delusional themes, and it is not to derogate him by treating him like a distrusted child. Such an assumption on his part again reflects his pathological thinking that he is worthless. The nurse's simple statement of her goal says several things to the depressed patient: It indicates her basic interest in him. It communicates her feeling that he is *worth* being saved, and it tells the suicidal patient that the nurse understands something of his inner thoughts and feelings. Thus, the hesitant nurse can see that her behavior, which on the surface may appear awkward and open to question, is really of benefit to the suicidal patient at several levels of communication.

PERSONAL HYGIENE
Cleanliness

To most psychologically and physically healthy people cleanliness of body, teeth, hair and clothing is taken for granted. Care of the body is so habitual that no particular thought is given to it. If the nurse is not especially cognizant of these necessities, she may lose track of the patient's physical condition until he actually reeks! This is hardly a healthful situation.

The depressed patient should be strongly encouraged to bathe. If he absolutely refuses, then the nurse must inform him that he will *be bathed* if he cannot or will not assume the responsibility. Obviously the patient should be given the option to cooperate before attendants forcibly bathe him. However, if it becomes necessary to provide assistance, sufficient personnel should be assembled prior to approaching the patient.

Sometimes after a patient has been forced to undergo such a procedure, he will recognize that sufficient strength is present to lift him bodily, and rather than go through such trauma again he will simply acquiesce. This is why it is imperative to have sufficient personnel assembled before one attempts to deal with the recalcitrant patient.

It is a particularly good practice to discuss with the attendants the meaning of their restraining acts. They are often made highly anxious by what they are doing and the patient's response to it, and their anxiety is reflected in their nervous laughing or unnecessary roughness in handling the patient. It is useful to discuss with the less educated staff the great fear that the patient feels. They should know that the patient does not refuse a procedure as an act of contrariness, but rather because he is terrified. They should know that the patient is literally fighting for his life. If the nurse explains to her staff that people do become uncomfortable when they touch others, especially if those others are nude or struggling, and if she encourages her staff to talk about the situation and to express their own feelings, she will notice that they are able to handle the patient in a more concerted effort with more group cohesion and a minimum of roughness. The result will be circular. The patient will be less frightened and will struggle less; therefore, the staff will have less need to react to the patient's anxiety.

When the patient is better and bathes willingly, this is a good opportunity to spend time with him. Especially for the female patient, the bath offers a marvelous opportunity for the nurse to talk with her patient while the latter is relaxed. If tubs are available, perhaps a bit of bubble bath can be utilized to promote a feminine sense of prettiness and well-being. Lying in a warm tub of water, relaxed and soaking, permits the patient to be comfortable and to ease intense anxiety for a little while at least. Most important, if the nurse is present, nurse and patient can share this small portion of the day that is as pleasant and relaxing as possible. It is wise to provide a chair for the nurse to sit on so she, too, can be comfortable. The nurse who is uncomfortable, busy and obviously anxious to return to her duties will communicate this to her patient. It is better if the nurse schedules the bath when she has time to rest and sit quietly with the patient.

Sleep

Sleep is a very important aspect in the treatment of any sick person. Much research is being conducted to explore the far reaches of the mind at rest. There will doubtless be numerous facts discovered about sleep in the coming years; we know already that it has a particular reparative quality which is necessary to the well-being of the human. It is known that prolonged lack of sleep can cause psychosis and even death.

Nursing attention has been given to the problem of insomnia in patients, both neurotic and psychotic. In patients in whom adequate doses of tranquilizers and soporifics have not caused sleep to occur, the presence of the nurse at the bedside for a sustained period sometimes will help to produce the needed rest. Sleep means different things to different people. To children sleep means separation from parents, possibly separation accompanied by horrible night terrors; for them sleep is not welcome and they will fight it. For the elderly person who fears death, sleep may be unwelcome, for he feels that there may be no awakening. For the delusional patient, sleep may mean unguarded periods in which "they" might ravage his vulnerable body. It is well to consider the use of sufficient tranquilizers during the day so that the patient experiences as little tension as possible. Nighttime sedation may be decided against in favor of warm baths, soup or heated milk, and the company of one who provides security.

Weaning the convalescing patient from sleeping pills is sometimes a problem. Some who use them come to believe that they cannot sleep without them. It then becomes the function of the nurse to help the patient to learn how to fall asleep. The patient who is able to do this without drugs is better able to depend upon himself. The relaxed nurse who can help her patient to relax completely before bedtime and who can provide a warm, safe environment may successfully influence her patient to sleep. The creative, resourceful nurse will use appropriately the measures that help children, because she will recognize that the ill patient is a regressed person. Some of the things that comforted him as a child may well have the same meaning now—warm liquid, softened lights, a cozy bed, the touch of a "mothering one."

Intake and Output

It is necessary to focus attention on symptoms caused by the depressed patient's physical retardation in order to understand some of his chronic physical complaints. He is subject to malnutrition and changes in normal bowel activity. The group of symptoms centering on retardation of gastrointestinal tract motility provides fertile areas for nursing intervention. Two measures which influence the activity of the intestines are physical activity and the character of that which is eaten.

Activity. Increasing the depressed patient's activity is not easy, but it can be accomplished by a consistent, firm approach. Chores assigned to the patient can be useful in that they not only provide activity that improves physiological functioning, but they also provide an opportunity for the patient to do something useful which, in turn, offers the opportunity for an increased sense of worth. Means of providing such opportunities will be discussed more fully under the section on psychological care.

Modification of intake. Gastric motility can be influenced by the quantity of food ingested at a given time. If smaller portions are provided, there is less to empty from the stomach. In addition, the miserable feeling of bloatedness is alleviated. It is difficult to have control over the types of food provided in large state hospitals, but in smaller private facilities the nurse does have the option to discuss her patient's problem with the institution's dietitian so that they can plan meals for the patient that are small but highly nourishing. Provision of bulk foods that are natural laxatives is also indicated.

Output. The nurse should also know about the bowel activity of her patient, for constipation is a chronic problem. It is a common one for the depressed patient and, once established, it is sometimes hard to alter. Laxatives and enemas breed problems of their own, once their use is begun. It is obviously better to modify the lower intestinal tract motility through appropriate food and physical activity than through the use of inert substances. If enemas must be resorted to, it is well to consider such preparations as suppositories or saline enemas. The depressed patient who is delusional may construe the long, rather uncomfortable procedure of the soapsuds enema as a punishment (which psychologically, and to a degree physically, it is) or as an assault (which it actually is), or even as part of a plot to destroy him. It is easier on the staff, equally effective and more therapeutic for the patient to provide him with a suppository or a small prepared enema that he can administer to himself after he has been given an explanation of its use.

Communications have been discussed before and they will be emphasized throughout the text. *Simplicity* of communication is absolutely necessary for the patient who cannot concentrate. It is required for the patient whose mind is bound down with obsessive thoughts he cannot control. The nurse must decide what it is that she wants to tell her patient. This means she must look at the actual message she wishes to communicate. She then pares her conversation to the bare minimum. Thus, regarding the use of laxative or enemas; she may say, "Mr. C., you have not had a bowel movement for three days. I know this must be uncomfortable for you and I have a laxative for you to use which will help you to move your bowels." For the neurotically depressed patient such a statement might evoke appreciation, irritation or a neutral acceptance of a fact. It does communicate the nurse's interest in her patient's well-being, in addition to the simple fact that a medical problem is being attended to. For the psychotic patient, who may think that he has no intestinal tract, or that he is dead from the waist down, or that the doctors and nurses are trying to kill him slowly and methodically, such a statement might evoke great anxiety. Again, the nurse's matter-of-fact, firm, but kind attitude is crucial. Should the patient argue, struggle or tell the nurse that he has no bowels, the nurse should respond simply but firmly that she understands (or is aware of) the patient's feelings, but she knows that he does have intestines and it is necessary to administer this medication.

If necessary, help may be utilized; however, should the situation arise, adequate personnel must be assembled before the nurse approaches the patient. They should restrain the patient quietly and matter of factly. This is certainly a poor way to carry out a procedure, but if it is necessary, it is far better than attempting to administer the medication with the patient struggling, resulting in the procedure's being done clumsily and requiring much time. Speed and efficiency should be bywords. The situation is similar to that of the pediatric patient who is approached for an injection. The inexperienced nurse might accede to the youngster's wish to "Wait a minute," or "Let me get a drink of water," or "I want to get up first." But the time used up does not lessen the frightening aspect of the situation; it really makes it worse by turning it into a longer, drawn-out procedure. It is far more humane to go in, announce what is necessary, do it, and then discuss it, permitting the patient time to react and to vent his anger on the agent of the painful or frightening procedure. In this case, what is good in the pediatric unit is also wise in the psychiatric unit.

ASPECTS OF THE PSYCHOLOGICAL CARE OF THE DEPRESSED HOSPITALIZED PATIENT IN A HOSPITAL SETTING

If the patient is being evaluated and treated by a psychiatrist, the nurse can add to her own impressions valuable information from the patient's history and record as it is developed by the doctor. She can ascertain from these documents, or through conference with the psychiatrist, information about the "critical period" in the patient's life, that is, the original pathogenic factor which triggered the depressive reaction. With this information the nurse can better understand the meaning of the patient's disease.

In many cases the nurse will discover that long past events supplied the psychological matrix for the subsequent exaggerated reactions which bring the patient to hospitalization. People are sensitized to traumatic events or losses from the past by insecurity and by unendurable situations of stress to which they were exposed as children. The precipitating cause of neurotic depression is usually more recent trauma, whereas that of psychotic depression can be more remote, with the patient making a meaningful connection (for himself) between the long past event and the present stimulus. What this means to the nurse is that it is usually easier to understand the events leading up to the reactive (neurotic) depression; it requires additional exploration and assumption to acquire a useful understanding of the psychotic patient's basic problems.

When the patient's physical needs have been met, the resourceful nurse will keep in mind that her patient needs recognition, meaningful attention, acceptance and activities that can promote his self-esteem.

COMMUNICATIONS

Whether in the hospital or in the community, the first requirement for the nurse who proposes to help a depressed individual is that she permit herself to react to the communications of the patient. The word communication has been used, rather than verbalization, because the depressed person may describe his hideous feelings through actions as well as, or rather than, words. The effective nurse must understand the world of her patient in order to empathize. She cannot help if her approach is sterile and bereft of feeling.

The effective psychiatric nurse is one who can characterize her patient in two ways: First, she sees him through the observable clinical symptoms he exhibits. The physical symptoms of the illness act as guideposts to the feeling state of the patient. Additionally, the effective nurse perceives aspects of her patient's being through an empathic awareness of him. This perception evolves from the nurse's awareness of her patient's feelings as they are reflected in both his resting state and his responses to the environment. Many nurses are not so effective as they might be because they limit their awareness of and responsiveness to the patient at the level of his observable clinical symptoms. The effective psychiatric nurse experiences the being of her patient in his totality. She responds to the clinical symptoms and to his feeling state; this is to say, she can communicate on a highly rational goal-directed level or she may choose to relate at a less well differentiated level prompted by her awareness of the patient's feeling state.

Laura R., 23 year old mother of a newborn, was admitted to the hospital after her husband realized that she was spending entire days weeping as she wheeled her child up and down the lanes of the park in an effort to quiet the child and encourage him to sleep. She needed tranquilizers and soporifics in order to sleep, and her days were a nightmarish morass of tears and frantic activity to ensure that her child would remain quiet. The admitting doctor diagnosed her illness as a probable postpartum depression.

The patient remained on a maximum security unit for the first three months of her hospitalization. She admitted to having made suicide attempts during her pregnancy. Now her condition was sufficiently unstable to require extremely close supervision. Laura's therapy went well. She was an intelligent person and gained insight rapidly into her underlying problems. Soon she was expressing great amounts of hostility. She argued a great deal with the nursing students and seemed unable to establish positive meaningful relations with anyone except her psychiatrist, whom she worshipped in a childlike way, and the head nurse on her unit. She saw little of the latter; however, the nurse tried to allot at least half an hour a day to Laura.

It was in occupational therapy that this patient made a pair of baby shoes for her young son. She planned to give them to her mother to take home to the child. When visiting day arrived, Laura went to the shop to get the shoes she had so painstakingly made. The therapist told Laura, regretfully, that she could not locate the shoes, but that she would search for them when time was available. The student accompanying Laura was baffled as she watched the patient's face crumple and turn deep red. She was frightened as Laura ran from her into the small bathroom and locked the door behind her. The nurse called the ward immediately and asked the head nurse what to do. The nurse came to the shop and stood at the bathroom door. She spoke quietly through the wooden wall. "Laura, it's me, Joanie. Can I come in? Don't be afraid."

Laura called out, "I am afraid. What are you going to do to me?"

"Nothing. I promise. Let me come in and be with you. There is no one with me. I won't hurt you." The door opened a little. The nurse stood still as Laura looked out, hesitated, and then opened the door wide enough for the nurse to enter.

The patient turned and walked to the corner of the little room. She slumped down on the floor, sitting with her back resting against the bare wooden wall. She began to sob. "They lost my baby shoes. They just don't know where they are. They made me make those shoes for visiting day and they did not care enough to put them away where they could find them. I'm just a meaningless blob. No one cares about me. They just want me to be good and do what they want." The nurse sat down on the floor opposite the sobbing young woman. She said nothing. Laura continued: "Nobody cares. I'm not anything but a big blob. They just want me to move around like an obedient robot. It does not matter if I have feelings. I'm just a thing. I hate them. I hate them."

The nurse sat and listened. She watched her patient and wondered what this incident meant. She began to speak when Laura grew more quiet. "We care about how you feel, Laura. We care very much. I think it is *you* who have felt like a meaningless blob because you have been sick. I don't think that you have known what you wanted to do, most of the time. It's good that you can tell me how you feel. I can see that you are very angry. It's good that you can get your feelings out in the open. What would *you* like to do?"

The patient looked at her and laughed. "I don't know. I've been such a hideous blob for so long, I really don't have any idea what I want to do. What can we do? Are some big burly attendants waiting out there to pounce on me when we go out that door?"

The nurse said, "No." She explained that no one was there and that she and Laura could leave together to go to the ward if Laura wished to. The patient seemed reassured and she got up and left the building with the nurse, her friend.

The incident is a telling one. The patient overreacted to a situation that might have provoked mild irritation in one who was better able to consciously experience her feelings and to express them. For Laura it was like a suddenly opened vent, allowing the content under pressure, her feelings, to come out explosively. This was bewildering and frightening for her and for the nursing student with her. The head nurse who was called did not immediately understand the situation. She was not afraid, however, and could sit down on the floor with Laura and evaluate the situation as she listened to the young woman.

The nurse was able to react empathically. She listened and she watched her patient. As she heard Laura's words, and witnessed how frightened, angry and bewildered the patient felt, she was able to assume, correctly, that this patient needed to be heard. She needed to be given the opportunity to shout out, if necessary, what it was that was bottled up in her. The nurse listened until Laura had finished; then she quietly added her own thoughts. Had the nurse observed this patient in crisis, only superficially, had she not heard her and assessed the importance of the event, the nurse might have acted out of her own anxiety and called for help as Laura feared. The patient might have been restrained and taken to the ward and sedated, which would have been contrary to her need at this juncture. The nurse watched; she listened; she was able to empathize and respond helpfully.

Building Meaningful Communication Patterns

The psychotic is often delusional. It is necessary to recognize the minute meaning of one's verbal and nonverbal behavior to this individual, because delusions feed further delusions and the process becomes quite unwieldy and antitherapeutic. To avoid this danger, it is well to try to understand where the patient is starting. This establishes a baseline. From this point on, the nurse tries to build meaningful communication patterns with her patient. This means that she must decide what she wants to communicate; then she tries to use words that mean the same thing to her and to the patient. When she has delivered her message, verbally or nonverbally, she then awaits some response from the patient that will indicate his understanding of her message.

The process is not easy, but it is exciting and rewarding. The psychiatric nurse is at the battlefront, struggling against those forces that have engulfed the patient. Her rewards are extravagant when such a patient shows improvement!

Mrs. P., a 73 year old society matron, was well known to the hospital. She was admitted periodically with a psychotic depressive episode. Her illnesses usually lasted a period of several months, and then she became well enough to resume her activities in the community, which were well known and highly advantageous to the poverty-stricken members of the town from which she came. Mrs. P. was extremely delusional. She described to the ward staff how her "insides rotted away, so that eating was not only unnecessary, but quite painful." Thus, this patient required tube feeding. She also refused to void and had to be catheterized at least once every 24 hours during the most flagrant period of her illnesses.

The nursing student on the night shift was elected to catheterize Mrs. P. She approached her patient's cubicle with some trepidation, but found the patient awake and seemingly lucid. "Mrs. P., I have come to take your urine from you since you are unable to void. I shall need some help, so if you can assist me, we will not have to ask for the other nurse to help." Mrs. P. seemed to listen. She said nothing, but looked expectantly at the young nurse as the equipment was unfolded and set out on the night table. The student asked Mrs. P. to maintain the position that was required and the patient did so. As the student proceeded with the catheterization, she spoke quietly to her patient. She told her when it would be uncomfortable and she indicated when the catheter was in place and that the urine was emptying into the provided receptacle.

Mrs. P. asked what time it was and the nursing student told her. She also told her the date and the day. She asked the patient if she had been able to sleep at all, and the patient replied that she had not. She told the nurse that she felt frightened and could not sleep. The student withdrew the catheter, removed the equipment from the bed and told Mrs. P. she would take the materials away and then come back and stay with her so that Mrs. P. could rest. After she had cleaned the equipment in the utility room, the nurse returned to Mrs. P.'s bedside. She sat in a chair pulled up to the bed and held the patient's hand until the latter was able to fall asleep.

The interaction between patient and nursing student was very meaningful. The nurse told the patient in simple terms what she proposed to do. The patient understood for she was cooperative in the procedure. As the catheterization continued, the nurse talked with the patient about what she was doing so that the patient's perceptions would not provide causes for further delusions. The patient apparently was comfortable with her night nurse, for she was able to tell her that she was frightened and could not sleep. The young nurse did not delve into the basis of her patient's fear, for she recognized that it probably involved complicated, stressful delusions. Instead, she offered to come back and stay with the frightened woman. Her offer was accepted and Mrs. P. was able to fall asleep, secure in the feeling that her nurse was there.

The nurse is in a good position to teach the depressed patient new types of responses that will enable him to express his negative feelings openly. This is very crucial to the individual who has bottled up much anger inside himself and who is unconsciously self-punitive. If the nurse is to provide the experiences that this type of patient requires, she will often be perceived as less than a sympathetic friend. She may be viewed negatively from time to time, but such a situation is also useful for the patient. It is not always necessary or even desirable to be a friend; rather, it is therapeutic to be strong but kind and not too permissive. The patient needs the strength of another person who can support him when he is weakened by the ravages of his superego. He needs to hear someone say, "It is important that you go to your therapy hour. I will not let you stay on the ward." When the patient awakens in the morning and is not sufficiently motivated to get up and begin the day, a useful nurse is one who insists that the patient get washed and begin the daily program. The depressed patient desperately needs an organized, planned schedule so that he does not decline to a state of vegetation.

Psychiatric nurses need to be excellent listeners. They also need to develop skills in conversing. The depressed patient sometimes has a keen mind and, once "turned on," he can generate interesting conversation, providing the nurse can help him to get started and then act as an audience. Psychiatric illness certainly does not preclude the presence of talent, skill and resourcefulness. Patients often display these valuable personality assets if given the opportunity, and such an opportunity enhances self-esteem. It can be an interesting treat for the person who happens to be listening.

ACTIVITIES TO MEET PSYCHOLOGICAL NEEDS

Assigned chores can be utilized by the resourceful nurse as an outlet for the patient's feelings. For instance, if there is need for aggressive feelings to be vented, an activity may be provided that requires the use of aggressive types of behavior. If the patient is in a stage of his illness in which guilt is verbalized, an activity may be provided that is demanding and seems punitive. The patient may then feel he has worked out his measure of punishment. Additionally, the successful completion of the task provides a sense of worth for work completed.

Occupational therapists are best trained to identify such activities, but in the absence of a skilled therapist, as in some state hospital situations, the nurse can provide chores such as bed making, floor polishing, bathroom cleaning and grounds policing. These activities utilize energy, they have meaning to the patient, and they provide recognition for work that does, in truth, need to be done. If occupational therapy is available, aggressive impulses can often be expressed through such activities as metal work, in which the patient has an opportunity to beat hard and long on materials that are not immediately malleable. Such an endeavor provides time to thrash out feelings. A depressed man said about the metal work he had done when he was very ill: "I hated going to the shop. I hated you for sending me. I died a thousand deaths each morning before I went, wondering how I would find the strength to walk to the shop, but after each session there, I felt surprisingly good. I was exhausted, but it was a good, clean fatigue. It did not feel like the sick, wrapped-up, suffocating feeling that I had from depression. While I hammered at the metal it was good. I raised that hammer and I slammed it down again and again. I did not think about it; it just happened. I liked the security of feeling as it happened over and over. The noise blocked out the sound of the horrible thoughts that never left my head except when I went to O.T."

Many years ago there was a question on the state board examination in psychiatric nursing that described a patient who was extremely depressed and ridden with guilt feelings. The question suggested four activities which could be prescribed by the nurse; they were reading, going for walks, polishing the floor and cleaning out the toilets. The last answer was the correct one. Those taking the examination that year were indignant when they discovered the correct answer. They felt that as nurses they could not subject a patient in their care to such a demeaning activity as cleaning toilet bowls. It took much thinking and discussion for them to realize that such a patient felt the need for derogating activity. He would probably be telling himself in many ways that he was not better than a toilet bowl; he would be ruminating about killing himself because he was so "dirty and ashamed and worthless." If he were assigned to a chore that was also dirty and demeaning, he would find it less necessary to derogate himself because others, external to him, seemed to be doing so. In a sense, his superego would no longer need to punish him because the nurse took over this function. Of course, she would also praise him when the chore was well done. As he verbalized less often about his worthlessness, she would be able to show him tangible evidence of his worth to her. She could then reassign him to a less dirty job, saying, *not* that he was good, or special, or anything that he could not possibly believe at that point in his illness, but that she needed his cleaning skills in some other area, such as bed making, or floor polishing, or another job that could be done around the unit, and one that would still use a great deal of energy. (Floor polishing is a good activity because it requires that the person push a mop back and forth repeatedly over the same area. Thus, the job does not require concentration that the patient is incapable of, but it does provide the reward of seeing a useful outcome, i.e., the shining floor.)

Bed making is not so good a task for the patient who needs repetition because the process of bed making utilizes many small, different motions. It is a better activity for the patient who is slightly less depressed and who would benefit from doing something in the company of another person.

Such recreational activities as volleyball, Ping-Pong, bridge and hiking are useful. They enable the depressed patient to use up energy generated by tension. In addition, they provide enough competitive activity to stimulate the expression, in sublimated form, of anger. Discretion must be used, however, in assigning the patient to a given activity so that he is not put in a position of competing without hope of success. It is often better to encourage team sports so that there is no negative recognition for an individual who has lost. If the hospital has a gymnasium the overactive patient can sometimes be sent there with an attendant to play "21" or simply throw a medicine ball.

Movies, TV and books further round out the patient's day. The nurse should keep in mind that her sicker patients may not have the concentration required to enjoy some of these diversions. For some women, knitting or sewing projects offer some relaxation. Like floor mopping, and other ward cleaning chores, simple knitting and sewing are rather monotonous and do not require concentrated effort. However, if these activities are being pursued, the incomplete work should be collected at the end of the session, for the needles provide lethal tools for the patient who may impulsively act out his suicidal tendencies.

WARD MEETINGS AS ADJUNCT TO MEET PSYCHOLOGICAL NEEDS

Ward meetings are another useful adjunct to therapy. Here the patient group can experience a sense of cohesion with others and have the opportunity for support from a peer group. In addition, patients experience the feeling of importance created when their views are elicited and heard. Such a forum provides a fine opportunity for the patient group to plan parts of their own program. Choices may be made available for activities and goals.

A crucial part of the patient's recovery involves the awakening of his own creative ability in order to break up the repetitive nature of his depression. Ward meetings or small group activities provide the milieu in which the patient can begin to experience himself as being productive. It is true that the depressed patient needs a carefully planned, well organized program; by the same token, he should not be so boxed in that there is no opportunity for personal expression. Creating an opportunity for the patient to help in planning activities is an excellent means for providing for the expression of personal preference. The program of a patient who is initially too ill to make such judgments should be revised at close enough intervals so that he is frequently consulted. Eventually he will be well enough to contribute. Such activity fosters decision making and responsibility. The latter are necessary for full recovery and a return to the community.

THE NURSING CARE OF THE DEPRESSED PATIENT IN THE COMMUNITY

Taking responsibility for the safe return of a patient to his optimal level of health through the concerted efforts of a health team is not only feasible but practical in many types of medical problems. For the psychiatric nurse who works with patients in the community, the goals must usually be altered. Among the many facts that make this necessary is the reality that there are not enough supervisory personnel available to make it realistic for a nurse, no matter what her preparation, to plan therapeutic intervention with the majority of her patients. The conditions under which the nurse and patient in the community work do not lend themselves to an endeavor in depth. The type of patient and the illness that will come to the nurse's attention also influence the kind of nursing intervention planned. If the patient is acutely ill and suicidal, it is likely that the local police will initiate an admission process to a hospital (this is the least desirable method of entry), or the patient may come voluntarily to a treatment facility and request care, or he may be admitted to a hospital on a commitment basis by a referring physician. At any rate, the acutely ill patient generally finds his way to a treatment facility.

The patient who remains in the community tends to be a person who is not living through the first, crucial onset of symptoms, but rather is one who has been ill for some time and has learned to live with his problems. This individual's adjustment may be marginal; however, he is able to maintain himself outside a hospital. Thus, the sick person who comes to the attention of the psychiatric nurse in the community is usually chronically ill. This means several things: (1) the person has been ill for an extended length of time; (2) his illness may be serious, but it generally is not of a life-threatening caliber; and (3) the person has made a number of conscious and unconscious adjustments to his illness. This is useful on the one hand and detrimental on the other, for the successful adjustments make the person more comfortable and less likely to give up his symptoms and his disease process.

These factors amount to the totality of an individual who does not represent an "ideal" candidate for psychiatric therapy. On the other hand, the nurse who sets her goals realistically will plan to help the patient to *modify* his reactions (behavioral) to his illness so that he can live more effectively within the community setting. Within this frame of reference, the nurse has her work cut out for her, and potential success is a probability.

It is foolhardy for the nurse to attempt to take on the care of an acutely ill, suicidally depressed patient in the community. Such an endeavor is likely to end with the death of the patient, for there are just not enough controls outside a hospital for such a person. The nurse who attempts such a "feat" needs to give careful scrutiny to her own motives. Only unconscious forces could influence such an ill advised venture.

The psychiatric nurse who is based in the community approaches the physical care of the depressed patient through health teaching. She is not available on a continuous basis, as is the nurse who works in a hospital, so that family, available neighbors or friends must be utilized in the patient's therapy. Again, the individual who is sick enough to let his physical condition deteriorate is usually in an institution.

For the unusual situation, for instance, an elderly individual who lives with his children, arrangements must sometimes be made for daily care. The nurse must talk with the family about the need for personal hygiene and then arrange a workable schedule with them. Such a program might mean that the elderly, depressed patient is helped to bathe late in the morning after the young children have been gotten off to school. It may mean bathing and grooming in the evening when the head of the household comes home and can be available for lifting and carrying. In other words, the nurse must think in terms of the household schedule. The typical hospital routine was established for the convenience of hospital personnel, and it need not, and in most cases should not, be superimposed upon the home situation.

Physiological complications are less likely to be observed in the ambulatory patient because these symptoms, i.e., the "vegetative signs," are seen only in very retarded patients. Such conditions are associated with acute processes and such patients are, advisedly, in hospitals. Should such an unfortunate patient be in the community, the nurse should consider referral directly to a hospital (if this is possible in her state) or referral to an agency or outpatient clinic which could make the initial moves to have the patient admitted to a treatment facility.

In planning the psychological care of the patient the nurse can identify the majority of her goals from the circumstances that bring her in contact with that individual. For instance, if the patient comes to a clinic seeking help for his blue moods or a chronic sense of depression, the nurse can assume that this individual is not satisfied, that he may be in pain, or that he may wish to change some facet of his life. At any rate, it is apparent that the patient is motivated to change. The individual who is referred by family, neighbors or friends may recognize the need for help, or he may be content with the status quo. The latter situation does not augur well for the efforts of the nurse.

In the referring situation the nurse will learn her first important facts about the depressed patient from statements from the sick individual himself or from others. The self-referring patient will attempt to tell the nurse what brought him to her. The referring "others" will also describe what it is about the identified patient that should bring him to the attention of the nurse. Such statements are likely to describe a person who cries a good deal, one who cannot sleep at night or an individual who worries about his physical health and cannot stop even though medical examinations show no abnormalities. The depressed individual who refers himself may speak of his chronic lack of energy, his feeling of pointlessness, or his inability to get up in the morning. A more sophisticated person might even characterize himself as "depressed."

With this type of patient the nurse should be particularly cautious. First of all, "depressed" might mean one thing to her and another to the person using the term. A continuation of the interview without asking for clarification of the patient's use of the label might lead to later disagreement when the nurse proceeds with one type of approach and the patient has a totally unrelated expectation. Next, use of labels is often an unconscious way of getting around painful feelings and thoughts. The psychiatric nurse who accepts the statement, "I am depressed," without asking for further clarification really does not learn anything about her patient. Labels are signposts; they provide a frame of reference. They may even push the investigator in the right direction as he begins a dialogue with the patient, but labels are only the beginning. "Depressed" frequently means, "I don't feel like myself. I am sad." It does not say anything about *why* the patient is this way. It gives no hint about how he is coping with his feelings, or what his thoughts are. The nurse-interviewer who accepts such a self-diagnostic label without seeking clarification has misunderstood her responsibility. Sooner or later she will realize that her data is sadly incomplete, and she will have to back track in order to fill in the details.

For the doubting reader, consider this mythical situation:

> The nurse reports to the agency staff that she has begun seeing a carpenter who has a reactive depression.

What does the staff now know about the patient? Think carefully. What facts have been given about the person who has just started treatment? Consider a different kind of report:

> The nurse reports to the agency staff that she has begun interviewing a 65 year old retired chauffeur who comes to the agency through his own referral. He claims that he cannot sleep at night, he has lost weight recently, food does not taste very good anymore, and his wife died a month ago.

In the first example, the staff members do not get a real sense of the new patient as a person. What is actually heard is a statistic for the monthly report—one more reactive depressive. The second report pictures an elderly person who has recently suffered a great loss. He describes his troubles as weight loss, change in appetite and sleep disturbance. From the recitation of problems, as the patient sees them, a more meaningful diagnosis can be made. Granted, it is the same diagnosis—depression—but it becomes a label, a shorthand method, for categorizing broadly the types of problems faced by the retired chauffeur. From such statements the nurse can begin to formulate a view of the patient based on his feelings and behavior. It is to these facets of the person that the nurse will address her efforts. Thus, the patient who claims that he cannot sleep offers hints that something keeps him from sleeping. The nurse will need to know what these things are. Is there a young baby at home? Are financial worries keeping the individual awake? Is the person kept up by fantasies that frighten him? Clarification of these issues will lead to further discussion.

It is crucial that psychiatric nurse and patient arrive at a mutual understanding of the patient's purposes in coming for help. Next, the two principals must arrange a plan that is mutually satisfying and meets the needs of both parties concerning time and place of meetings, length of sessions and remuneration, if this is a factor. The nurse is then ready to instruct the patient concerning the way they will work together. Generally the nurse tells him that what is said between them will be kept confidential by her. She explains the importance of the patient's honesty (as well as her own) in their communications, and encourages the patient to talk about those things that seem pertinent to him and to his problem as he sees it. The nurse usually needs to explain to the uninitiated patient that she will not be giving him answers or demanding that he change his life style, but that the two of them will try together to find solutions for the patient's predicament.

Basically the same goals that the psychiatric nurse identifies for the care of the institutionalized depressed patient will be those of the nurse in the community, for the underlying problems of the patient are the same. This means that recognition, acceptance and a sense of self-esteem will be fostered by the nurse's behavior. The psychiatric nurse will try to identify situations in which the patient might have used more effective means of expressing himself. This goal is a rather sophisticated one for the beginning practitioner and should not be attempted until the patient shows some awareness of the maladaptiveness of his behavior patterns and indicates a willingness to try new approaches.

Thus, the initial nursing care plan will include gathering data about the patient—his history, his present life style, his relationships with others, his picture of himself. During this process the patient will describe in greater detail how he perceives his problems. As the nurse listens and begins to formulate a picture (clinical impression) of the person who is talking to her, she should check her perceptions by asking if what she thinks is actually true.

> Mr. T., a truck driver for a large brewery, came to the community mental health center because he was not feeling his usual self and thought that the clinic might be able to help him. He described his life as quiet. He lived alone in a multiple dwelling where he had resided with his wife until her death a year prior to the initial interview. Mr. T. found it sufficient entertainment to go to a "neighbor lady's" house about once a week for some beer and a card game. Mr. T. reported that he worked regularly and was regarded as an old reliable employee. He had two grown sons who were married and lived away from the city. Mr. T. did not see them often and did not appear very interested in them.
>
> The patient complained of feelings of apathy. He did not really enjoy his work anymore or his weekly visits to the lady friend. He slept poorly and always felt tired. In addition, the meager meals he was accustomed to fixing for himself were no longer palatable to him.
>
> The nurse interviewing Mr. T. was not clear about the reasons that brought him to the agency at this time. Because he obviously spoke with difficulty, she did not want to frighten him by asking a question for which he might not have an answer. She felt that it might be better to strengthen the relationship first. This being her decision, she asked him if he would like to come back and talk again. He agreed and the next appointment was set.
>
> Mr. T. arrived promptly for his second appointment. He seemed more comfortable in his recitation, and the nurse felt more at ease with him. She asked him how he had felt the past week and he said, "better." She then requested him to continue with his discussion from the first interview. As Mr. T. went over essentially what he had reported before, the nurse felt it was safe to interrupt and ask for clarification of her observations. "Mr. T., I have been listening to your words and watching your expressions and I am getting the impression that you are unhappy with your life. Is that so?"
>
> The patient nodded mutely. Tears welled up in his eyes. There was a long silence before the nurse interrupted it by encouraging her patient to continue with his story. "You were going to tell me about your sons and their families. . . ."
>
> Mr. T. began to speak haltingly about them and their separate lives in other states. He described them as people who were far away

and uninterested in him, and he in them. Mr. T. again mentioned his deceased wife as the person who kept the family together. Since her death he and the boys had not had reason to communicate. Mr. T. did not continue his discussion of the family, but mentioned his satisfactions with work. He described himself as a valued employee and a trusted "unofficial" officer of his employer.

The nurse realized that Mr. T. had switched subjects, but she noted his tears and the obvious difficulty he had in discussing his family. The time was drawing to a close and she permitted the conversation to move to "safer" more comfortable ground. When the time was up she said, "The time has gone more quickly today, Mr. T. You've told me about your family and some of your feelings toward them. I've heard also that you like your job and take much satisfaction in it. I'm sure you are a valued person in your position. Shall we meet at the same time next week? Perhaps it would help to talk a bit more about your sons and your feelings toward them."

The interviews continued for three months. Mr. T. spoke more and more of his sons. He described them as not caring about him, and he showed increased affect as he repeatedly spoke of them. It became apparent that the deceased Mrs. T. had been the connecting link between the sons and father and that with her death any closeness was shattered. Mr. T. was angry at his children and unable to face any but the most positive feelings toward his dead wife. As the interviews continued, the patient showed increased evidence of sorrow and anger. He cried often and freely when he was talking about his family. At the same time, Mr. T. was experiencing increased pleasure in his daily living. It was in the fourth month of interviews that Mr. T. mentioned quite casually that at the time he began to feel "bad," he was considering asking the lady friend to marry him. The nurse was surprised at this disclosure and asked why Mr. T. had not mentioned this before.

"I don't really know. I guess I just didn't think of it," he said.

The nurse felt that this added bit of data helped to round out the picture of Mr. T.'s illness and his reasons for coming to the clinic. When the nurse and the patient had spent considerable time discussing Mr. T.'s feelings, his eyes began to grow watery. It had been established between them that sometimes Mr. T. felt great sorrow, but that almost as often he was angry and felt helpless. The nurse had asked aloud what Mr. T. did about these feelings and toward whom they were directed. Mr. T. admitted that he felt angry at his sons and usually he felt great sadness about his wife, but occasionally he thought maybe he was angry at her too.

Feeling that a fairly secure base had been constructed for Mr. T. to learn new avenues for the expression of his feelings, the psychiatric nurse asked him: "I wonder if your thoughts about marrying Mrs. C. made you too uncomfortable? Could your anger at your sons and your mixed feelings about Mrs. T. have anything to do with your feeling so bad?"

The patient looked puzzled and the nurse said nothing more. "I am not sure I understand you," he finally said.

"What I am wondering is if your warm feelings toward Mrs. C. and the prospect of marrying her brought back to you, perhaps more forcibly, your angry feelings toward your sons and the mixture of love and anger that you feel toward your dead wife? Sometimes when we contemplate embarking on a new life—in your case, a new partnership—we feel the need to first 'put the house in order.' I wonder if your bad feelings and your inability to sleep or enjoy your food could be the result of trying to put *your* house in order, but not being able to get all the pieces straightened out without help."

Mr. T. looked thoughtful. He sat quietly and looked at the floor and then at his hands in his lap. "I don't really know. Maybe so. I don't feel particularly bad anymore. I sleep. I eat. I watch television and I've even been thinking about going around to C's (the lady friend's) house."

The nurse listened to Mr. T. and she felt more confident of her perceptions. Mr. T.'s depression had lessened as was indicated by his decrease in symptoms. He was thinking of renewing his relationship with Mrs. C., which spoke well of his future satisfactions. He reported satisfactory completion of his daily work and described himself in this role in positive terms, which indicated his continuing sense of worth. The nurse felt that their work together had indeed helped Mr. T. to break free of the problems that threatened to engulf him and he was now on the verge of being able to continue without help. She looked at Mr. T. and smiled. "I'm glad you are feeling better. I think you will continue to improve, and soon you will be able to stop coming here. Let's talk a little about the sorts of things that you can do in order to keep yourself feeling well."

The rest of the interview was taken up with identification of feelings and means of expressing them more directly than Mr. T. had been accustomed to doing.

In the last few interviews, the nurse focused almost exclusively on Mr. T.'s growing ability to express himself. She praised his growth and assured him that it was important that he allow himself to *feel* his anger and his sadness and that he needed to be able to communicate these feelings to the people with whom he associated. The nurse also took each appropriate opportunity to point out to Mr. T. his strengths and to elicit from him responses which indicated his acceptance of them as part of himself.

The psychiatric nurse in community practice may not always encounter her patient in an office setting. She may find it necessary to go into the home. In the case of a housewife, it is useful for the interview to be conducted in the setting where the problems arise, for this gives the nurse an opportunity to assist her patient where the latter experiences the majority of her problems. She can support the patient in her efforts to grow. Being with the housewife and helping her in the home offer an ideal setting for promoting the patient's sense of worth and her self-confidence. As she is able to perform more adequately, she feels better. In the home she can talk, express herself, air her thoughts aloud, and have the opportunity to hear the nurse correct distortions, seek clarification on issues that are unclear, and help the patient to understand problems that are not initially understood.

The psychiatric nurse interviewing in the community must ascertain the reasons for a patient's coming for help. She translates these reasons into basically behavioral terms, i.e., "can't sleep, can't eat, can't get up," and so forth. Her efforts will be directed to changing this behavior. Means of accomplishing these behavioral changes usually involve teaching the patient to recognize and express his feelings, helping him to gain a more realistic self-image, and fostering in him the urge to assume a better living style.

REFERENCES

1. Arieti, S.: Manic-Depressive Psychosis. *In* Arieti, S.: *American Handbook of Psychiatry*. New York, Basic Books, Inc., 1959.
2. Deutsch, H.: Melancholia and Depressive States. *In Neuroses and Character Types*. New York, International Universities Press, 1965.
3. Fenichel, O.: *The Psychoanalytic Theory of Neurosis*. New York, W. W. Norton and Company, 1945.
4. Gutheil, E.: Reactive Depression. *In* Arieti, S., (ed.) : *American Handbook of Psychiatry*. New York: Basic Books, Inc., 1959.
5. Huston, P.: Psychotic Depressive Reaction. *In* Freedman, A., and Kaplan, H. (eds.) : *Comprehensive Textbook of Psychiatry*. Baltimore, The Williams & Wilkins Co., 1967.
6. Laughlin, H.: *The Neuroses*. London, Butterworth & Co., Ltd., 1967.
7. Mendelson, M.: Neurotic Depressive Reaction. *In* Freedman, A., and Kaplan, H. (eds.): *Comprehensive Textbook of Psychiatry*. Baltimore, The Williams & Wilkins Co., 1967.
8. Redlich, F. C., and Freedman, D. X.: *The Theory and Practice of Psychiatry*. New York, Basic Books, Inc., 1966.

SUGGESTED READING

Custance, J.: The Universe of Bliss. *In* Kaplan, B., (ed.) : *The Inner World of Mental Illness*. New York, Harper and Row, 1964.

This account is highly recommended because it describes the real feelings and perceptions of a patient in the midst of his manic-depressive illness. The description is actually terrifying because the reader must immerse self in the "craziness" of the writing in order to understand it. It is highly recommended, because the student will leave the topic knowing the syndrome is not a group of sterile symptoms.

Engel, G.: Grief and Grieving. *Am. J. Nursing*, 64 (No. 9) :93, September, 1964.

Dr. Engel is considered an authority in the field of grief and his article covers much of the information known about the process. Reading this article will provide the student with basic knowledge and an opportunity to read directly the work of a recognized authority in the field.

Hillyer, J.: Reluctantly Told. *In* Kaplan, B., (ed.) : *The Inner World of Mental Illness*. New York, Harper and Row, 1964.

Another fine account of depression as actually experienced by the patient. This paper, while not horrifying like Custance's, does provide the reader with the empty feeling of the depressed patient. It is well written and easy to read.

Neylan, M. P.: The Depressed Patient. *Am. J. Nursing*, 61 (No. 7) :77, July, 1961.

This article provides a substantial, though fundamental, survey of the nursing perspective on depression. For the reader who does not assimilate easily through literature, this is a particularly good selection because it gives the necessary information clearly and concisely.

Robinson, L.: The Depressed Patient. *In* Robinson, L.: *Psychological Aspects of the Care of Hospitalized Patient.* Philadelphia, F. A. Davis, 1968, Chapter 7.

This short article focuses on the depressed patient in the general hospital setting. It is suggested because it permits the student to think beyond the confines of the psychiatric institution.

Rykken, M.: The Nurse's Role in Preventing Suicide. *Nursing Outlook,* 6 (No. 7): July, 1958.

The writer provides a thorough discussion of suicide. She presents the phenomenon as an entity in itself, rather than as the end point of another disease. Her presentation is extremely readable and is filled with facts that the competent psychiatric nurse will want to know.

Shneidman, E. S.: Preventing Suicide. *Am. J. Nursing,* 65 (No. 5) :111, May, 1965.

Dr. Shneidman has earned the recognition of the psychiatric world for his in-depth study and efforts in the area of suicide. His publications on the topic are numerous. This article is literally filled with information which will be of great value to those who might encounter the potential suicide. Says the author, "All that is required are sharp eyes and ears, good intuition, a pinch of wisdom, and ability to act appropriately, and a deep resolve."

Thompson, C.: Analytic Observations During the Course of a Manic-Depressive Psychosis. *In* Green, M. (ed.) :*Interpersonal Psychoanalysis, the Selected Papers of Clara M. Thompson.* New York, Basic Books, Inc., 1964.

Though the information offered in this paper is not strictly in the educational province of the nursing student, it is suggested for the student who might be exceptional in the area of psychiatric nursing. Dr. Thompson is a particularly gifted writer, and her presentation is both interesting and informative. It permits the reader a view of the process of psychoanalysis. At the same time it deals with a topic, manic-depressive psychosis, that is appropriate to the student's interests.

chapter 8

THE PATIENT WHO IS UNABLE TO REACH OUT

It is sometimes frustrating to care for the mentally ill; occasionally it is exasperating. For each of us it is frightening and anxiety-provoking as we encounter the human experiences in our patients that we suspect or know are ours as well. This latter situation is one which all psychiatric caretakers encounter sooner or later, for we are all human and those feelings that assail the mentally ill individual are really little different from the experiences of all human beings, except in quantity and quality. Thus, the nurse who listens closely to the endless monologue of her "crazy" charge may feel a terrifying sense of loneliness as she realizes the quality of her patient's isolation. Her reaction is not to the patient's experience but to the awakening of her awareness of her own potential for aloneness. The nurse who allows herself to experience this dreadful feeling is sharing a human agony with another person. Through it she can better understand both the patient and herself; likewise, she can better go about the business of providing the sense of community that the patient who is isolated and terrified needs.

As Harry Stack Sullivan, a psychiatrist particularly expert and innovative in the care of the schizophrenic, wrote, "We are all more human than otherwise." He was reminding the generations of psychotherapists who would follow him that patients are people, as nurses and doctors are people, and that the best way to understand less rational or verbal patients is by recognizing in them and in ourselves the commonality of our human experiences.

It is suggested that the reader remember these words, because the following pages will discuss a problem that is probably new and may be particularly frightening. We will be exploring inner life. For some, their defenses will be so strong that the grimmer visions will not be recognized; for a few, the gifted who might be sufficiently free and secure enough to risk it, the exploration will bridge the gap between rational sanity and irrational psychosis, permitting the nurse to dip into the world of her lonely patient and to risk the boundaries of self in reaching out to a lost human being who cannot find his way back to the outer world. We shall be learning about the outcasts of society who struggle against loneliness and the fear of rejection. Some defend themselves adequately with only occasional lapses into their inner worlds; some dwell most of the time apart from the rational world around them. A few inhabitants of this lonely, terrifying world protect themselves poorly; they dwell constantly in a place of their own creation where others can rarely follow and where only they can experience their pains. "Ambulatory schizophrenic," "hospitalized," "leading a marginal existence"—these are descriptions of very desolate people who have in common the characteristic of aloneness. They may live amid other people, but they are unwilling or unable to relate to them.

The call girl who barters with her body but does not divulge her name; the young child who stands in the corner of a ward in a state hospital unable to say more than, "Bird, bird, bird, bird"; the man who struggles each day to trust his psychotherapist enough to utter the words that crowd his thoughts—all these people carry a similar diagnosis. They share an underlying problem as well. These lonely, frightened human beings are called schizophrenic. They may be further divided into subclassifications of simple schizophrenia, hebephrenia, catatonia or paranoia, depending upon their symptoms; however, they are basically human beings who have been hurt to the point of psychic mutilation. Their earliest experiences were unlikely the warm, security-providing ones that healthier people take for granted; rather, their pasts are suggestive of inadequate, impersonal or even hostile relationships. They were not permitted, as infants, to sense the warmth, the benign closeness of a mothering one who nurtured them and permitted their painful growth to maturity; they did not know they could falter, enjoy again the safety of mother's warmth, and try once more. A schizophrenic patient once described this basic situation wistfully as the "snug harbor" she could never have. She said the harbor for her small boat was filled with reefs and shoals, and once she could find her way out of it, she never wished, nor would she have been permitted, to sail back in, for the drawbridge had been lowered.

ETIOLOGY

The causes of schizophrenia are still widely disputed. Literature abounds on the topic, but none is truly conclusive, although several schools of thought describe good theoretical bases for the disease. Most prevalent presently seems to be the theory that schizophrenia is an illness of withdrawal, based on severe early trauma. The proponents of this believe that the lack of warmth and a giving relationship in infancy leaves the patient hungry for dependency but unable to experience warmth from others because he is unable to identify it. The personality does not mature to the stage of the differentiated ego. In other words, the schizophrenic cannot distinguish "me," the ego, from "not me," which is the external world.

The reader who has studied biology may be able to understand this dynamic picture more easily by considering the lowly amoeba, a single-celled organism with a cell membrane surrounding it that separates the organism from the environment. In the case of the schizophrenic, this protective membrane is not felt. The "psychic protoplasm" of the individual flows into that of his surroundings; he feels open and vulnerable. He cannot separate himself from that which is near and seems to threaten him. Thus, in later, active illness, the patient fears engulfment by close relationships. To prevent such occurrences, he maintains lonely isolation.

Some students of schizophrenia[2, 3, 6] believe this entity is a disturbance in communication. They regard the family of the schizophrenic patient (more often the mother) as ill. Thus, communications with the prepsychotic child are distorted. The future patient receives messages from the mother with two or more possible meanings, all of which are reasonable and could be acted upon. The possible meanings of her message are so dissimilar, however, that they create a highly anxious situation for the child who is unable to select the proper response, that is, the response he feels will gain mother's approval. A familiar and descriptive phrase for this situation is "double bind." The following example describes a situation in a prepsychotic's interaction with his mother in which one overt message is given while another, covert one, is simultaneously sent: A well meaning, though cold, mother says to her son, "Come here dear, I must kiss you." The child hears her say, "Come," but he sees that she is recoiling from his touch. Her teeth are clenched. The child hears, consciously, that he should come, yet he senses preconsciously (with complete accuracy) that mother really wants him to stay away. The preschizophrenic child who receives the majority of his messages in this way must make a response, because his psychic survival depends on doing that which will gain mother's approval. To resolve his dilemma, he tunes out his own perceptions of the overt communication. In effect, he disowns his ego—that agency of the mind responsible for his hearing of and decoding messages—so that he can react. The ultimate fear of engulfment is finally realized because the schizophrenic has now given up his prerogative to be stimulated and to respond, via his own ego, to the environment. To resolve his dilemma, the child withdraws.

Therapists of this theoretical school believe that treatment involves the schizophrenic's relearning a system of communication. He must, in effect, form a trusting relationship with the therapist in which he can again experience and respond appropriately to all his perceptions. He must be able to communicate with the therapist as to his perception of himself and the environment. Finally, with the help of the therapist he differentiates that which is real from that which is not. Such a task requires an enormously stable and open therapist who knows himself well, for the schizophrenic patient will often sense that which is not yet conscious to the therapist. In order to protect the patient and to help him to develop a differentiated ego that he can depend upon, the therapist must be prepared to acknowledge that which the patient senses to be in existence.[11]

There are researchers who are convinced that schizophrenia is inherited; some feel that the disease is biochemically based. One group of workers feels that the cause is a combination of the factors already discussed. There are those who believe that "schizophrenia" is actually a label for a combination of diseases. Thus, it can be seen that, as in other disease entities previously discussed, many answers are not yet known. However, patients continue to present with a group of symptoms labeled "schizophrenia." Psychiatric nurses must be trained to care for these people, offering them better chances to find their way back to reality.

DYNAMICS OF THE DISEASE

The schizophrenic patient is a highly sensitive, lonely individual who perceives himself as vulnerable to psychological threats from the environment. As such, he is constantly watching, constantly ready to identify danger before he is hurt. The ambulatory schizophrenic may be in an arrested or even mildly ill state in which his ego, though weak, functions adequately so that he can, most of the time, distinguish himself from the outer world and repress his inner world. (In this sense, the ego is like the cell membrane of the amoeba mentioned earlier. The membrane protects the self from the environment and also from the inner world, or unconscious.) In such a patient, then, the ego is strong enough to monitor the environment and to control the actions of the individual in response to it. Periodically this individual may need to retreat into a more frankly psychotic state, but for the most part he is able to maintain himself, through constant vigilance against danger, by living a marginal life in which he never permits himself to become close to anyone. People who live this kind of life are often found among migrant workers, hobos, prostitutes, and the alcoholics of skid row, and among the creative artistic population as well.

Schizophrenic illness does not always lead to uselessness and a noncontributory existence. Great artists such as Nijinsky, the dancer,

Van Gogh, the painter, and Robert Schumann, the composer, were all victims of schizophrenia who used their illness as a steppingstone to their inner, creative worlds. One might wonder how the psychotic experience could be so utilized. Laing, a British psychiatrist, describes the condition as one which "entails a loss of the usual foundations of the 'sense' of the world that we share with one another. Old purposes no longer seem viable; old meanings are senseless; the distinctions between imagination, dream, external perceptions often seem no longer to apply in the old way. External events may seem magically conjured up. Dreams may seem to be direct communications from others; imagination may seem to be objective reality."[8] Laing also writes that psychosis need not be all breakdown because it can be break*through*. It can mean freedom and renewal as well as enslavement and psychic death. Psychosis seems to have meant freedom for some creative individuals; it has given them the opportunity to unfetter their minds and, in effect, to produce masterpieces. It is believed that the creative schizophrenic makes use of his unrepressed thoughts in their original primary language.

For many schizophrenics their illness has meant the inability to carry on in the world around them. They are not creative; indeed they are unproductive.

TYPES OF SCHIZOPHRENIA

The least ill-appearing schizophrenics are termed schizophrenic, simple type. These people appear to respond like a nonpsychotic individual at times, while at other intervals they react inappropriately to stimuli and seem unable to communicate in a manner that is rational and meaningful. Their symptoms tend to be less florid than those of other types of schizophrenics. Like the others, however, they tend to need greater defense against their vulnerability than is provided by loneliness and seclusion. In addition to the physical conditions of their lives, they further isolate themselves by focusing on their inner worlds. Other types of schizophrenic patients, namely, the catatonic and hebephrenic, display more florid behavior. The paranoid schizophrenic will be presented in the discussion of projection.

The catatonic schizophrenic is characterized by either extreme lassitude or extreme psychomotor agitation. In the former state the patient may be mute or almost stuporous; he may be found standing or sitting motionless for long periods of time. In the catatonic state the patient may exhibit "waxy flexibility," which is a condition in which the patient's limbs may be placed in any position and the patient will maintain that stance.

In extreme psychomotor agitation the catatonic patient talks and shouts almost continuously. He may be destructive, and his movements must be controlled since he might injure himself or others. Ultimately this behavior may lead to the patient's death from exhaustion unless he can be calmed.

The hebephrenic patient, whose symptoms symbolize the most deteriorated of the schizophrenic conditions, is markedly regressed to a point of primitive, unorganized behavior. His responses are grossly inappropriate. Such a patient often grins and grimaces. The hebephrenic is regarded as the most regressed of the schizophrenic patients; he is known for his silly behavior. The prognosis for the hebephrenic schizophrenic is extremely poor.

THE LANGUAGE OF THE SCHIZOPHRENIC

Schizophrenic individuals tend to live with their fantasies, their fantasized companions and their own languages. The latter are of great interest to nurses, because it is possible to observe so much of the schizophrenic's life, pain and progress toward health through his language.

The language of schizophrenia often sounds foreign to those who hear it. To the sick individual, his language has very precise meaning, no matter how cryptic it may sound to others. The terms "neologisms" and "word salad" have been used in connection with schizophrenic language to describe the creation of new and meaningless words. Current literature and psychotherapists who are students of communication believe that all communications from schizophrenics are meaningful, and that the meaning of the messages is known to the patient.

Primary process, the language of infancy, is utilized by the schizophrenic in much of his communication. It sounds unfamiliar to the listener's ear because it is composed of thoughts disguised through displacement and condensation, which make the message difficult for the listener to understand.

Condensation is a mechanism that telescopes an entire thought or picture into a single symbol. It is a type of schizophrenic shorthand. For example, one of the most familiar symbols is the human breast, which signifies warmth, comfort, food and affection. To observe condensation and primary process thinking in the normal context, the reader need only recall the response of the young infant who observes a pacifier, a bottle or the mother's breast. Immediately the child responds with a happy, excited expression (unless he is satiated). The infant is responding to several implicit meanings—all telescoped into the single symbol.

In an actual clinical example of condensation, we observe Miss O., a 54 year old schizophrenic patient. She once told of her deep devotion to the ward psychologist (whom she did not know). It became clear that the psychologist, who had a short and bushy beard, reminded her of her grandfather, whose hair had looked similar. The grandfather had been a source of kindness, understanding and affection. During her stay at the hospital the patient had observed the psychologist as he passed through the ward. His bushy beard reminded her of the warm moments she had shared with her grandfather and of the many good qualities he possessed. Thus, she formed an attachment to the psychologist.

In this example displacement is also observed. The girl identified the personality of her grandfather in the psychologist. She then transferred her feelings from her relative to the psychologist. Thus, the feelings evoked in one frame of reference were refocused on another object or person.

A second example illustrates a negative outcome. Martha, a 42 year old housewife, was seen every week in a community mental health center by a mental health aide. The patient had been followed weekly since her release from State Hospital where she had been hospitalized for one and a half years. Martha was a quiet factory worker who enjoyed being alone and worked best in a job where she could be by herself. One day, after her mental health aide had suggested that the interval between their meetings might be lengthened to two weeks, Martha went back to the factory where she worked and hit her supervisor when the woman requested that Martha submit a stock inventory to her in two weeks.

The two situations were not similar; however, Martha transferred her feelings of anger from the mental health aide to her supervisor at the factory. She reacted to the suggestion of the aide as if it were a rejection. She was unable to deal with her feelings directly, and when the supervisor requested an inventory in "two weeks," the reaction to the aide was impulsively acted out toward the supervisor. In this example, Martha transferred her feelings through the vehicle of primary process. Utilizing the words "two weeks" as a stimulus, she condensed the entire situation with the mental health aide and acted upon it with her supervisor.

REGRESSION IN SCHIZOPHRENIA

As in other psychiatric disorders, the patient who is schizophrenic is severely regressed. He must cope in a world for which he is ill equipped because he has little or no functioning ego. Therefore, he tests reality poorly. Delusions and hallucinations are the result of his inability to differentiate between memory traces, sensory experiences, and actual current events. The profoundly ill schizophrenic is like a young infant; he is highly narcissistic. To him, everything that occurs in the life space around him is in some way related to him. (The reader should recall that the young infant cannot at first differentiate between himself and mother's breast. He does not recognize that the breast appears as a result of his cries. It is a developmental task for the baby to recognize that the pains of hunger, the lack of warmth, and fatigue end because he as an independent being signals that these conditions exist.) The situation is similar for the profoundly disturbed schizophrenic. He feels that all conditions around him are related to him in some way, as elements caused by him, or situations impinging upon him as the result of his existence. Like the infant, the schizophrenic is convinced of his omnipotence.

> When she came on duty in the morning, the head nurse always saw Janet T. curled up on the floor by the door to the ward. The nurse attempted to speak to Janet and to get her to come back to the dayroom, but she never succeeded; however, the male attendant was always able to persuade her to come to the dining area for hot coffee once the head nurse had disappeared from sight.
> When Janet had become better integrated and was able to describe some of her feelings, she told her therapist that she felt a great fondness for the head nurse. It angered her, however, that the nurse left her at night. Janet felt deserted. In the mornings she waited by the door to make sure her nurse would return; however, the only way she could be sure of protecting the nurse from her rage and potential violence was to become almost stuporous and lie on the floor.

This is a good example of the kind of thinking that the schizophrenic utilizes. The patient felt great ambivalence toward her nurse. She both cared for her intensely and hated her for her perceived rejection. She was convinced that her hatred was so forceful that she would actually harm the object of her love. This danger was guarded against by becoming stuporous, thereby rendering herself incapable of harming the nurse.

PROJECTION IN SCHIZOPHRENIA

A symptomatic hallmark of schizophrenia is the appearance of hallucinations and delusions. Again an analogy can be made to the young infant in whom, it is conjectured, hallucinations occur with regularity. It is believed that early signals of hunger in the infant create a tension which is reduced by the infant's reactivation of a memory image of the breast (or bottle, as the case may be). The schizophrenic patient, profoundly regressed, narcissistic like the infant and highly vulnerable to psychic assault, gratifies many of his needs by projecting them and the wish for their gratification outside himself. The results are hallucinations and delusions. Though the immediate productions may sound highly nonsensical or devastatingly frightening to the observer, *if that person can contain his own anxiety so that detailed observations are possible,* it will usually be learned that the projected thoughts, that is, the hallucinations and delusions, are stimulated by the patient's present experiences. They are generally related to his immediate needs and the persons in the environment who can gratify those needs. Often the stimuli for hallucinations are the activities and emotional responses of those with whom the patient has a close relationship.

The presence of delusions that are basically persecutory or grandiose characterizes another type of schizophrenia called the paranoid type. The typical paranoid patient is suspicious, guarded and reserved. Sometimes he is markedly hostile and acts aggressively. The paranoid patient typically does not manifest his illness until middle age. He is a person who is usually intelligent, and in those areas of his life where delusional thinking does not predominate, he is able to conduct himself appropriately.

Mr. R., a chronically ill paranoid schizophrenic, who had been hospitalized for 15 years was heard talking to a newly admitted boy. "You will have to learn to stay out of that rocking chair because it belongs to me. I am Jesus Christ, son of our Lord, agent of the Pope. I am at a loss to eliminate those transgressions upon the working. . . ." Though this message was garbled, Mr. R. clearly wished to have the rocking chair for his exclusive use.

In the next example, we see a persecutory delusion in an acutely ill man in a general hospital. The onset of this patient's illness was sudden and the cause evident. In this latter case, the prognosis is good.

> Mr. C. was a 56 year old house painter who had been admitted to the intensive care area after open heart surgery for mitral valve stenosis. He was comatose for three days postoperatively, though his condition was considered good. When he awoke, Mr. C. was told of the successful outcome of his operation. He did well until the 10th day postoperatively, when his temperature spiked and he was found to have some pneumonia in the right lower lobe. The patient was put on a hypothermia blanket and given other supportive care. On the evening of the 11th day the patient (who had a tracheostomy) wrote a note to the nurse telling her that "they" had been there talking about him and that "they" were plotting to harm him. The nurses were unable to persuade Mr. C. that his thoughts were erroneous.
>
> The liaison nurse in consultation with the intensive care staff was able to demonstrate that Mr. C. had been very frightened by the sudden turn for the worse in his condition. This, added to his understandable anxiety concerning the open heart surgery, plus his lack of sensory stimulation in the intensive care unit, compounded a great problem he could not deal with adequately. These conditions combined to cause a short but frank psychosis.
>
> In this state when he could not adequately distinguish his own body boundaries (the reader who has seen the post-operative open heart patient can more easily imagine this predicament because of the numerous tubes, catheters and gadgets that are attached to such a patient to monitor him), the patient easily misidentified visual

and auditory cues. He probably did see a group of doctors or nurses talking. They may even have been discussing Mr. C.; however, they were not plotting to harm him. This interpretation was delusional. It was probably fostered by a weak ego in a regressed, physically ill man, who perceived the hospital unit much as a child would. He could not control what was done to him and this set of circumstances nurtured the seeds of a delusion that harm would come to him. In the delusion itself was the wish to be the center of attention. Mr. C. had been terribly ill and he undoubtedly wanted to feel the care and concern of those around him. Unlike the schizophrenic patient, Mr. C. did not maintain his delusion over a long period of time. The nurses told him repeatedly where he was and who they were. They assured him that they were interested in his getting well and that, indeed, he *was* recovering. By the 15th day, Mr. C. was oriented once more and was able to talk clearly about his "funny thought."

AUTISM IN SCHIZOPHRENIA

The severely ill schizophrenic may be autistic. This means that he is intensely occupied in studying and responding to elements within himself. Autistic behavior involves the patient's attention being directed to his own feelings, his fears and his delusions, and to those factors in his environment that he can manipulate in order to gratify his needs, thereby stopping his pain temporarily. The autistic patient does not respond readily to those around him. He is extremely preoccupied with his inner world, the people who populate it, and the language he invents for his created people. One can understand how the schizophrenic has come to be thought of as infantile and highly narcissistic.

PORTRAIT OF THE SCHIZOPHRENIC

The schizophrenic is seen as a person who has been severely traumatized at an early age. As a result, he has great difficulty distinguishing himself from the world around him. In order to protect his ego boundaries he has become a highly sensitive individual who is apt to misinterpret various stimuli. The more grossly ill schizophrenic utilizes several mechanisms to maintain whatever stability he has. Condensation, displacement, projection and regression are the mental mechanisms commonly associated with this disease process.

THE NURSING CARE OF THE SCHIZOPHRENIC PATIENT IN AN INSTITUTION

Acutely ill schizophrenics who are sufficiently symptomatic to be admitted to mental hospitals are there for one of two reasons or a combination of both. The patient in a state hospital is usually admitted because he has become so grossly disturbed that he cannot be contained in the community and family. The acutely ill schizophrenic found in a private hospital is there because those responsible for him and to him believe that the therapy available there is worth the monetary expenditure, that is, that psychotherapy will have a curative effect. Because treatment of the schizophrenic is usually prolonged, it is expensive in terms of time, money and human endeavor.

The role of the psychiatric nurse in the state hospital differs from that of her colleague in a private institution. Both nurses are dealing with a very sick person who is severely handicapped. In the private hospital, however, therapy is generally provided by a psychiatrist. In both settings the nurse's first responsibility is for the patient's physical well-being. When this primary concern has been dealt with, that is, when nursing care reflects effective observation of physical needs and facilitation of intervention, then the nurse is ready to integrate into her total approach her plans to meet the patient's psychological needs.

PHYSICAL NEEDS OF THE SCHIZOPHRENIC PATIENT

The patient sometimes has no desire, or perhaps freedom, to care for his own alimentation, elimination and personal hygiene. Therefore, the nurse must be an accurate observer and an organizer who can plan and provide for these necessities.

The nurse must identify the required behaviors, be they bathing, eating or sleeping. She will then communicate her thoughts to the patient. If the patient is able to comply, there is no problem. If the patient is unable to accommodate because of delusions, imagined power struggle or physical incapacity, the nurse must be prepared to be firm. Patients who cannot care for themselves are afraid, but when they see that others are strong and firm and able to care for them, they tend to be less frightened.

Eating

Eating can be a very real problem. Intake of nourishment is necessary for survival. It is not typical of the schizophrenic to stop eating in the hope of causing his own death, but he may not eat for fear of being poisoned. One can interpret such a delusion in many ways. The patient may feel that some particular person is persecuting him, or that a large group are trying to harm him. Such an idea may indicate the patient's need for a sense of importance. On the other hand, the patient may be partially correct in his interpretation of certain cues that have informed him that someone is trying to destroy him; likely, it was a significant person in his past who was unable to survive psychologically if the patient did develop and become independent. On the other hand, such a delusion may be a projection of the patient's own murderous fantasies.

There can be many interpretations for the patient's not eating. The nurse's initial concern, no matter what the interpretation, is to provide necessary nourishment to keep the patient alive. Some workers have found it of value to eat with the patient. At times this is enough to convince him that he will not be harmed. Occasionally if the nurse tastes the food before giving it to her patient, this will alleviate his fears. For a few patients, tube feeding may be necessary. When this procedure is required, it is useful to have the tube passed by a third party, such as the administrative resident on the ward, who is not directly involved with the patient's psychotherapy. This is done in order to prevent the patient's feeling that he is being assaulted by "his" doctor. The actual feeding may be administered by the nurse or the therapist. Whoever gives it should try to communicate that the procedure is done in order to sustain life, rather than as an assault. Tube feeding is actually an encroachment. The patient is literally having two foreign substances (tube and food) pushed into the confines of his body. For a patient who desperately fears engulfment and being taken over, this procedure is very traumatizing; however, when alimentation is at stake, just as when other issues of physical versus psychological well-being are considered, the physical problem takes priority.

Personal Hygiene

Personal hygiene can often provide another arena for pitched battle. On the surface it appears that the patient is simply obstinate and wishes to remain dirty; however, this is usually not the case. All behavior is meaningful, although similar behavior may have different meanings for different patients; one cannot readily generalize. It can be said, though, that schizophrenic patients who will not care for themselves have elaborate delusions regarding bathing and/or the equipment used for that purpose. Sometimes patients report, when they have improved, that while quite psychotic they thought bathing was dangerous, that it would remove some of their psychic abilities. Many of the delusional blocks to personal hygiene involve the individual's bodily integrity and the possibility of encroachment on it. Again, if it becomes necessary, bathing must be accomplished forcibly.

Explanations need to be honest; they must be simple and firm. No mentally ill patient should be told a lie; for the schizophrenic, such a maneuver is particularly poor practice because this individual is so uncannily able to sense the real nature of the environment around him. After all, he is practiced at picking up preconscious signals, for this has been his defense against the assaults of significant people in his childhood. He has leaned heavily upon this skill to protect him all his life. Untruths are not only morally and ethically bad, but they reinforce the schizophrenic's illness, which, in effect, dictates that he not listen to the real, functioning ego that tells him what is occurring around and to him. Thus, when the patient correctly identifies the nature of a situation, and the "healthy" people around him say in effect, "What you feel is not so, but this is the case," it reinforces those early lessons which represent the illness for which he is now hospitalized. The situation reinforces the notion that the patient's sense of "I" is erroneous; what he feels is not so, and in order to be rid of his "I," he must simply switch it out or stop recognizing its presence. Obviously this is antithetical to the whole plan of psychotherapy.

Janice, a 40 year old former high school librarian, had been severely disturbed for several years. She created many problems on the ward because of her impulsive and disruptive behavior. Each day when it was time for baths, she became assaultive, screamed obscenities and made it impossible for bathing to be accomplished without the aid of several attendants.

While Janice and an attendant were walking through the fields one day, the attendant, who was particularly interested in this patient, asked her why she behaved this way each morning. Janice replied that "they" were trying to electrocute her. She knew the murderers would finally "zap" her if she were not vigilant.

The attendant thought about Janice's reply and she reviewed the patient's record in an effort to decode the message. It was noted that Janice had had electroconvulsive therapy (ECT) eight months previously.* In that particular institution, ECT was administered early in the morning and baths were given prior to it. The attendant felt sure that Janice had generalized from the schedule surrounding the shock therapy to the bathing program in her present unit. The attendant discussed her hunch with the head nurse. They agreed that the patient should be asked to validate their interpretation of her behavior. The attendant took Janice for a walk outside of the ward. "I am glad we could go for another walk, Janice. I've been thinking of what you told me last time about your fear of being electrocuted. You had mentioned that if you were not vigilant, you would be 'zapped' by the murderers."

Janice grinned and looked embarrassed. She made a motion to cover her ears with her hands.

"Let me talk to you. I listened to your words. Listen to mine too. They won't harm you. They're only words. I think that you expect to have electroshock therapy every time you have a bath. I guess I'd fight too if I expected that to happen to me whenever I got clean. We aren't going to spring any treatments on you, though. I shall help you to wash if you like and no one else will be there. I simply want you to get clean. It doesn't feel good to be sticky and smelly."

Janice looked at the attendant. Her face appeared thoughtful and calm.

---

* See Chapter 11 for a discussion of ECT and other somatic treatments.

The next morning the same attendant approached Janice and told her matter of factly that it was time to get clean. She promised that after the bath the two could go for a walk outside. Janice undressed quietly. Her hands shook with a fine tremor, but she did not falter. The attendant helped her to bathe and then to dress and took her outside. The ward staff watched in amazement as Janice reached for the attendant's hand as they walked out the door.

Physical care of patients is a necessity. It offers a unique opportunity for the psychiatric nurse to establish a relationship with the patient who is unable to trust another. The nurse, through her ministrations, demonstrates to the patient that she not only is concerned but that she actually *will take care of the patient.* Within the boundaries of the caring relationship there is realistic proof of the nurse's motives. The suspicious patient does not need complex delusions to understand the presence of this person. When the patient has been adequately cared for ("mothered"), the relationship can sometimes be stretched to envelop other kinds of motives and objectives. They will be explored further.

All schizophrenic patients live in a state of partial regression to early phases of their development, but they live simultaneously at the level of their chronological age. As one writer so aptly described it, the schizophrenic does "double bookkeeping"; he lives two sets of lives. The psychiatric nurse can choose the simpler route and give custodial care. If, however, she is interested in dynamic nursing and the progress of her patient, she is cognizant of the fluid state of her patient's ego. She adjusts her relationships with the patient accordingly. She may be supporting the intact segment of the patient's ego at one point and yet at another be giving the same patient great amounts of blatant mothering and love in an effort to reach that other segment of the patient which is severely regressed. The work of Schwing[10] demonstrates the wisdom of such an approach. In the pages of that writer's book the reader sees unfolded the amazing push toward health made by grossly disturbed schizophrenics when they have the opportunity to interact on a regular basis with a kindly, warm and giving woman over a long period of time.

The reader has hopefully developed a mental picture of the schizophrenic as an individual who may be either immobilized and physically unable to respond or so mobile that he cannot accommodate to the demands of the environment. Such an individual must have assistance in accomplishing the simple tasks of daily living.

The first focus of the nurse, then, is toward nurturing, i.e., feeding, grooming, touching and holding, companionship, reassurance and, when necessary, control. Through these functions the patient comes to understand that the nurse's motives are mothering and caring. Beyond these activities the nurse can evolve other therapeutic activities with the schizophrenic patient. Major among these should be working together to understand one another's communications.

This is a terribly difficult task for one who has been trained to perceive messages in a particular manner, as has the schizophrenic. However, if the nurse has been experienced by the patient as a *real* person, as one who can be trusted and relied upon, then the more formidable task can be successfully undertaken.

PSYCHOLOGICAL NEEDS OF THE SCHIZOPHRENIC

The psychiatric nurse who undertakes the task of gratifying the schizophrenic patient's needs must be willing to set aside a period of time on a regular basis to be with her patient. Once this time interval is decided upon, the nurse *must* make good her word. At first she offers just her presence, expecting nothing in return. It is foolhardy in working with a schizophrenic to set short-term goals that will involve long-term changes. Thus, the nurse who expects her catatonic patient to greet her by name by the end of the first week of interviewing may become frustrated and angry when the deadline draws near. Schizophrenics are like dieters; they will not accept the goals of the therapist unless they, too, have committed themselves. Just as the fat person must want desperately to lose weight before he is willing to give up his calories, so the schizophrenic will not relinquish any of his symptoms until he is convinced that his pain will lessen by his doing so. To talk, to recognize and to correctly identify means the possibility of rejection or disclosure. No schizophrenic will take this chance until he feels safe with his therapist. Thus, the nurse may have to spend many hours demonstrating her capacity for kindness and sincerity.

One's kindness, her capacity to help and her sincerity can be translated through tolerance of inappropriate behavior, acceptance of violent affect, reliability and consistence, and through the demonstration of empathic understanding. At times the patient will actually *need* to withdraw. The sensitive nurse will allow this to happen; she will permit the schizophrenic patient to set the pace of the relationship.

> Bobbie Y., an 18 year old high school student, had been committed to the hospital at the age of 16. He was observed at that time to spend many hours in his room. Prior to admission his parents and sister were unable to draw him into conversation. One evening his sister found Bobbie in the cellar watching blood spurt from his arm. The boy kneeled before a laundry tub with his slashed limb hung over the wringer. His sister ran to him screaming, "Bobbie, what have you done?"
>
> The boy watched her. His lips turned up in a wistful smile. "God commanded me. He said, 'Let there be blood in My name.' I know he wanted me to kill Dad, but I thought I'd try this first." The girl screamed, "Oh no," and ran, horrified, from the bloody scene. The panic-stricken family called the family doctor and soon

Bobbie, sutured and bandaged, was dispatched to the psychiatric hospital.

Bobbie's first two years of hospitalization were marked by severely disordered behavior. He was grossly delusional and had to be watched constantly for suicidal attempts. The boy did not respond to shock therapy. Formal psychotherapy was also without appreciable benefit.

At the beginning of Bobbie's third year of hospitalization, a clinical specialist was assigned to the building where he resided. She took an interest in the lanky young boy who stood each day by a metal plaque which reflected his image. She observed him as he touched its cold surface with gently questioning fingers. The nurse read Bobbie's history, obtained the ward administrator's approval, and then approached the youth to tell him of her interest in helping him. "Bobbie," she said one morning, "I am Miss Van Allen, a nurse. I should like to come talk to you every day at this time. I hope that you and I can look at some of your problems together and find some answers to the questions that trouble you."

"My name is Mr. Clark and Dr. Lowell. You are Dr. Allen. You can open the gate for me."

"No, Bobbie. Only your doctor can do that, but you and I can work together to make you well enough so that you can be discharged."

"I am the devil."

"You must think you are very bad," said Miss Van Allen, "but I doubt that you are. I should like to see you tomorrow, at this time. Perhaps we can talk more about your feelings of being bad."

"I am God."

"I don't understand, Bobbie. You just told me you are the devil. Now you tell me that you are God. Can it be that you are letting me know that you are both good and bad? If that is so, Bobbie, you are describing me, too, and most other people. We all act good and bad. We all have good thoughts and ones that we fear are bad. I do have to go now. We shall talk again tomorrow."

The nurse has approached Bobbie for their initial contact. She has explained her identity and her business as simply as possible. The patient, in return, has tried to describe something of himself. Miss Van Allen listened and tried to interpret his message.

The following day when Miss Van Allen came to the ward, she found Bobbie on his bed masturbating. She stood by the bed momentarily but the boy gave no sign of recognition. "I am here, Bobbie. I am going to sit in the chair near your bed for the half hour we have together this morning."

The boy stopped masturbating but did not look at Miss Van Allen or indicate that he had heard her. At the end of the appointed time the nurse indicated that she was leaving but would return the next day.

Miss Van Allen returned for six days at the planned hour. Bobbie no longer masturbated, but he did remain mute. Periodically he stole glances at the nurse, indicating nonverbally that he was aware of her presence. The nurse did not break the silences often, knowing that they are of value and do not represent vacuums.

She tried to concentrate on her patient and to understand the meaning of the long periods of quiet. Several times she indicated that it must be frightening to divulge one's innermost feelings to another person. Aside from this statement, greetings and goodbys, she did not offer conversation. On the seventh visit Bobbie touched her arm as Miss Van Allen unlocked the door to the ward. "Jesus Christ spoke to Dr. Clarke. He said that you would come back. He knew that they couldn't frighten you with the growling white wolves." Bobbie looked directly at the nurse. Though his body seemed stiff and unrelaxed, the boy's eyes reflected a pleading expression.

"No, Bobbie. I wasn't frightened. I would not desert you. Remember, I told you I would be here every day with you. Did you think your thoughts were really going to frighten me away?"

This exchange marked the beginning of a long and fruitful relationship for nurse and patient. There were many weeks of highly symbolic communication interspersed with short periods of silence. The nurse continued to build the relationship, however, using the boy's words as indications of his feelings. She often had to listen for several hours to begin to piece together the threads of a feeling theme, and then it was necessary to ask Bobbie if the proposed meaning was correct. Sometimes it was; at other times he indicated that she had misunderstood. Basically the nurse tried to put herself in the position of being a bridge to reality, to relations with others. She indicated her acceptance of Bobbie as a person with strong, though often ambivalent, feelings. She told him time and time again that his "bad" feelings were not bad at all, but merely human. She reminded him that all people have such feelings.

When his communications seemed obscure, Miss Van Allen told him so. She indicated her desire to understand him. Occasionally when she felt that a seemingly obscure message was becoming more clear, she would ask him for validation. Eventually, when Bobbie welcomed her visits and was able to tell her so, the nurse asked Bobbie if he could not perhaps say out loud what he wanted and what he feared and disliked. At this phase of their work together, the patient was ready to form other relationships with more staff on the unit and so his social circle was enlarged.

The story of Bobbie had a happy ending. He made good progress and was assigned to psychotherapy with one of the residents. At this time the ward nurses formulated nursing care plans for him in conjunction with his therapy. Supportive therapy of the schizophrenic in treatment is more characteristic of the nurse employed in a private treatment facility. Considerations in formulating such plans are several.

Short-term Goals

It is helpful for the nursing staff to arrange goals for the patient in terms of short-term, intermediate and long-range. Short-term goals are those objectives which can be accomplished in the shortest time interval, and usually they must be done before the patient can move on through other types of behaviors. In the case of Bobbie, a short-term goal was for the patient to permit himself to be in contact with the nurse. He was so anxious on the second contact that he masturbated. However, as the nurse returned repeatedly and was not daunted by his behavior, the patient began to tolerate her presence better.

Intermediate Goals

An intermediate goal might be for the patient to express his feelings in whatever mode he felt able. This objective could not be reached before the patient could tolerate the person whom he would learn to trust sufficiently to share his painful, and often unacceptable (to him), thoughts. This goal would involve behaviors on the part of the nurse that would permit the patient to draw closer to her. Included in these would be the actual physical caring for the patient in such a way as to be a mother substitute. Permitting the patient to use the nurse as a substitute object for his hostility is another nursing behavior which is appropriate in this phase of the work.

Long-term Goals

A long-term goal for the patient would be his becoming able to communicate in less highly symbolic language, so that his meanings could be more clearly understood by those with whom he communicated. To reach this objective the patient would need to trust another and to communicate often and fully enough that the other person could become familiar with his symbolic representations and characteristic modes of thought.

Another long-term goal would be to assist the patient to identify the types of living situations that had caused him great anxiety and to help him to learn to reduce his own tension before his ego began to shatter under the impact of the forces impinging on him. This goal, of course, could not be accomplished before the short-term and intermediate ones were completed.

RELATING TO THE SCHIZOPHRENIC THROUGH ACTIVITIES

Nursing care plans should include activities that bring the patient into contact with staff in a manner that fosters the patient's self-confidence. The activities should be so designed that they assist the patient in evolving and maintaining an identity.

As was said earlier, schizophrenic individuals are very regressed people; they tend to be highly narcissistic. Bleuler characterized this type of patient as *autistic, apathetic, ambivalent,* and *associatively loose.*

The worker who stops to consider the kind of human being who manifests these characteristics realizes that the schizophrenic is a person who is extremely self-centered, unlikely to be able to reach out to those around him, afraid to try for outside contact, and easily in flux. This is indeed the case. The individual who is diagnosed as schizophrenic finds it difficult to the point of impossibility to reach out to someone to say, "I want help," and to commit himself to whatever aid is available. In structuring a plan of activities for such an individual, the nurse can provide many opportunities for reaching out to another, opportunities for the patient to experience the warmth and gratification of receiving and, finally, the opportunity for the patient to help himself and have a sense of accomplishment in independent endeavor. The latter, however, is a long-term goal and should be preceded by an extensive experience in receiving.

For the severely regressed patient, verbal communication is difficult and much that is communicated must be done on a nonverbal basis. The nurse, through such activities as feeding, clothing and bathing, shows in a maternal type of situation her caring, concern and warmth. Though being touched is for some schizophrenic patients a completely unbearable experience, for others it communicates many of the messages of caring that are necessarily translated into nonverbal terms. Another useful avenue is found in the feeding process. Like the young child whom the schizophrenic so profoundly resembles, the patient is oftentimes gratified by sweet things. Some workers have achieved success by frequently visiting their secluded or voluntarily isolated patients with a small gift of sweets, e.g., a piece of candy or a cup cake. It is conjectured that such an act signifies to the schizophrenic the bringing of affection and goodness. One cannot simply bring the sweet and perfunctorily offer it; rather it is presented as a gift from the caring nurse to her patient whom she sincerely desires to feed and care for.

> Mr. T., a 61 year old man, was transferred from the state mental hospital to the surgical service of a general hospital for cholecystectomy. The surgical nurses requested consultation with the liaison service. Mr. T. was not particularly verbal prior to surgery, though he did indicate awareness of his surroundings and was cooperative. For several days postoperatively he responded normally, i.e., he responded when spoken to, coughed and turned as requested, and asked for the bedpan when it was needed.
>
> The liaison nurse was called on the fourth postoperative day. The patient would not respond; he refused to open his eyes and lay curled up in the fetal position. The staff nurses were concerned because the patient refused food and would not talk.
>
> It was decided by the liaison nurse in consultation with the staff nurses that one aide would be assigned to this man as much as possible. She would make no demands upon him, but would make his bed with him in it, offer the urinal on a regular basis, and provide the patient with a liquid diet, i.e., soups, juices and milk, that he could drink through a straw.

At first there was no sign of behavioral change in the patient; however, after two days of constant care from the aide, Mr. T. was observed to peek around at the other patients in the ward. He sucked when a straw was placed in his mouth. The aide began to encourage him, but she did not make demands. After several more days Mr. T. kept his eyes open, except when addressed directly by other members of the staff. He took his diet well and, when switched to a regular diet, fed himself. It was the impression of the ward staff that Mr. T. reacted most directly when the aide offered him nourishment through the straw.

In a more typical case, the writer worked directly with a young schizophrenic girl for several months. The patient, a 16 year old, was diagnosed as catatonic. She was mute and kept taking off her clothes. As a result, she was secluded in a room by herself. Each day the nurse would visit with her for a half hour. When the nurse happened to mention candy one day, the patient indicated interest. The following day the nurse brought two pieces, one for herself and one for the patient. This provided a beginning, and each day thereafter the patient looked for the candy. It provided a link between the two. When the patient first communicated, it was in an effort to thank the nurse for the sweet.

Food can become a vehicle for communication. In these early experiences with the nurse, the patient learns that the nurse is more similar to himself rather than to the dangerous, rejecting or indifferent people of his past. He perceives that she comes because she cares about him. At times she also extends from herself small tidbits, such as candy, which are an extension of her sweet and affectionate feelings for him. Both Schwing[10] and Sechehaye[12] have reported successes with such approaches.

When the schizophrenic patient is able to tolerate the nurse and can receive her visits without undue stress, more complex activities can be added to the program. It is likely that the patient who depends on the consistent and caring approach of his nurse will attempt to imitate (identify with) her in some ways. Like the young child, his ego is weak and he is searching for his own identity. In the early stages of his treatment, as he allows himself to give up those identities which he has created out of his symptoms, he will attempt to find characteristics for himself which are more ego syntonic, i.e., more appropriate to his real being. Because he depends on his nurse and accepts her, he is likely to assume various characteristics of the nurse. These primary identifications should be met with warmth and approval.

Sue followed her nurse around the ward much of the day. She often asked those who passed her, "What's my name? Who am I?" Her expression was one of a baffled lost soul. One morning the nurse left her cap on the desk in the office. Sue took it and placed it on her own head. She told those who saw her, "See, I am Mrs. Roberts." The nurse assured her that she was Sue, but that she was very much liked by Mrs. Roberts and that she could do some of the same things that the nurse did if she wished to help. Sue agreed and was given the task of helping Mrs. Roberts put away the ward supplies. The patient, who had previously paced the hall or gazed into space most of the day, took part in the activity until it was completed. She looked quite pleased, and each member of the ward staff went out of her way to praise Sue for her effort and to thank her. Sue began to assist the nurses each morning. She would not work alone at an assigned task, but when the nurse worked alongside of her, she continued the job until its completion. After several weeks of "joint" effort, the patient was able to concentrate on an assigned task and to complete it without the nurse's assistance.

When the patient is able to try activities that do not center on the presence or support of his nurse, social activities can be instituted that permit the patient self-expression. Activities involving the creative arts are particularly suited to this purpose. Such things as painting, clay modeling and activities utilizing music permit the schizophrenic an opportunity to express his feelings openly and with great freedom. Dance therapy, a relatively new area of treatment, is highly regarded.

As the patient becomes more reliable in his responses and "public behaviors," his nurse can plan with him for trips outside the hospital grounds. Shopping expeditions, movies, walks, and so forth, help to break up the monotony of institutional life. Planning for an expedition outside the hospital walls is useful in several respects. Not only does it offer diversion, but also a realistic opportunity to make plans and to implement them. This, of course, is a way of utilizing ego functioning. When the plans are implemented the planner has a chance to see that what he has organized comes to fruition. Such a procedure helps the individual to see that he can manipulate his environment and that it will respond in a predictable way. For the person whose life has been ordered by others for any length of time, as happens in a mental hospital, this is a good experience. Finally, such outings are useful because they act as reinforcers of behaviors that the schizophrenic must accept. For instance, the patient who hallucinates frequently and either talks with the hallucinated phenomena, or postures and gestures, will not be tolerated long in the civilian community. The patient will have to come to terms with the possibility of ostracism. If outings are rewarding to the patient, and the opportunity for them hinges on acceptable behaviors, then the patient is more likely to give up the unacceptable behavior. This is roughly what conditioning is about. The desired behavior is identified; the patient is rewarded or reinforced when he performs acceptably.

Tim asked the ward administrator if he could go to town when the ward meeting was over. The doctor asked the patient group if they thought Tim should go. Denise stood up and said angrily: "You can't go out today, Tim. You stood at the window all morning playing with yourself and talking to nothing. The people in town are going to think we're all crazy if you go in the stores acting like that."

Several other patients looked as if they wanted to speak. The doctor called on Bob. "Well, I think he should be allowed to go. If he wants to go badly enough, he'll have to act like he's well enough to go."

The head nurse said: "I think Tim should stay on the ward today because he seems anxious. I think perhaps Tim would not have good control over his feelings today; however, we could plan on permitting him to go out tomorrow, if he feels that he can handle it."

The doctor asked the group what they thought. All agreed that the nurse's plan was a good one.

The nurse who works in a state mental hospital has far fewer opportunities to plan and to implement therapeutic programs for her patients than does her colleague employed in a private setting. The latter, because of better facilities and additional staff, can realistically plan to spend more of her time with one patient. For the state hospital employee, realistic nursing plans will usually focus on group work. Discussion of such programs will be explored in the chapter on problems of the mental hospital.

THE NURSING CARE OF SCHIZOPHRENIC INDIVIDUALS IN THE COMMUNITY

As has been discussed previously, physical care for patients in the community is not the problem that it presents in those patients who are sick enough to be institutionalized. Instead, the psychiatric nurse caring for patients living in the community has the opportunity to concentrate on the psychological aspects of the nurse-patient relationship. In the case of the schizophrenic, the nurse needs to focus first on establishing the relationship. In this particular situation she will have to demonstrate to the patient that she is *worth* the patient's risking his psychic safety. That is, the patient must accept that this new individual will not harm him by rejecting or engulfing him. Much as in working with the hospitalized patient, the nurse will have to structure her dealings with the ambulatory patient in such a way that he has great psychological freedom. He needs to know that he can come and go as he deems appropriate and that the nurse will not falter; that is, the patient can set the pace. If he needs to retreat temporarily, the nurse will not chase after him but will remain predictably in her appointed place awaiting his return when he feels able. Beside the physical element, the patient must discover that he can say what he thinks and feels without fear of recrimination or rejection. When these basic tenets are understood by the patient, the relationship can bear the weight of closer involvement.

At such time as the schizophrenic has learned to trust the nurse, he has also identified her as a unique individual unlike the persons in his past who have harmed him. He has been able to recognize another human being who has characteristics different from those he normally attributes to those with whom he has contact. This is not a small lesson for the schizophrenic to learn! Now he is ready to examine some of the causes of his anxiety that becomes so severe he must decompensate. This is not easy, but it is the only opportunity that the patient has to protect himself from future psychosis. Thus, inquiry and exploration are required. This work is best done at such a pace and in such a way that the patient's anxiety is not significantly raised during the investigatory effort. There are ways and means to maintain a loosely relaxed environment. The places where the work is carried on and the activities that are done concurrently act as relaxers. Thus, a young mother who is being interviewed might work more comfortably if nurse and patient talk over the breakfast table and have a cup of coffee. The adolescent is likely to enjoy conversation at a neighborhood drug store or while walking in a nearby park. An elderly person would feel refreshed by sitting outside on the porch or in the backyard. Aside from the advantage of helping to keep the patient relaxed because he is in his normal "nonsick" environment, such a setting also helps to reinforce the nurse's identity as a unique individual. She is less easily stereotyped in an informal setting.

The nurse and patient can then begin to understand the patient's daily living problems at a slow, cautious pace, always refocusing in various ways on the realities of the present relationship between the two. The nurse may choose to see her patient twice a month. This decision will depend on the patient's availability and the nurse's caseload. Twice a month is considered a realistic schedule, however, because it permits for relatively close scrutiny (allowing the nurse to observe the threat of decompensation before it actually occurs) and it also lets the patient have infrequent enough sessions that he can feel independent and take advantage of the maximum amount of freedom. With such a basic program, appointments can be increased if the patient becomes more frightened, delusional or anxious. Appointments can be decreased if the patient requests it or he seems to be managing his life in an efficient and gratifying manner. (The patient who is being followed by an aftercare agency attached to a hospital should be seen at least monthly if he is on psychotropic drugs.)

In bimonthly interviews it is wise to permit the patient to lead the discussion, bringing up whatever topics he chooses; but the nurse should also listen for hints of his feelings concerning the matters he describes. If she hears that his feelings about the topic are unclear or negative, or if he seems anxious, the nurse should ask about this, suggesting that this is the message she is hearing. The patient then has the option to deny it, indicating his inability to deal with the feelings at that point (unless, of course, the nurse has been wrong in her perception), or he can begin to explore the situation, looking for validity in the nurse's observation or reasons for his feelings.

Martha, the 42 year old housewife and factory worker described earlier, was seen by her mental health counselor every two weeks. After Martha struck her supervisor, she was fired. The situation was very frightening to Martha, and she came directly back to the mental health center. It was decided to admit her, probably on an overnight basis, to the center's residential unit in the University Hospital psychiatric section. It was arranged that Martha's counselor would visit her that evening. When she arrived, Martha, with tear-stained face, was waiting for her by the door. "I don't know what happened. She was talking and I hit her. I just don't know what came over me."

The counselor said, "Hello, Martha. I'm sorry to have to be seeing you here. Are you very upset?"

"I'm afraid. I don't know what has happened. They're taking over my mind again."

"No," interrupted the woman's counselor, "no one is taking over your mind, Martha. You and I know now that the 'they' are your thoughts that you don't like. They are part of you, though. You are like me and like other human beings. We have thoughts we like and thoughts we don't like. But there is no 'they' controlling you. Only *you* control you." The mental health counselor smiled. "Come on, and try to tell me what happened to you today. Let's go sit down in the corner over there." The two women approached an overstuffed couch and sat down.

Martha turned to the counselor and said, slowly, "I remember leaving you earlier today and returning to the factory. The supervisor came in and told me to have a report for her in two weeks. Then I hit her."

"You must have been quite frightened, or perhaps very angry, to make it necessary to hit her."

"I guess so," said Martha, with a puzzled look on her face. "I can't imagine why, though. She's been awfully nice to me."

"Had anything happened on the way back to your job after you left me?"

"No, . . . I don't think so. I had to wait for a long time for the bus. There was an old lady standing on the corner with me. I sort of felt like kicking her."

"You must have been angry while you waited for the bus."

Martha grinned, "Sounds that way, doesn't it?"

"What do you suppose made you feel this way toward the lady at the bus stop and later toward your supervisor?"

"I don't know. You are so nice to me I hate to be any trouble."

The mental health counselor listened to this seeming non sequitur in the conversation. "Martha, could it be that I was not very nice to you today? Is it possible that you have been very angry at me?"

Martha looked anxiously about her. She arose abruptly saying in a cold voice, her eyes looking straight ahead of her, "Excuse me. I have to go to the bathroom."

"I'll wait here for you, Martha."

The patient left the room. While she was away, the counselor tried to reconstruct the interview in order to understand what had occurred. Martha had been waiting at the door. She appeared anxious and apologetic. She had recognized her counselor, however, so her contact with reality had been rather good. (The anxiety that had provoked her act, or was a consequence of it, had not been great enough to shatter her ego functioning.) Martha had then blurted out that "they" were taking over her mind again. At this point the counselor had stopped her and pointed out the meaning of "they." She had said this because Martha had seemed in good contact and the counselor thought that, because of this and the trust established in their relationship, Martha could tolerate the correction. Indeed she had. The counselor reinforced her statement by saying that Martha was like herself and other human beings. She had feelings that she liked and others that she did not like. At this point the counselor invited Martha to look with her at the events that led up to the patient's admission to the unit.

The conversation had established that Martha had indeed felt strongly about *something* at the time that she left her afternoon appointment with her counselor. The latter then asked if this was true, suggesting that Martha's anger may have been originally directed at her. Martha seemed to respond with a non sequitur, saying that the counselor was so nice. The latter listened to the statement and it seemed to her that it was not a non sequitur at all but a direct response to the counselor's question. Perhaps Martha was unable to admit her true feelings and had instead labeled these feelings as her thoughts of gratitude. The counselor felt that Martha was really quite angry at her and was unable to tell her. She realized that she was, in effect, a symbol or representative of other people in Martha's past who had treated the patient in a way that angered or hurt her. The counselor waited. She tried to be aware of her own feelings. She recognized her anxiety and identified the source as Martha's having left the room and, in effect, having left *her*. She knew that she could not follow the patient because the woman needed the psychological space to withdraw as necessary. The counselor waited.

After about 15 minutes had elapsed, Martha reappeared. She came into the room, stopping in front of the counselor. "You told me I could not come back every week."

The counselor did not immediately understand the statement. She tried to reconstruct the original situation. . . . Of course, it was their last meeting when she had suggested that Martha lengthen the time between their appointments to every two weeks. She tried to keep her expression as noncommittal as possible, permitting the patient to express more of her own feelings without receiving the nonverbal message that she was being patronized, rejected or unheard. The counselor said, "Martha, did you feel that I was sending you away from me when I suggested you come every two weeks instead of weekly?"

"You did, you did," the woman sobbed.

"I can understand your feelings then. No wonder you wanted to kick and hit. You thought I was sending you away and that I did not want you anymore. That is not what I meant, though.

What I wanted to tell you, and I guess I did it poorly, was that I thought you were doing very well and that you could begin to take more responsibility now. I wanted to tell you that you've been a good worker and have overcome many of your problems and I thought you did not need me as much as before. . . . I think very highly of you, Martha."

The patient had sat down on the couch. She perched near the edge as far from her counselor as she could. The counselor said nothing more. She looked at her patient trying to recognize some sign of Martha's acceptance or rejection of the message. There was none.

"Martha, I wonder if you are still angry at me. Do you suppose you could tell me when you feel strongly about something I have said or done? Could you learn to let me know instead of hitting other people? After all, it's me you feel this way about, not your supervisor or the lady who waits with you for the bus."

"It is very hard," said the patient. "I feel stiff like cardboard."

"It is always hard to do something new for the first few times. It is like breaking in a new, stiff pair of shoes, but the shoes may turn out to be your most comfortable pair after the stiffness is worked out of them."

Martha looked at her counselor and said, "Don't take my sanity from me."

"It's been a tough day for you. Let's let this rest for now. I shall be here tomorrow, and we can see if you feel well enough to leave here and we can talk to your doctor."

"Thanks," Martha said. She looked relieved as the counselor arose from the couch. Together they walked to the nurse's station where the counselor left Martha and went to write up her report for the ward staff and the psychiatrist to see.

The preceding interview has been reported to show how the counselor (who might have been a nurse) helped the patient to explore the reasons for her actions and feelings. At the same time the counselor tried to maintain the level of anxiety, i.e., not permit it to increase by pointing out the similarities of the two people's feelings. In addition, she allowed the patient to introduce material that she felt able to identify. When the patient became too anxious and needed to withdraw, the counselor did not follow. This permitted the patient to retreat to a safer position. When she was able to return, the counselor was there, indicating that she was not rejecting Martha and was not injured by Martha's feelings. As a result, the two individuals were able to explore together Martha's real feelings and the situation that had evoked them. In this way Martha was given an opportunity to develop a more effective way of expressing herself.

REFERENCES

1. Artiss, K. (ed.): The Symptom as a Communication in Schizophrenia. New York, Grune & Stratton, 1959.
2. Bateson, G.: Schizophrenic Distortions of Communication. *In* Whitaker, C. A.:

   Psychotherapy of Chronic Schizophrenia Patients. Boston, Little, Brown and Company, 1958.
3. Bateson, G.. Jackson, D., Haley, J., and Weakland, J.: Toward a Theory of Schizophrenia. *Behavioral Science,* 1:251, 1956.
4. Brody, E. B., and Redlich, F. C. (eds.): *Psychotherapy with Schizophrenics*. New York, International Universities Press, 1952.
5. Haley, J.: The Art of Being Schizophrenic, *Voices,* 1:133-147, 1965.
6. Jackson, D.: Comments in Whitaker, C. A.: *Psychotherapy of Chronic Schizophrenic Patients*. Boston, Little, Brown and Company, 1958.
7. Jackson, D. (ed.) : *The Etiology of Schizophrenia*. New York, Basic Books, Inc., 1960.
8. Laing, R. D.: *The Politics of Experience*. New York, Pantheon Books, Random House, Inc., 1967.
9. Lidz, T., Fleck, S., and Cornelius, A.: *Schizophrenia and the Family*. New York, International Universities Press, 1966.
10. Schwing, G.: *A Way to the Soul of the Mentally Ill*. Translated by Rudolf Ekstein and Bernard Hall. New York, International Universities Press, 1954.
11. Searles, H. J.: *Collected Papers on Schizophrenia*. New York; International Universities Press, 1965.
12. Sechehaye, M.: *Symbolic Realization*. New York, International Universities Press, 1951, p. 195.

SUGGESTED READING

Books

Dixson, B. K.: Intervening When the Patient Is Delusional. *J. Psychiatric Nursing and Mental Health Services,* 7 (No. 1):25-34, January-February, 1969.

This is a readable, lucid presentation that will aid the student as she explores nursing approaches to this difficult problem in the nursing care of the schizophrenic.

Flynn, G.: Hostility in a Mad, Mad, Mad World. *Perspectives in Psychiatric Care,* 7 (No. 4):152-158, 1969.
   Nursing Intervention in Hostile Behavior. *Ibid.*
   The Nurse's Role: Interference or Intervention? *Ibid.*

This article and the panel discussions which have been published in Perspectives in Psychiatric Care offer the reader a valuable experience in terms of understanding how psychiatric nurses view hostile behavior and the nursing approaches to it. The articles are all presented in the same issue and so are easily retrievable.

Fromm-Reichmann, F.: *Principles of Intensive Psychotherapy*. Chicago, University of Chicago Press, 1950.

Though the topic of this book is not immediately relevant for the nursing student, the text is still heartily recommended because it says so much that is true about the schizophrenic patient as a person. It also permits the reader a glance at Dr. Frieda Fromm-Reichmann, one of the eminent psychoanalysts and specialists in the treatment of the schizophrenics in the twentieth century. The book is small and very readable.

Greene, H.: *I Never Promised You a Rose Garden*. New York, Holt, Rinehart and Winston, 1964.

This autobiographical account of an adolescent schizophrenic's illness and her treatment at Chestnut Lodge by Frieda Fromm-Reichmann is a near classic that should not be missed by anyone. For the basic student the book gives a lucid first-hand account of how it really feels. For the reader with more historical interests, the book gives a marvelous opportunity to see the fantastic Reichmann at work. In and of itself, this book is good reading. It goes quickly and effortlessly, and the reader learns much about psychiatry without even trying!

Hill, L. B.: *Psychotherapeutic Intervention in Schizophrenia*. Chicago, University of Chicago Press, 1955.

Again, the stated topic is not pertinent to nursing students; however, the book is so interesting and so informative that it would be only insular to say that this is not for nurses because it is not nursing. Actually, this volume, like the Fromm-Reichmann, offers much that can be applied to nursing therapy.

Mellow, J.: The Experiential Order of Nursing Therapy in Acute Schizophrenia. *Perspectives in Psychiatric Care*, 6 (No. 6):249-255, 1968.

The article is difficult to absorb in its entirety; however, for the above-average student it provides an unparalleled opportunity for the reader to "see Dr. Mellow at work." Such an experience will be meaningful for the student who proposes to enter graduate study in psychiatric nursing. Dr. Mellow has created a role for the nurse therapist, and she has written widely about her work. The material is highly exciting and relevant to all nursing in psychiatry.

Parker, B.: *My Language Is Me*. New York, Basic Books, Inc., 1962.

Again, a book is presented which permits the reader to experience schizophrenia with a patient who, this time, is an adolescent male. The book is interesting, though the focus is ofttimes on communication in the schizophrenic process rather than other aspects. The boy who is portrayed is treated as an outpatient, in contradistinction to the main character in Greene's book.

Probst, M. E.: Helping the Schizophrenic Patient Enlarge his Perceptual Field. *Perspectives in Psychiatric Care*, 5 (No. 5):236-241, 1967.

A very interesting and readable account of one nurse's experience in treating a schizophrenic patient. The article affords a good review of the subject of perception as well.

Schwing, G.: *A Way to the Soul of the Mentally Ill*. New York, International Universities Press, 1954.

If the student has not explored the valuable pages of this book before, this should be done before the subject of schizophrenia is left. Nowhere is there a better described manner of treating the patient than by Schwing. Nowhere is her unique approach shared except in this volume. This is a small but timeless text that no serious nursing student of psychiatry can afford to miss.

Sechehaye, M.: *Autobiography of a Schizophrenic Girl*. New York, Grune & Stratton, Inc., 1951.

This classic is the story of a young girl who was severely ill. She was extremely regressed and unable to make contact. The therapist takes the patient into her own home. This book is particularly interesting for students interested in the analytic approach and in symbolism in schizophrenia.

Tappan, C. B.: A Program of Resocialization for a Long-term Regressed Schizophrenic Patient. *J. Psychiatric Nursing and Mental Health Services*, 6:334-335, November-December, 1968.

This brief account of the therapeutic activities planned for a chronic schizophrenic patient is concise and readable. It gives the student an opportunity to see what might be done with a patient for whom social recovery is more realistic and shows in-depth insight.

Ujhely, G.: Nursing Intervention with the Acutely Ill Psychiatric Patient. *Nursing Forum*, 8 (No. 3):311-325, 1969.

The author is an excellent writer and experienced nurse. She has provided the reader with a lucid, practical discussion.

chapter 9

PSYCHIATRIC NURSING IN A LARGE STATE INSTITUTION

Historically, state mental hospitals have been huge, outmoded plants which have sprawled across acres of countryside, isolated from the rush and anonymity of the urban population. They have been complexes of uniformly bleak buildings which housed one to two thousand patients, cared for by staffs of far smaller proportions. The patients could be broadly characterized as acutely ill or chronic.

Until the advent of community mental health centers, which brought with them the philosophy of hospitalizing the acutely ill only until their crises were over, such patients could look forward to a hospitalization of up to two years. They regarded the hospital as a haven which was of temporary nature. They were, however, oriented toward their eventual discharge. The larger group of patients were, and still are, those human beings whose symptoms have resolved into a way of life. They have adapted to the life style of "inmatehood" by committing themselves to the hospital as a social environment. Chronically ill patients, whose hospital lives may extend from five years to a lifetime, experience the hospital as a total institution which provides for all their needs. It gives them food, shelter, physical protection, clothing and medication, all wrapped up in a package of anonymity, hopelessness and monotony.

Today some of this picture is changing. Because of public interest generated by the news media, through funding from state and federal sources and implementation by the expanded utilization of human resources, the traditional image of the state mental hospital is changing. From the East Coast to the West, new innovative programs for the treatment and rehabilitation of the mentally ill have sprung up. The effects of smaller housing units with warm looking exteriors and interiors have been studied. Results show that interpersonal interaction was favorably affected. Locked wards have been opened as studies have demonstrated that patients would behave as they were expected to; thus, if the staff expected more integrated levels of behavior and they *treated* patients as responsible people, responsible behavior was maintained.

Creedmoor State Hospital, Long Island, New York, has established a multiple family therapy program which is reported to be effective in the treatment of schizophrenic patients. Here the patient and his family are exposed to other families containing a schizophrenic member. All present have an opportunity to better understand their own problems by observing them in each other. At Boston State Hospital many creative innovations have been inaugurated, among them the Home Treatment Service and the extended use of volunteers. Atascadero State Hospital, a maximum security facility in California, has instituted a comprehensive program of change.

The professional journals abound with enthusiastic reports of effective change and improvement in the care of the mentally ill. Germane to most of these reports is the decentralization of huge plants and the unitization of smaller divisions so that individuals and small groups of patients become more visible. This, in turn, creates the opportunity to develop treatment *plans* for *people* rather than a custodial *regimen* for the *masses*.

In many state hospitals, however, there is still much need for change. The hierarchies of these institutions represent small societies in which there is a strong caste system. Communications tend to go from the top downward, with no reverse flow. Poor communications result. The social caste systems of these hospitals are usually rigid. Though the institution exists for the patient, he is relegated to the bottom of the status structure. Those people who have the most contact with him and provide his daily care, the attendants, are the least educated and least motivated of the groups in the administration hierarchy.

The locus of power is in the attendant in the traditional state mental hospital. The attendants are the "key carriers." They are often people who have less than a high school education, and are actually "unskilled" laborers. Often they hold down two jobs simultaneously in a losing struggle to maintain families on inadequate wages. Such a life style is terribly taxing, and the attendant usually shows stress from it. Aside from his many realistic problems and inadequacies, however, the attendant has often experienced life situations similar to those of the patient, and this puts him in a position to understand and to be able to empathize with the individual under his care. The attendant who likes working with people and is able to communicate this is often able to do significant work with patients because of his ability to understand the dimensions of the problems as they are experienced by his charge. These workers are geographically closest to the patient. They have the most contact with him, both physical and psychological.

Those patients who admit themselves voluntarily or are committed by the court to the typical large state mental hospital come because they are very sick and cannot afford the dynamic therapies that would be available in private facilities. One does not find patients in such institutions who are mildly neurotic. Instead, the observer will find psychotically ill schizophrenics, acutely depressed individuals with suicidal ideation, sociopaths and drug addicts who have run afoul of the law, alcoholics who have come to the attention of the law or whose families simply cannot tolerate their behavior any longer, and those people who have chronic organic problems. In the latter group are found the elderly of the United States society who can no longer be responsible for themselves and whose families have died off or simply refuse to care for their aged and infirm members. (See Chapter 13.) The institutions to which these individuals are brought are often characterized by their vastness, emphasis on custodial care, mass handling of patients, institutional rigidities, apathetic tone, and the perpetuation of the hopelessness of the patient's outlook. These ills are caused by the institution's large size and the unfavorable staff-patient ratio.

The nurse who comes to work on an acute service in the traditional state mental hospital faces situations similar to her colleague working in the community agency setting. In addition, she must usually deal with the problem of large numbers of patients and an inadequate and untrained staff. For this nurse, her therapeutic objectives will be those already identified in previous chapters. Her manner of implementation, however, must of necessity follow along the lines of that set up for chronic services. The latter is the subject of this chapter.

THE CHRONIC SERVICE

The nurse who chooses or accepts employment as a staff nurse on a chronic service unit is not only rare, but courageous. She is probably an unusually bright and innovative nurse. The right person in the job has the potential to have a wonderful experience and, at the same time, to accomplish many things that will help to move patients from chronicity to discharge. Most fundamental are modifications in the actual physical structure of the ward. The nurse coming to her new unit will likely see a group of mute, messy people in the drab uniform of that particular hospital standing in corners or against walls, or sitting on benches staring unseeingly ahead of them. An occasional patient will be seen lying on the floor under a bench, or curled up in a corner. Ocasionally a patient speaks to an attendant; rarely do patients speak to each other. The chronic ward often has a musty smell which is composed of dampness, urine and feces. All in all, the appearance of the ward is most uninviting.

In her initial approach to such a setting, the nurse must observe carefully those who share the ward—patient and staff. She will give them the opportunity to observe her. During this initial period of "sizing up" and acceptance, the nurse communicates her willingness to listen and to absorb. State hospital wards are not used to leadership from registered nurses. Both patients and staff will need time to adjust. Patients will wonder if their comfortable existences are to be tampered with or even shattered. The attendants who have run the wards without the guidance of a registered nurse are likely to feel resentful.

Any staff members who have oriented their activities around controlling patient behavior, defining circumstances that require the punishment of patients and, generally, carrying on the ward routine with a minimum of effort, may be quite resistant to the hint of new and innovative ideas. It is more economic of time, in the long run, to make haste slowly. When the staff members are ready for change, it will be indicated by their beginning to question the nurse, to include her in discussions, and to elicit her opinions in flexible matters. When these cues are evidenced, it is appropriate to begin instituting changes on the ward. Before anything is done, however, the staff should be carefully oriented to the objectives and the means by which the goals will be obtained. Obviously a cooperative staff will be one that is sold on the practical nature of change. Thus, the nurse's work as a leader entails selling proposed projects.

ENVIRONMENTAL CHANGES

It is easiest and most practical to focus first on the physical characteristics of the ward. Since the area is typically unclean, drab and institutional looking, such a focus is justifiable. Also, it is inanimate, so that no one person or group will feel that they are being attacked. Lastly, ward improvements are reasonably easy to accomplish. They can be made quickly so that staff and patients will be aware of the pleasant aspects of change from the outset. One need only obtain administrative approval and then find the means to implement changes.

The rearrangement of furniture is easily accomplished. Where chairs stand side by side in long dismal lines, small conversational areas can be formed by breaking up the lines of chairs and setting some of them around tables, or simply pulling a few chairs around in semicircles. Such arrangements encourage eye contact between the people who are seated. This is a first step to breaking up isolation and autism.

If paint can be obtained, it is worthwhile to identify among the patients and staff members those who can help to paint the ward. Such a project cannot be started immediately but should be discussed in a ward meeting and planned by patients and staff together. The project is a realistic and practical vehicle for bringing patients and staff together in a common, visible effort. The outcome of the group effort is twofold: it enhances the "new look" of the ward, and it provides more pleasant surroundings. More subtly, it shows the patients that the staff are willing to work *with* them. The painting project indicates a new kind of role for the staff which deviates from their more traditional "key carrying" function. Further, it allows the sicker patients an obvious mode through which to identify with healthier people, i.e., everyone paints.

If administrative approval is forthcoming, travel posters or other bright colored pictures may be placed on the walls. Mirrors and calendars are also useful; beside their esthetic value, mirrors help patients to accept their identities, for they can actually *see* themselves. In some back wards, patients have not viewed their own faces in 10 to 20 years! It has been noted that patients who can see themselves over a long period of time tend to improve their personal hygiene.

Calendars are extremely useful in chronic wards because time has lost its meaning to the majority of patients. They act and react to a set of stimuli developed around a fixed routine, i.e., get up at 5:30 A.M., go to breakfast at 6:30, return to the ward and clean up until 8:00, and so forth. Few people think in terms of, "It is the 4th of July; today is Independence Day." The use of the calendar offers a subtle reminder of the ways of the outside world. This is particularly helpful for patients who will eventually be remotivated and rehabilitated. Such individuals must again become familiar with the world they have left behind.

Plants and small animals are wonderful morale boosters on the ward. Birds, fish or even rabbits provide something alive and different in the patient area. They offer a focal point around which patients can observe and discuss. Also, they provide a need for caretakers. Patients are used to being cared *for*. It is interesting and useful for them to find a real object for *their* caring, i.e., ministrations.

Another area in which patients can take part is by making rugs for the floor. If several patients can be motivated to make these in occupational therapy, the ward will look warmer and less institutional, and the patients can take pride in their contributions.

STAFF DEVELOPMENT

The typical staff provided to manage the wards are nonprofessional, relatively uneducated, underpaid and imbued with a tradition of custodial care. They are, like their patients, bored and isolated from other staff by virtue of their positions in the hierarchy. To bring about change through the attendants on the unit, change must first involve the attendants themselves.

The psychiatric nurse who embarks on such a course must first prepare her staff. Such work takes time—perhaps six months to a year. Initially the nurse must be on the ward. She wins her staff by working alongside of them, listening to them, being open to their communications. In the early stages she wins their trust by not instituting changes for which they are unprepared. Thus, she waits and acquaints herself with the mechanical operation of her unit. When the nurse feels fully acquainted with the ward's daily problems and the staff have accepted her, she is ready to proceed. Initiation of daily staff meetings provides an arena for the hearing of one another's ideas, criticisms and triumphs. It allows for an anticipated time, each day, when problems can be thrashed out. Most importantly, the staff can begin to feel mutual support and a sense of identity. The large state institution engulfs not only patients but staff as well. It is useful, therefore, to provide a situation in which the ward staff members can experience themselves as a small group with definite character and importance.

The nurse who acts as chairman of the group may schedule the time, initially, for the reporting of patient progress and plans for daily care. This, in itself, begins to break down the old traditional kind of expectations of custodial care because the leader is saying in her behavior that change in patients is expected. Individualized care which will be modified from day to day is going to be given. Such an approach is a vast departure from the past. When the group is able to make contributions in this area, then the nurse is ready to introduce the next change. She can begin to tell the attendants about the patients they discuss each day. To prepare for this, the nurse will have to go back to the patients' histories and find the reasons for hospitalization, the diagnosis, and the progress notes written. This will, again, be new and innovative, for charts are not often read in chronic areas. Behavior is observed and accepted or punished. There is little evidence that typical attendants know or are motivated to find out the "whys."

After the nurse has demonstrated the usefulness of knowing why behaviors occur, some of the attendants are likely to become more interested in their work. It would be foolhardy to promise that this simple maneuver will cause radical improvement in *all* members of the ward staff, but the change it will foster in *some* of the members makes it a worthwhile expenditure of time and energy. Those who can be interested in simple dynamics should be encouraged, for an informed staff will lead to a wiser, motivated staff who care. Just as in the nurse's student experience, the attendants should not be exposed to a lecture of dry, uninteresting facts and labels; rather, the nurse must familiarize herself with a patient's history and then tell her staff about the patient as a human being with problems in living. Labels, i.e., diagnoses, are only a form of shorthand. They serve to place the patient in a category for which the doctor can efficiently plan care. Labels do not take into account the uniqueness of the patient and his particular problems. When the staff have heard about patients for several weeks, in terms of the latter's human situations—similar to those of the attendants who care for them—changes will again be observed in the staff. They will be observed to be approaching patients in terms of their humanness, rather than in terms of their symptomatic behavior. When the nurse begins to hear her staff discussing patients as people, it indicates that the step has been a success. From this point on, it should be indicated to the staff that patients will be presented each day and discussed in terms of their progress, with possible further alterations in their treatment plans.

As staff members become able to talk about the patients they see as individuals, it is time to introduce the topic of written descriptions. This is often a traumatic event for those who either cannot write or are ashamed of the poor written communications they produce. Such feelings will come out in the group meeting, providing the nurse has created a climate of freedom and acceptance in which the staff can express their real feelings. The nurse chairman of the group needs to listen to the fears of her group members and then enlist their aid in planning how patient progress can be duly noted. It may be suggested that several of the staff be assigned to the charting each day, perhaps for a week at a time. If this is the solution, then the rest of the staff would report their findings for the day to those assigned. If it is the group consensus that each attendant will chart, then the group must be supported in their initial efforts.

It is assumed that the staff, at this point, are ready to talk meaningfully among themselves, to experience themselves and their patients as people who are working together for common good; the staff should feel satisfaction in their projects. The nurse may now discuss in the daily staff meetings the kind of observing and charting that will be useful. She needs to help the staff to understand the usefulness of descriptive writing. She might point out to them that the statement "Mrs. White had her usual day. She hallucinated in the corner" tells little of this patient's actual experience and gives few clues to the staff for their future work with Mrs. White. Instead, plans can be better formulated if the attendant notes under what circumstances Mrs. White began to hallucinate as well as what she did that led the observer to believe that she *was* hallucinating. Thus, a useful entry on the patient's daily report might say: "Mrs. White awoke when the lights were turned on this morning. She washed, ate and dressed without assistance. When some patients were taken off the ward for a walk, Mrs. White watched the door as they filed out and then she walked to a corner of the room where she gazed at the wall and her lips moved quietly."

From this description, it might be theorized that Mrs. White had an awareness of feelings about the departure of a part of the group. She may have been angered or disappointed that she was not taken with the group. Perhaps she was simply bored and went to the corner and began hallucinating (if she actually was doing that) because there was little stimulation on the ward. With this type of descriptive report, Mrs. White might be studied more carefully, and nursing plans for her might be formulated based on the possible meaning of her noted behavior.

Concurrent with this step, the staff is ready to have a new type of assignment. Again, innovation must come through staff preparation. In the daily meeting the nurse brings up the plan to assign a small group of patients to each member of her staff. She should ask the group if there are preferences for patient assignments, because the groups formed will be long-term groups. Any attendant who feels great repugnance or fear toward any patient should not need to work with that patient for a long period of time. The attendants need to explore the wisdom of group assignments. They are instructed about the progress that is expected when patients begin to form small group identities (much as the staff did when they first began their meetings) and when they are placed in a group situation somewhat similar to that of the family.

With permanent group assignments the patients can look upon their attendant in a "den mother" or "den father" relationship. The attendant becomes not only the caretaker and the protector but also the wellspring from whom flows new ideas, recognition for achievement, comfort and security.

WARD PROBLEMS

Staff of long-term institutions are used to thinking of chronicity as synonymous with intractability. Such thinking arises from staff frustration when a gamut of approaches has been tried and the patient still does not respond. In order to alter this concept, change must be seen. Change will be observable in the environmental manipulations listed previously. Improvements in the patient population will evolve more slowly as a result of variation in the ward population.

One of the most basic understandings that staff and patients must acquire is that *behaviors can change*. Once patients have been divided into small groups with an unchanging group leader, attention can more easily be focused on the behaviors that need alteration.* Social re-

---

* See Chapter 11 for discussion of small group formation and management, i.e., group therapy techniques.

motivation requires alertness to situations and flexibility of approach that allows for change in activities; it also requires imagination.

Incontinence

One of the most fundamental behavioral changes to be achieved should focus on incontinence. If the ward is not to smell, if patients are to gain a feeling of pride in themselves and their surroundings, then it is necessary to establish continence in the patient group. The method is not startling or new. It simply means that the patient is taken to toilet at stated times throughout the day when it is likely that he may need to evacuate the colon or bladder. A routine is established and it is followed rigidly. Regular times for toileting should come upon arising in the morning, directly after breakfast, prior to lunch, shortly after lunch and, again, before dinner. The last time should be at bedtime. It is rare that all patients on a given ward are incontinent. If there are some who are continent, these patients can be utilized to toilet the incontinent ones. Patients can be utilized profitably in the improvement programs of other patients for other activities as well, such as feeding, bathing, and perhaps reading to those who are unable to do these things for themselves. Such activities not only offer assistance to patients who require it, but also provide an opportunity for those who are involved to be gratified by caring for others. It shows better socialized patients that they are needed and are valued by the group. As incontinent patients begin to evacuate in the appropriate place at the correct time, they should be praised and their accomplishments should be recognized through formal vehicles such as parties, prizes or desired expeditions.*

Eating Habits

When incontinence is no longer a ward problem (and this situation can be surprisingly quickly altered), other priorities in habit training should be established. Among the most common problems are personal appearance and eating habits. These facets of the patient's life can best be changed through example and, again, routine. Eating habits can be improved more readily if staff members are willing to eat with their patients. If possible, the group leader should eat at least one meal per day with his group. All appropriate silverware is placed on the dining table. The patient group is encouraged to communicate their expectations to recalcitrant members. Again, good behavior is rewarded.

Personal Appearance

In the matter of personal appearance, several maneuvers are practical. First, whenever possible, patients should be permitted to

---

* See page 182 for discussion of specific behavior modification techniques.

wear their own clothing. It is unusual for chronic patients of long tenure to own their own clothing, but if such apparel is available, it should be reserved for the patient to whom it belongs. This is part of one's identity, and every effort must be made to establish and solidify that concept. For women the use of cosmetics can be reinforcing. Sometimes church groups seek projects, and if the ward makes known their need for cosmetics, they may be obtained from this source. Occasionally a cosmetic company will contribute a quantity of its products. If make-up can be obtained from any source, its use is likely to spark interest among female patients and will reduce their apathy and discouragement and help them to feel more optimistic. The use of cosmetics is therapeutic because it reinforces interest in personal appearance.

ACTIVITIES TO ALTER REGRESSION

Small Group Activities

The small groups with their leaders should identify projects and goals for themselves. The programs established are individualized and aimed at meeting patients' needs. It is these few philosophical objectives that make the program new and innovative.

Small groups of patients are treated. They are treated *in* the group, not *as* a group. This arrangement makes the best use of a staff that is too small. The goals established in the group are individualized. They point up a patient's needs, not those of the staff, or those of the administration. In other words, all activity is focused around the small group of patients and their leader. If the group seems ready for outside activity, i.e., each member is continent and able to behave within an anticipated range of behaviors, then walks or shopping expeditions to neighborhood stores can be planned. When the group wishes and it is possible, trips to the hospital canteen are useful as rewards and incentives for future progress. Walks to the hospital library are good, if there is such a place, or to the chapel. When two or more groups seem ready, intramural sports can be planned. Volleyball is a good game for team effort. It permits lots of exercise and offers opportunity for various members to demonstrate athletic skill. At the same time mistakes can be made and glossed over without making any individual patient look culpable. Simple games of catch are appropriate for those patients who have poor coordination or for whom team activities are undesirable.

When small groups are well integrated, they might plan with their leader for trips to town. Such expeditions require careful planning and perhaps the borrowing of other staff members to help to chaperone. Such adventures are highly useful for patients whom the staff hope to rehabilitate with discharge in mind. Group discussion is useful in preparation for such junkets to relate how money is used in the area, i.e., bus fares, and so forth, to decide where the travelers will go and to discuss what they are likely to encounter while off the hospital grounds. Church groups are, again, helpful in projects such as this, for the church women are often willing to lend a hand with chaperonage. Of course, trips of this type require clearance from administration and they should not be planned in detail with the patient group or even suggested until permission has been granted. Thus, patients are saved disappointment if permission is not obtained.

A final suggestion is the use of heterogeneous groups. Better levels of behavior will be obtained if they are expected. When heterogeneous groupings are made, the better integrated patients expect higher levels of behavior from their more regressed counterparts. The effect of staff in this respect is expected; however, patients themselves are valuable as "prompters" for their peers' behavior. This is doubly valuable, for it communicates to the patients that there is a community of persons and interests of which they are a part. It is another way of perceiving the message that others care. Such activities help to dispel the stagnant atmosphere of the chronic ward. The use of occasional parties and dances to which patients from other wards are invited is still another mode of reward. When patients are continent, aware of personal appearance and talking, it is useful to utilize the group meeting as a place to plan parties, dances and other activities. The patients should be permitted to decide what kinds of affairs they will have, who will attend, and the themes of the occasions. If possible, occupational therapy can be involved, and the patients can make decorations and perhaps bake some of the refreshments.

Remotivation Techniques

As has been mentioned several times, it is extremely useful to have patients plan for their own activities and take major responsibility for implementing those plans. This allows for, and encourages, group interaction. Also, the use of initiative and a sense of responsibility are fostered. Small group meetings can be instituted as soon as patients have been in their assigned groups long enough to recognize the other members and their leader.* Though some patients may be mute, the group should be scheduled to meet at a regular time each day so that the habit is formed. The leader may wish to use techniques of remotivation at first if the group is quiet or mute. To do this, the leader will choose a topic for discussion. He will need to assemble materials illustrating his topic so that the group can actually see, feel or taste what it is that is being discussed. At first the subject should be simple. If the group is male, such topics as trains, automobiles or weather may be of interest. Pictures, poetry about the subject, or even small matchstick models can be passed around. The leader who reads a poem or story about the

---

* See Chapter 11 for discussion of group selection, preparation and group dynamics.

subject may be able to show illustrative pictures to the encircling group. He will ask simple questions of the patients such as: "Do you like the train?" "Who in this group has been on a train?" "Where did you go?" *Simple topics, simple presentations* and *simple questions* are the key to the technique. Patients who have not conversed for many years will not be ready for long, complex thoughts or statements. They need practice with rudimentary communications. When this has been forthcoming, they can move on to more complex subjects, such as planning for group projects. The following is an excerpt from a social remotivation group led by an attendant. The patients are six women between 45 and 73 years of age. The average length of hospital stay is 27 years.

Leader: Today, we are going to talk and think about babies. I have brought a short poem to read. (She proceeds to read about the cuteness and cuddliness of babies as they sleep, when they eat and when they are bathed.) Now I should like to show you pictures of babies. The first one I am passing around is a little baby with red hair. . . . Jane, what is the baby in the picture doing?

Jane: The baby is crying.

Leader: Has anyone in this group had a baby?

Another
Patient: I had a baby. I had a daughter. She's grown up now and has babies of her own.

Leader: Mary, do you like to see babies?

Mary: No. (She looks away from the group. The leader knows that she is dealing with a patient who has been mute for many years, so she does not press for more response from her at this time.)

Leader: While I pass this next picture around, I would like to hear about other people's experiences with babies.

Rita: I haven't seen a baby for many years. They make me nervous. I don't like to hear babies cry.

Leader: Do babies crying make other people in our group nervous? (Others nod their heads hesitantly.)

Jane: My little nephew used to pour oatmeal on his head when he was two years old. He always thought it was so funny. He'd sit up and laugh and laugh. (She smiles quietly to herself.)

Leader: You must have lots of pleasant memories about him, Jane. What do some of the rest of you think about babies? (Mary smirks at the leader.)
If none of you want to say more about babies, I'd like to read you another short poem, this time about a baby doing something different. (The leader reads the poem which is about a baby anticipating the presence and smile of his mother. When the poem is finished the leader asks the group if they enjoyed the reading. All but Mary say they did. The leader then says:) We've had a good poetry reading session today. Before we stop and have hot chocolate, can we decide on a topic for Friday's group

meeting? (A patient suggests clothes. It is agreed on by the group and they then adjourn to the dayroom for refreshments.)

The use of food during or after the remotivation meetings reinforces the pleasurable aspect of the meetings. This memory lingers on in the patient's mind, helping him to be courageous enough to come for the next session. Patients should never be put in the position of being stressed by requests for responses they cannot make. Rather, the skilled leader is one who waits for cues pertaining to the patient's readiness and then seeks responses from him.

Ward Meetings

When several small groups are verbalizing well, i.e., are able to hold at least short discussions, it is time for the groups to meet together one or more times per week for ward meetings. This is a big step forward. Now the group can begin to form a larger group identity. It is useful to invite the ward resident, or administrator, to one of these meetings each week on a regular basis so that administrative approvals can be acquired as patients plan for future activities or make alterations in present ones. Also, ward projects can be developed in these meetings and assignments for small responsibilities within the larger project can be given to individuals or small groups of patients. The following is an excerpt from a ward meeting of 50 men between the ages of 32 and 74. The average length of hospitalization is 29 years.

Nurse:	Good morning, gentlemen. It is 9 A.M. and time for us to begin the ward meeting. I have several announcements to give you. . . . Mr. Harris, the barber, will be here this afternoon between 2:30 and 3:30 if anyone wants a haircut. Miss Dibble from the library has called to say she would like some volunteers to help her unpack several cases of new books this afternoon and, last, we were very lucky when we took our complaint about the coffee to the dietary department. They promised to look into the matter, and we shall have a report back for you as soon as they call us. . . . Now, who has something to report?
John:	If Tim don't stop takin' my shoes at night, I ain't goin' to be responsible for what I do. . . .
Nurse:	Does anyone else want to say something about this problem? We've heard a lot of complaints from John about this.
Howard:	I think we should kick Tim out of here. He does nothing but start trouble.
Tim:	Go to hell.
Frank:	Come on, boys, Tim is sick. He don't know what he's doin' half the time.
John:	You sure know enough to make my life miserable at night.

Nurse: Can you tell us what happens around here at night, John? For those of us who aren't here that late, I think we need to have a little better picture of the things that go on after evening activities.

John: Well, we all git ready for bed when Mr. Trout (evening attendant) tells us to. Everybody gits in bed like he says to and then, after the lights go out, there's Tim in somebody's bed or takin' their clothes or something. . . . I git so angry, I don't know what to do.

Nurse: Can someone else tell us of their experiences with Tim? . . . Has anyone else had any trouble like John?

Sam: He don't bother me much at night. I socked him good last time he got in my bed and started messin' 'round. I told 'im, "Tim, if you come messin' around me agin, I'm goin' to beat the living tar out of you" . . . and you know what? He ain't been nowhere near me since.

Tim: Go to hell.

Lawrence: I don't blame Tim. It's lonely around here at night . . . and scary too. I don't mind Tim getting in my bed. I hear strange noises at night and I'm frightened.

Howard: Ah, Larry is scared of his own shadow.

Attendant A: What should we do about Tim at night? Should we make him sleep in the quiet room?

John: I sure don't want to be the one who put Tim in the quiet room. I think I'll just slug him like Sam did. . . . He sure don't bother 'im no more.

Nurse: What does the rest of our group think we should do? Tim, do you want to say anything about this? (No one offers a comment.)

Nurse: Tim, do you get into other people's beds?

Tim: Yeah, sometimes when the voices tell me to. . . . I get in beds sometimes.

John: You better sure as hell stay out of my bed or I'm goin' to give your "voices" a big bloody nose.

Tim: Go to hell.

Nurse: I suppose we all agree that Tim should stay in his bed after lights go out. I can sympathize with Lawrence who feels frightened at night. . . . I wonder if Tim feels scared too?

Bobby: (Blurts out.) Shut up, shut up. I'm not scared. (Attendant A. gets up, approaches Bobby and rubs his shoulder.)

Nurse: I think being scared is something we all feel sometimes. I wonder if it would help the people who feel scared in the evening if we left a lamp lit on the small table outside the nurses' station. How do you feel about that? (Lawrence, Tim and Bobby nod vigorously. The others do not seem interested.)

Nurse:	Let us try that for a week and then discuss the problem again. . . . Now, let's turn to the project we began discussing last week. As you know, the majority of you have been going to your jobs for at least a month now and working very hard. You have done your jobs well and we promised a special treat for all this work. What is it going to be?
Fred:	Can we go to a movie in the village?
Sonny:	Naw, I don't want to see no movie. Let's have a party.
Tim:	Go to hell.
Howard:	How about having a ward dance and inviting the C cottage ladies?
Nurse:	All right, gentlemen. We have three suggestions— a party, a movie, and a ward dance to which we should invite the C cottage ladies. Let's take a vote. (The patients raise their hands to indicate their choice.)
Nurse:	It looks like the majority of you would like to have a dance. That means lots of preparation. Can we form committees to get ready? (Most of the patients nod their heads in the affirmative.)
Howard:	I want to be in charge of inviting the guests.
Frank:	Howard always gets his way. I want to help invite the girls, too.
Mark:	(Hesitantly.) Could I help with decorating the ward?
Attendant A:	Our group would like to be in charge of the food. We have permission to walk into the village and we could pick up some things at the grocery store.
Nurse:	Gee, it sounds like we have lots of enthusiastic workers. Let's form our committees and put people in charge of them. Then let's decide on a date for the dance and see if that is okay with Mrs. Parker (division supervisor). (Most of the men were assigned to committees, leaving out only those few patients who did not seem interested or who were still too ill to take responsibility in these areas.)

It can be seen that much group interaction is generated as a ward project is planned. As the dance plans evolve, more and more group activity will ensue. At the same time enthusiasm and pleasant expectations will grow. The ward staff will reinforce the idea that this project is a reward for the hard work and diligent efforts of the men themselves. Thus, responsibility will be reinforced in the minds of the patients. For some, the planning, the implementation and the actual social affair will be an end in itself; for others, it will be another step toward social rehabilitation and a move closer to discharge.

BEHAVIOR MODIFICATION

Much has been said in the previous sections on habit training and reinforcement of ideas. These concepts have been developed into a technique known as behavior modification. The advocates of this type of therapy believe it is useful, for it is practical and efficient. Through behavior modification a patient or group of patients can be conditioned to utilize a new response or set of responses to a given stimulus. Though there are detractors who argue the ethics of imposing conditioned behavior on patients, the technique, based on learning theory, has gained wide acceptance in private practice, hospitals for the mentally ill and institutions for the mentally retarded.

Those who use this method believe that mental illness is actually a set of learned responses and that the aberrant behaviors observed in patients are not symptoms, but the actual disease process. Behavior modification advocates feel that they have altered the disease process when they have brought about a new response in the patient's behavior. To do this they identify four factors: the behavior to be altered (or extinguished), the desired behavior (response), a reinforcement (reward) for the new behavior, and a program (or schedule) for reinforcement.

The behavior to be changed may be any type of response which is maladaptive for a given patient or group of patients. Such things as hallucinating, masturbating, assaultive behavior or lack of attention to personal hygiene are examples of behaviors which can be altered by this method. The desired response is that behavior which will bring about more gratifying results for the patient. A reinforcer is something that the patient likes and which he will regard as a reward; reinforcers are as individual as the patients themselves. For one patient, reinforcement might be food, for another it could be a special privilege, for still another it would be as simple as a touch from the person working with the patient. Reinforcers selected from the environmental context of a state hospital ward might be such things as speaking to the ward doctor or chaplain, going to the canteen or staying in one's room to sleep, read or play records.

Responses which are reinforced after each occurrence are the easiest to extinguish or remove. This is probably because reward is expected after each conditioned response. If the act is not followed by the reward, the learner has no reason to persist in the response. Schedules that utilize intermittent reinforcement are less easily extinguished, but they take longer to become learned. Schedules that reinforce in an irregular intermittent fashion are the best means of creating behavior that is likely to remain stable. It is likely that intermittent reinforcement is particularly effective because the learner never knows when he will be rewarded; thus, he maintains the conditioned behavior for many trials (or occurrences) while he anticipates the reinforcer.

Example 1

Judy is a 40 year old hebephrenic schizophrenic who has been in the hospital since her 23rd birthday. She is assaultive, obese and dirty. When staff members take her to be bathed she attacks them and creates a situation that makes her personal care a catastrophic event. It was decided that the first response to be learned was one of cooperation when summoned to the bathroom. To accomplish this, Judy was placed under careful observation for several days to see if there were any particular staff member whom she seemed to prefer. One attendant was noted as having a less negative relationship with this patient than others on the unit. The attendant began to carry small pieces of candy, and when she was near Judy, she said "hello" frequently and smiled at the patient. When the patient made a friendly gesture toward the attendant she was given a piece of candy. This was done each time Judy gave a friendly response. After six days Judy was noted to respond positively to the attendant whenever that staff member approached her. (The attendant was never put in the position of having to coerce or punish Judy in any way.) When the response was well established, the attendant was put on day duty. She was assigned to supervise the bathing of several "good" patients. Judy was invited to go with her attendant to "help" her with the supervision. Again, when Judy walked to the shower room with the attendant, she was given a piece of candy. (At this point, Judy was still being bathed by other staff members and she was grossly uncooperative.) When Judy was observed to enter the shower room freely, the attendant was ready to start the next phase of the plan. As they stood together in the shower room she suggested to Judy that Judy might like to wash herself without the other attendants present. The attendant (who had observed Judy's particular likes and dislikes) suggested that, if Judy took a good shower, the two of them might walk to the village drugstore for a soda. Judy looked dubious but agreed to try it. The first shower was a less than cleansing one. The patient was in and out of the water within two minutes and little soap had been used. The attendant told her that the shower was not as thorough as was necessary to go out walking in the village, but perhaps the next day's would be better. However, Judy was rewarded with a piece of candy for her effort.

The next day the patient entered the shower readily. The attendant stood nearby to offer assistance. When it seemed that Judy was going to repeat her performance of the day before, the attendant asked if Judy would like some help so that she would get clean enough to walk into the village. The patient nodded eagerly. The bath was accomplished without further ado, and the reward was given that afternoon. In the ensuing weeks, cleansing showers were always rewarded with candy, sometimes with a stroll into the village. At the end of 90 days, Judy had apparently given up her assaultive behavior and was willing to bathe with the supervision of a chosen few.

Example 2

Ben is a 30 year old catatonic schizophrenic. According to his chart he has not spoken to anyone for many years. The ward nurse decided that she would like to try to break through Ben's mutism. The nurse watched Ben for several days at different times. She studied him to find if he gave any signs of awareness in any particular situation. She noted that Ben seemed to become more tense when he was washed and dressed in the morning. He relaxed and appeared less "ready to resist" when he was left alone. The only time that Ben seemed interested in the world around him was when the porter came through the ward each day to deliver the mail. Thus, the nurse collected her data through observation.

She asked the porter to stop near Ben's chair the next day when he brought the mail. The porter did so when the mail had been taken to the nurses' station. Ben curled up in his characteristic pose of defense. The nurse beckoned the porter to her. She asked him to repeat the move the following day, though this time she asked him to take his bag with him. The nurse watched the following day as the porter, carrying his mail pouch, approached Ben. Again, the patient curled up, but he studied the bag before withdrawing. Now the nurse felt that she had observed something significant. Again she asked the employee to stop by Ben's chair on his rounds. For the next two weeks the porter stopped by Ben's chair each day. He put down his bag, stood away from it, and said, "Hello, Ben." The patient continued to ignore the porter, but each day he looked longer at the mail pouch. Eventually the nurse asked the porter if he would take an envelope (that she supplied) from the pouch and hand it to Ben.

The porter did this for a week. At first Ben would not take the envelope directly from the porter but would retrieve it if the man left it within reach of him. Ben did not attempt to open the envelope. The nurse observed that each day the porter was able to come closer to Ben to deliver her envelopes. Finally, the day came when Ben actually looked up as the porter entered the ward and walked toward the office. He watched until the porter came out again and approached him. The nurse watched with glee as Ben extended his hand for the anticipated envelope. This time the porter was instructed to tell Ben he would see him tomorrow.

The envelope that the nurse now placed in the porter's pouch contained a piece of paper upon which she had written, "I am glad that you care enough to want to read your letter from me. Miss Williams." Ben continued to take an envelope each day for several days before he tried to open one. Finally he did, however, and he read its contents. Ben made no observable response. He did, however, open the envelope again the following day. This time it said, "I am glad you are opening your letter. Tomorrow there will be a pleasant surprise in your envelope. Miss Williams." The next day, Ben met the porter at the entrance to the ward. He held out his hand for his letter. When it was forthcoming he grunted and shuffled off to his corner, opening the letter as he went. Out of the envelope dropped a pencil, a piece of blank paper, and a piece of candy.

Ben looked at the paper and pencil, dropped them beside his chair and quickly ripped the paper from the candy and ate it. As he did this, he looked furtively toward the nurses' station. That afternoon Miss Williams approached Ben. She said, "Hello," and offered him a piece of gum, but Ben curled up in the corner and refused to acknowledge her presence. She realized that her patient was not yet ready to deal with her directly.

On succeeding days the porter went faithfully to Ben each afternoon and delivered his envelope containing a short message from Miss Williams. Finally, on a Friday, the note enclosed read, "If you would like candy on Monday, you will have to indicate this by writing the word candy on the enclosed paper." Ben read the note, looked quickly toward the nurses' station, and awkwardly grasped the enclosed pencil. He painstakingly printed the word "candy."

The following Monday, Ben left the note under the door to the nurses' station. He did not look at anyone, but dropped his message and returned to the corner that he regarded possessively as his own. When the porter came, Ben looked up expectantly, knowing that his envelope was in the pouch. The porter, now familiar with the project, winked at Ben and handed him the awaited communication. He said, "See you, Ben." The patient looked at him and smiled. The mail was duly delivered Tuesday, Wednesday and Thursday. A note in the envelope Thursday said, "Tomorrow if you want candy, you must ask the porter for it."

On Friday the staff of Ben's ward waited expectantly. The porter also waited and wondered. He felt a little afraid, for he did not know what was going to happen. Miss Williams had assured him that it would not hurt Ben if he was denied his daily envelope and candy. She explained that if Ben was unable to comply with the request the porter should continue with his usual routine of saying "hello" and "goodbye" and then go on his way until the next time he came.

The porter delivered the mail at the station. Then he turned to Ben and walked to his corner. Ben looked up at him and waited. The porter stopped in front of the silent man. "Hello, Ben." Ben looked at him. His eyes studied the eyes of the porter before him. "Candy, please. . . ." The porter found himself hiding a big smile. From the window of the nurses' station, Miss Williams also suppressed a grin and the urge to run out and hug both Ben and the porter. All on the ward who knew what was happening were filled with delight at the milestone that had been achieved this day in the life of one catatonic patient named Ben.

The end was not in sight, but a good beginning had been made. It would be some time yet before Ben would be able to transfer his trust from the faithful porter to Miss Williams, but this would come when Ben was ready to talk directly to the nurse. By the same painstaking steps that moved Ben from mutism to uttering a meaningful sound to the porter would come the bridge to Miss Williams. From there he would be taught to speak, at first haltingly, then with facility, to others.

Token Economy

A specific type of program of behavior modification is called token economy. This type of program is becoming widely used where behavior modification is advocated. In a token economy program, the nurse switches from her customary role to that of a "behavioral engineer." She helps her patients to learn techniques that they can use to control their own environments in such a way that positive responses are elicited from others.[5] In the token economy program, certain behaviors are rewarded with tokens which in and of themselves have no value, but which can be traded for commodities or privileges. In the first application of a token economy to a psychiatric ward, Ayllon and Azrin[1] "reinforced serving meals, cleaning floors, sorting laundry, washing dishes and self-grooming. Reinforcement consisted of the opportunity to engage in activities that had a high level of occurrence when freely allowed."[5]

It was learned from early observations that such occurrences as being able to rent an available room, selecting people with whom to dine, passes, and so forth, could serve as reinforcers. Thus, it was learned that those who wished to shape or modify behavior should look to the patients for effective reinforcers. Those activities that they involved themselves in when permitted freedom were the best sources of reward. In token economy, the reinforcers are "earned" through purchase with tokens.

At Eastern State Hospital in Washington a modified version of other economy systems and behavior modification programs is employed. Plastic tickets are used as tokens. The tickets are earned by patients for performing certain activities such as morning care, morning chores, ward duty assignments, housekeeping duties, and for attending and participating in groups, working on occupational therapy assignments, doing errands for the staff, attending school, recreational activities, church, doing personal correspondence and laundry, and for socializing with other participants. Tickets are redeemable for buying meals and tobacco. Watching TV or hospital movies and attending dances are privileges that can be purchased. "Fines doubling the regular price are levied if program participants do not pay for activities in advance, or for some other infringement of the Budget Plan regulations. Anyone earning fines of five or more tickets a day is placed on restriction for three days.[16]

The Kennedy Youth Center, in Morgantown, W. Va., a residential treatment center for juvenile delinquents, also utilizes token economy. A student earns points having cash value, one cent for one point, for doing well in school and at daily chores. He may use this money, which averages about $2.50 per week, to buy snacks or may save for a trip home. He may buy recreational activities and pay rent. Status and privileges are emphasized in order to give reality training. The new trainee has the least commodious living arrangements. As he earns points, he may move to better rooms. To live there, he pays higher rent. Additionally, he may discard the center's uniform and wear his own clothes. Also, he can go into the adjacent town on escorted trips.

An "honor student" lives in the best accommodations, for which he pays the highest rent. He has expectations placed on him in terms of the work he does with other trainees. He wears his own clothes, does not have to report to his room before midnight, and is given an alarm clock and is expected to awaken himself. Additionally, he is given a chance to go home on furlough and later is granted one-day passes into town. Occasionally such a student is allowed to hold an outside job. Most important, he becomes eligible for parole. The center is proud of the results. Rather than instilling behavior through fear and physical force as happens in most penal institutions, the trainee conforms to rules and learns internal controls because he is part of a system that pays off, i.e., the token economy.*

Mental hospitals that utilize behavior modification usually find it particularly helpful in chronic areas. Socially acceptable behaviors are taught first. When patients are performing acceptably in this area, work is the next behavior introduced.

Work is an important facet of the adult patient's life; he needs to do something useful. If he does it well, he needs to be rewarded, for such is the way of the outside world to which he will return if rehabilitated. Work roles should be assigned according to the ability of the patient to carry out the task. Thus, an elderly woman should not be required to get down on the floor to scrub; however, it might be appropriate for such an individual to be the clothing sorter, the food server, or the person who watches the incontinent group for signs that one of them needs to be taken to the bathroom.

The job assignment is not to be equated with a chore. Rather, it is a bona fide work responsibility. Being assigned to it should elicit a feeling of pride in the patient, who is given praise and recognition for the good work done. It is very important for the staff member to offer an assortment of jobs and to rotate these assignments from time to time so that boredom or obsessive concern does not become associated with the work. (One does not improve the lot of a patient who is responsible for the cleanliness of the shower for six years but who thinks of nothing else during his waking hours!) Also, work should not be an end in itself, but should reflect the mode in which people in the outside world create and maintain their lives. Payment for services should be instituted on the ward. Remuneration can take many forms, such as cigarettes, privileges, scrip for use at the canteen, candy, gum, a trip off the grounds with chaperonage, or tokens, if that system is used. Payment may be defined by the patients as a group in the ward meeting. If their ideas are feasible, they should be implemented.

It is well to keep in mind that sometimes patients on chronic wards are retardates. For these patients, activities must be geared to

---

* The Sunday Sun, Baltimore, Maryland, May 23, 1971.

their specific competencies. Likewise, payments for their work should also be planned around things that they will enjoy. Simple games, candy and coloring books are useful to keep on hand for them. Though it looks strange, at first, to see an elderly adult coloring or playing with a simple childish device, it should be borne in mind that this adult actually has the mental apparatus of a young child, and his payments for services must be geared to the mental apparatus housed within the adult body.

REFERENCES

1. Ayllon, T., and Azrin, N. H.: *The Token Economy*. New York, Appleton-Century-Crofts, Inc., 1968.
2. Belknap, I.: *Human Problems of a State Mental Hospital*. New York, McGraw-Hill Book Co., Inc., 1956.
3. Brazinsky, B., Brazinsky, D., and Ring, K.: *Methods of Madness: The Mental Hospital as a Last Resort*. New York, Holt, Rinehart, and Winston, Inc., 1969.
4. Dunham, N. W., and Weinberg, S. K.: *Culture of the State Mental Hospital*. Detroit, Wayne State University Press, 1960.
5. Frasner, L.: Token Economy as an Illustration of Operant Conditioning Procedures with the Aged, with Youth, and with Society. *In* Levis, D. J. (ed.): *Learning Approaches to Therapeutic Behavior Charge*. Chicago, Aldine Publishing Co., 1970, pp. 75, 76.
6. Goffman, E.: *Asylums*. New York, Doubleday & Co., 1961.
7. Greenblatt, M., Levinson, D., and Williams, R. (eds.): *The Patient and the Mental Hospital*. Chicago, Free Press of Glencoe, 1957.
8. Levinson, D., and Gallagher, B.: *Patienthood in the Mental Hospital*. Boston, Houghton-Mifflin Co., 1964.
9. Levis, D. J. (ed.): *Learning Approaches to Therapeutic Behavior Change*. Chicago, Aldine Publishing Co., 1970.
10. Mowry, R. S., and Fairweather, G.: *Social Approaches in Treating Mental Illness: An Experimental Approach*. New York, John Wiley & Sons, Inc., 1964.
11. Scheff, T. J.: *Being Mentally Ill: A Sociological Theory*. Chicago, Aldine Publishing Co., 1966.
12. Schwartz, C., and Schwartz, M.: *Social Approaches to Mental Patient Care*. New York, Columbia University Press, 1964.
13. Saasz, T.: *The Myth of Mental Illness*. New York, Paul B. Hoeber, 1961.
14. Von Mering, O., and King, S. H.: *Remotivating the Mental Patient*. New York, Russell Sage Foundation, 1957.

Journals

15. Beal, E., Sutton, I. W., Ognjanov, V., and Hughes, D.: Nursing Care Approaches for Operant Reinforcement with Psychiatric Patients. *J. Psychiatric Nursing and Mental Health Services*, 7 (No. 4):157-159, July-August, 1969.
16. Cavens, A., and Williams, R.: The Budget Plan: Behavior Modification of Long-Term Patients. *Perspectives in Psychiatric Care*, 9 (No. 1):14, 1971.
17. Ellsworth, J. R.: Reinforcement Therapy with Chronic Patients. *Hospital and Community Psychiatry*, 20:238-240, August, 1969.

SUGGESTED READINGS

Eddy, F., O'Neill, E., and Ostvachan, B.: Group Work on a Long-Term Psychiatric Service. *Perspectives in Psychiatric Care*, 6 (No. 1): 1968.

This is a *very* pertinent presentation of the role of nurses and aides as group leaders on a chronic service. The discussion is lucid and describes many of the practical details which might interest a worker in such an environment.

Galioni, E. F., Almada, A. A., Newhall, C. M., and Peterson, A.: Group Techniques in Rehabilitating "Back-Ward" Patients. *Am. J. Nursing*, 54 (No. 8): 1954.

This article presents the experimental work done with a large group of chronically ill patients. Much of the push toward better integrated behavior seemed to be influenced by the staff's attitude.

Goodman, L. R.: Regression—Some Implications for Nurses in Large Public Psychiatric Hospitals. *Nursing Outlook*, 10 (No. 4): April, 1962.

This is an excellent article because it provides in a concise, lucid style many valuable hints for modification of regressed behavior through nursing intervention.

Hayes, J. S.: The Psychiatric Nurse as a Sociotherapist. *Am. J. Nursing*, 62 (No. 6): 1962.

The author maintains that psychiatric nursing has paralleled the development of psychiatry. Patients are no longer expected to remain in hospitals forever. If they are to return to society, the psychiatric nurse's role is to facilitate such a move.

Lamb, J. T.: Freedom for Patients in Mental Hospitals. *Am. J. Nursing*, 68 (No. 3): 1958.

This article presents the outcomes of an experiment in which locked ward doors were opened and patients were encouraged to make group decisions.

McCown, P., and Wurm, E.: Orienting the Disoriented. *Am. J. Nursing*, 65 (No. 4): 1965.

This is a highly readable account which will be valuable to the student who is interested in behavior modification.

Morimoto, F. R.: The Socializing Role of Psychiatric Ward Personnel. *Am. J. Nursing*, 54 (No. 1): 1954.

The writer, a nurse researcher at Boston Psychopathic Hospital, describes the results of a study done at that institution. It showed that staff were not active enough as "socializers" on the ward and so they did not take full advantage of their potential as therapeutic agents.

Pope, J.: The Changing Scene of Psychiatric Nursing in a State Hospital. *Perspectives in Psychiatric Care*, 5 (No. 4): 1967.

An interesting account concerning the process of change in one institution.

Pullinger, W. F.: Remotivation. *Am. J. Nursing*, 60 (No. 5): 1960.

This is an *excellent* "how to" article on remotivation technique. It is highly recommended to anyone wishing to try behavior modification.

Ruhlman, R. G., and Ishijama, T.: Remedy for the Forgotten Back Ward. *Am. J. Nursing*, 64 (No. 7): 1964.

This article provides a good description of poor ward conditions prior to the initiation of a therapeutic program which brought about many positive changes. They, too, are identified and described effectively.

Books

Schwartz, C., and Shockley, E.: *The Nurse and the Mental Hospital*. New York, Russell Sage Foundation, 1956.

Though not a current publication, this volume is still relevant to the nurse who wishes to practice in an inpatient setting.

Stanton, A., and Schwartz, M.: *The Mental Hospital.* New York, Basic Books, Inc., 1954.

The hospital described is *not* the typical sprawling mental hospital for the public, but a small institution known for its psychoanalytically oriented therapy with schizophrenics. The book is highly recommended because of the detailed analysis of hospital life that it provides.

Dunham, N., and Weinberg, S.: *Culture of the State Mental Hospital.* Detroit, Wayne State University Press, 1960.

The student who is interested in the state mental hospital will find this volume useful as a source for comparison with the institution in which she works or studies.

VonMering, O., and King, S. H.: *Remotivating the Mental Patient.* New York, Russell Sage Foundation, 1957.

This book is a classic for all who plan to work with chronically ill patients who have been institutionalized for long periods. It should not be overlooked.

chapter 10

COMMUNITY
MENTAL HEALTH

Community mental health focuses primarily on prevention. It is an exciting field that encompasses new broad-reaching concepts and complex foci. It concentrates not on individuals and specific mental illnesses, but on groups; indeed, on whole communities. Included are such groups as schoolchildren, shopkeepers, factory workers, neighborhood dwellers, church congregations and transients. Rates of disability are studied, as are factors in the community characteristics which influence mental health and illness.

Community mental health nursing and psychiatric nursing in the community are not synonymous. The latter occurs when the nurse, either public health, school, industrial or clinic based, finds herself following a psychiatric patient outside the confines of an institution. The nurse may be employed in a public health agency at the local or state level and may have, among her other cases, some patients with psychiatric problems. The nurse working in a hospital-based clinic might also find herself seeing patients in their homes or neighborhoods as a means of maintaining the clinic's contact with them. Indeed, some psychiatric residential treatment facilities encourage their staff nurses to establish therapeutic relationships with patients while they are hospitalized and then to see the patients in their homes when hospitalization is no longer necessary. Such an arrangement is valuable because continuity of care is maintained. In any of these transactions, however, the focus of the psychiatric nurse (or the public health nurse utilizing psychiatric nursing techniques) is to promote recovery in her patient or group of patients. To accomplish this goal she utilizes psychotherapeutic techniques such as the one-to-one or group relationship. She is oriented toward the use of chemotherapy and, if necessary, protracted residential care.

The nurse in the community mental health center utilizes group techniques also. Additionally, however, she relies on the help of non-professional workers whom she trains and supervises. She spends considerable working hours evaluating the *potential* therapeutic needs of community residents by studying the stresses under which they live and their means of coping with them. When acute and incapacitating mental illness occurs, the nurse looks to residential facilities for brief intervention. Community mental health is a many faceted specialty which is highly complex. In order to understand it, one must be aware of the origins of the movement.

BACKGROUND OF THE COMMUNITY HEALTH MOVEMENT

ADOLPH MEYER

Psychiatry in its infancy was unready to operate in the community, but the roots of this movement were laid quite early. At the beginning of the twentieth century, leaders in the field, such as Adolph Meyer, were advocating the unification of many caretaking agencies in a single geographic area containing a mental hospital. Meyer envisioned these agencies—schools, police and welfare—as conducting an integrated program of prevention, treatment and aftercare of the mentally ill who had been hospitalized. Psychiatrists, according to Meyer, would be utilized primarily to educate other types of workers such as police, teachers and social workers so that they might provide the actual care needed by the "catchment" area population.* Meyer's program was not implemented because there was not sufficient support, nor were there appropriate personnel available. However, attention has been focused on isolated segments of the plan.

CHILD GUIDANCE CLINICS

At the same time that Meyer proposed his plans, clinics were being established to diagnose and treat the diseases of children; they were to investigate factors influencing the growth and development of the young

---

* A "catchment" area is a geographic designate containing community members to whom the community mental health center is responsible for delivery of health services.

and hopefully to decrease adult illness by detection and treatment in childhood. The clinics utilized a psychiatrist-psychologist-social worker team.

Though the program was well planned and ambitious, it failed. The planners of the children's clinics realized that they were woefully under-staffed for such an ambitious undertaking, and soon the clinics were encountering only a small segment of the community population. They ceased to focus on the prevention of disease in the total community and operated no differently than other facilities for the treatment of children.

MILITARY PSYCHIATRY

After World War II traditional psychiatry again felt the impetus of change. This time the community mental health movement was given a powerful thrust by personnel who had successfully worked in the military programs for delivery of mental health services. It had been demonstrated in the military that large populations could be monitored and treated through the utilization of nonmedical personnel; that is, that soldiers could be treated by their superior officers. Dependents who gave evidence of psychological problems could also be reached through intermediaries. Thus, the military psychiatrist found himself treating many more patients indirectly through the use of nonprofes-sionals. Additionally, group work was emphasized. The one-to-one con-cept gave way to new and successful techniques that utilized less time than traditional modes of therapy. Also, personnel who were indigenous to the area were utilized. Finally, the military programs influenced a movement toward the breakdown of isolation from the public. Psychia-trists came out of their ivory towers down into the squalor where mental disease is bred. More and more the community mental health philosophy was heard and felt. "Treat mental illness where it is, when it is. Pre-vention obviates the need for treatment."

ADVANCES WITHIN TRADITIONAL HOSPITAL SETTINGS

Advances were also made within traditional mental hospitals. The concept of a therapeutic milieu was born. Such leaders as Maxwell Jones in England reported astonishing successes when patients were allowed freer communication with their own group, the staff and the community. This was facilitated through "open" wards and frequent meetings of all those living and working on the ward. Residential treat-ment facilities tried to augment their therapeutic programs by providing urban centers where former patients could contact workers without having to actually return to the confines of the hospital. Rehabilita-tion programs were established, with the focus on preparing patients to live effectively in the community. Finally, the hospitals made provision for partial care of patients. It was noted that some mentally ill did not need 24-hour care. Instead, they could be maintained on nighttime boarding, day care or, in some cases, hospitalization over the weekends. Through these programs patients could work and maintain contact with their families.

THE JOINT COMMISSION ON MENTAL ILLNESS AND HEALTH

In 1955 Congress directed the establishment of a Joint Commission on Mental Illness and Health. The Commission was charged with the task of evaluating the human and economic problems of mental illness and its treatment. The group was asked to identify methods that might lead to the development of preventive programs. The Final Report, *Action for Mental Health,* of the Joint Commission was published in 1961. This report recommended that prevention and treatment services be instituted on local community levels.

President Kennedy delivered a message on Mental Illness and Mental Retardation to the Eighty-eighth Congress in 1963. As a result of that legislative body's deliberations and the words of Kennedy, the Community Mental Health Centers Act and other measures were passed. They provided federal support for projects initiated at the state level to improve state hospitals, institutions for the mentally retarded, and support for inservice training. In all, Congress appropriated $8,000,000 to underwrite comprehensive state hospital health planning. The passing of this legislation produced a flurry of activity. Current facilities had to be evaluated; needs and resources of communities in relation to the current facilities were investigated. Out of this activity, recognition of the need for training of personnel was noted. Plans for refurbishing and expansion were made by individual states which kept in mind that the five "basic" services of the community mental health center would have to be evidenced if, indeed, federal funds were to be awarded. The five necessary services established by law were: (1) inpatient services; (2) outpatient services; (3) partial hospitalization services, such as day care, night care, and weekend care; (4) emergency services, available 24 hours a day; and (5) consultation and educational services, available to community agencies and professional staff. It was the prerogative of the individual center to design the means by which it would meet each requirement. Within each area such programs as diagnostic services, rehabilitation programs (including vocational placement and training), educational programs, and pre- and aftercare services were developed for clients. For staff training, research and evaluation programs were organized. The plans for community mental health centers were ambitiously comprehensive. Some states were able to implement them; the start of other centers was withheld until personnel could be trained and more effective plans formulated.

THE COMMUNITY MENTAL HEALTH
CENTER TODAY

The community mental health center is a *system* of services and a set of attitudes organized to accept and meet the responsibility of mental health care for all the members of a designated population.[13] Community mental health programs attempt to deliver the type of service required by the client without causing disruption to his life, i.e., without removing him from his work, family and community. Ozarin writes that the community mental health center must be responsive to the needs of the people it is to serve. The best program is one in which the community is involved. If the center program is to be relevant to the needs of its citizens, there must be an open channel of communication. This is accomplished by interaction and joint planning with community members and other social institutions that serve them, i.e., schools, police, health resources, social agencies, churches and citizens.[11]

Besides direct services to the community inhabitants, another important part of the work of the center is to prevent mental illness through consultation with nonpsychiatric personnel working in the community who are in a position to detect and work with persons or groups who are at "high risk," that is, likely to become mentally ill. Still another goal is to offer support to community programs already established to create an environment conducive to mental health; an example of this is a "Golden Age Club," which is geared to the needs of the aging population.

The community mental health center often grows out of a situation in which several agencies have been working together on an informal basis. Often these agencies are sharing the same patients, each agency providing a service which the patient needs and which is not available through the other agencies. In such a situation it is not uncommon for a majority of five required services to pre-exist. With the addition of one or two services, the center is formally organized and can apply for federal funds. A typical case is one in which a state hospital sends its recently discharged patients to an aftercare clinic near their homes for drug therapy supervision and monthly monitoring by some representative of that clinic, such as a social worker or nurse. If the clinic can gain access to several beds in a nearby hospital for short-term admissions, or if it can staff a unit in the state hospital itself, the conglomerate can then usually staff the remaining services without difficulty. The state hospital, which has previously been a focal point, becomes an incidental along the road to recovery, and the community setting becomes the anchor point that patients (or clients, as the centers prefer to identify them) and the health team see as the place to maintain those who become ill. As the center becomes more effective, the focus shifts from disposition of the ill, i.e., short-term hospitalization and return to the community, to maintenance of health and prevention of illness.

San Francisco provides one of many models for a community mental health program. The city is divided into five districts. All citizens live within one of the five catchment areas. A team of workers in each area is responsible for the mental health needs of the people in its area. The center itself (or system of services) is composed of four detention wards, two treatment wards and a follow-up clinic at San Francisco General Hospital. The facilities, which pre-existed before the community mental health center, were reorganized as a mental health center and crisis intervention model, and replaced an earlier diagnosis and disposition goal. Interdisciplinary teams provide comprehensive and continuous care. They focus on resolving crises which lead to the need for emergency hospital treatment. Each clinic unit is assigned to one of the five identified catchment areas. Care is given through satellite clinics in the community which are separate from the county hospital.[13]

A center in New York utilizes the Bronx State Hospital for its inpatients. The center itself, called the Dr. Martin Luther King Jr. Center, serves 55 square blocks in a low income area of the central Bronx. The health team at King delivers all health services to an assigned group of people living in a designated number of blocks. Originally the program provided medical care primarily and the teams were composed of a public health nurse, several family health workers, an internist, a pediatrician and a lawyer. When, in January 1968, the King area became part of the Bronx State Hospital catchment area, the psychiatric staff of the hospital began to provide psychiatric consultation services. There are currently eight teams established in the King center. Six of these teams have a consulting psychiatrist or clinical psychologist who is also on the staff of the Bronx State Hospital. He attends weekly team meetings in which problem families or households are discussed. In the meetings the consultants attempt to highlight and clarify the psychopathological aspects of the households being discussed. They may also take part in team clinical sessions by interviewing patients directly in the presence of the referring team members.[10]

Community mental health centers are as varied in their design and programs as they are numerous. There are a total of 245 centers now in operation in the United States. When all funded centers become operant, approximately 60 million people will be served.[11] The organization of these centers also varies; however, it has been noted that "central responsibility is essential to assure continuity of care within a comprehensive range of accessibility and available services. The most

effective model of organization utilizes a single program director reporting to a governing board whose membership is representative of all the
affiliating agencies which make up the center."[11]

Responsible to the program director are persons charged with the
running of one or more aspects of the program. Under them are social
workers, nurses, other medical personnel and an array of paraprofessionals such as drug counselors and mental health technicians. Drug
counselors are often individuals who are ex-addicts or persons particularly
interested in helping the addict. They receive their training through
on-the-job experience and close supervision. Mental health technicians
are trained in two-year community college programs and are prepared
to counsel clients over short spans of time, helping them to redirect
their coping efforts toward more effective patterns of living.

Many centers also utilize community members in their work. They
are usually housewives who are also trained on the job and who are
expected to follow their clients into the neighborhood itself. By using
well prepared staff to train, supervise and consult with personnel who
are not professionally educated, the community mental health team is
able to reach many more individuals. Ozarin noted that centers serving
low-income areas and using local residents as mental health aides find
that the responsiveness of the center to local mental health needs is
enhanced. Such workers are able to establish relationships more easily
with the clientele, who are often reticent in dealing with professionals.
With utilization of nonprofessionals, however, ethical questions are
raised concerning the identification of jobs that can be handled by the
nonprofessional versus those which should be dealt with by the professionally trained. It has often been a focus of concern to those interested in health care delivery that the poor receive less care by qualified professionals than do the financially well off. Answers to this question are not forthcoming at this time, and it is likely that community
mental health centers will continue to use nonprofessionals unless professional manpower becomes abundant.

PRIMARY PREVENTION

The concept of primary prevention is central to the operation of
the community mental health center. It can be called a keystone
around which the entire mental health movement pivots. Primary
prevention involves decreasing the rate of new cases of mental illness by counteracting harmful factors before they have had a chance
to produce illness. A healthy population is the goal. Such programs
as maternity and family-centered clinics help to prevent mental illness
by recognizing and trying to influence the relationship of family members. It is known that healthy adults are more likely to develop from
children who are given the opportunity to be raised in specific, healthful
ways. Thus, the maternal and family-centered clinics attempt to in-

fluence such vital phenomena as the mother-child relationship. Discussion groups for parents are established in which free communication is encouraged and parents can report their problems in child rearing and can expect support and guidance. Such discussion groups are also formed for teachers, policemen and others who are in contact with growing children.

The discussion groups are generally led by a member of the community with the assistance of a professional member of the community mental health center. Other groups reached by the professional worker are day care and nursery program personnel, welfare workers, public health nurses, vocational and marital counseling agencies, legal aid societies, social centers, adult education groups, unions and industry-sponsored programs, church and pastoral groups, and Golden Age groups. The goal is the same throughout—to support mental hygiene practices and to offer guidance to those groups whose members are likely to experience stresses that can lead to mental illness.

An important facet of primary prevention is *crisis intervention*. It is theorized that individuals grow through a continuous process of meeting situations, coping and resolving. When one copes effectively, growth takes place; when one fails, growth does not occur. Thus, it is theorized that if mental health workers can offer support at a time of crisis, further growth can occur and mental health will be fostered. Primary prevention means the prevention of mental illness when symptoms appear. It emphasizes mental health *maintenance* rather than illness prevention.

The following case illustrates the use of crisis intervention in maintaining mental health by the support and further development of coping mechanisms.

> A call came into the center at 2:30 A.M. It was issued by the police precinct and asked for support as they answered a complaint of domestic disturbance in the neighborhood. A team was dispatched to meet the police at the given address. When the cruise car and its occupants arrived and had been joined by a team from the crisis intervention service, the four people entered the apartment building. It was dimly lighted, filled with fetid odors of dirt, urine and grease, and the narrow hallway revealed a cluster of sleepy-eyed people standing behind half-open doors, watching. Screams and baritone threats were heard from above, along with sounds of thrown objects hitting the walls. A hurried explanation from the gathered group indicated that Mr. Brown was having the "usual Saturday night" with his woman, Lillian. They had shared the upstairs flat for several weeks, having rented it on a weekly basis. With the couple lived Lillian's three children from previous liaisons. The neighbors described Mr. Brown as one who kept to himself except for Saturday night when he really "put one on." It seemed that he and Lillian had been going at it for several hours, getting progressively louder, and throwing more and more objects.

The two policemen led the way up the dark stairs. The mental health workers climbed hesitantly behind them. They were greeted at the upper landing by a garbage can pitched out the narrow doorway. The first policemen kicked the door open wider. He called in, "All right, knock it off or you can calm down in the cooler." The shrill screams continued. He shouted this time: "All right! I said knock it off!"

A small dark-skinned woman with stringy hair and shredded wrap-around emerged. She stared at the quartet. The tall, muscular man behind her was evidently Mr. Brown.

"Got a complaint, mister," said the vocal policeman. "The neighbors say you two are keeping them up with your screaming and fighting. Now what's going on?"

Lillian stared sullenly at the law officials. She looked at her man and seemed to snarl. "He can't treat me like any old piece of garbage. He's keepin' me and my kids in this fire trap and runnin' around with some high yellow. I ain't stayin' here while no rats runs over my kids' faces."

The other policeman and the center workers looked nervously around them. There was little furniture to be seen. The first policeman said, "Can we talk about this here, or are we going to have to go in to the station to get it straightened out?"

Both Lillian and Mr. Brown nodded vigorously. "No, sir. We can talk about it right here."

"Okay. Let's sit right down here and talk." Lillian took the only chair; the policeman who had first entered the room leaned against the wall and addressed himself to the occupants of the apartment, the other officer and the mental health team who now sat on the floor. "Mr. Brown, Lillian, I am Officer Scott and he is Officer Bennett. The other gentleman and that lady are Mr. Williams and Miss Mayer from the Community Mental Health Center. They came along because they thought maybe they could help you."

Lillian interrupted the officer, "I don't need no help. I need a man who's comin' home Saturday night without no load on. I need a place for my kids that ain't got roaches and rats runnin' around it. I need to git away from this stinkin' hole." She glared at Mr. Brown.

"Is that what you were trying to tell Mr. Brown tonight?" asked Miss Mayer.

"You're damned right. That's what I was sayin'," the Negro woman replied.

"We can see that you are pretty outraged at him. Is there more, or don't you think he understands what you've said?"

"He don't understan' nothin'," said Lillian. "If'n he cin git away with this crap," she said, waving her arm in a half circle, "he ain't goin' to do nothing about it nohow. Long as I has the food on the table and the clothes washed, he jes don't care nohow." Mr. Brown stood impassively as Lillian accused him.

Mr. Williams, the other worker, spoke, "Mr. Brown, Lillian sounds like she is pretty upset. . . . How do you see all this?"

The muscular man looked at the floor and then over to Lillian and finally at the worker. His eyes were shiny and brimmed with tears. "I don't want no trouble. I works hard. I works regular. I pays the rent. This woman ain't got no count to yell like that. She can jes move right on out."

Lillian began to sob softly as the man spoke. Miss Mayer walked over to her and put a hand on her shoulder. "It gets hot and miserable when it's summer and the roaches and the rats are running around and there's no one to help out with the kids. We'd like to help you both if we can. How about it? Can we have some coffee and get together on some ideas?" The six people sat together, drank coffee, and talked.

Eventually the policemen left. The workers stayed for several hours and listened as Lillian and Mr. Brown talked about their problems, their misunderstandings and, increasingly, of their affectionate feelings for one another. When the conversation dwelled on positive feelings, when Lillian's fury seemed drained, the workers from the mental health center arranged to meet the couple the following day in the center itself. Then they left, hoping that the tranquility they had brought would extend through the night. As a result of that call from the police, the center registered Mr. Brown and Lillian as clients. The former was encouraged to join an adult group that met at the neighborhood recreation center once a week. Though the group gathered for sports, it also encouraged discussion. The men who came soon found that others there felt tired, discouraged and without hope. The group leader helped the men to speak about themselves and, as they did, the group supported them.

Lillian was seen several times for individual treatment by Miss Mayer. She was able to describe her anger and her hopeless feelings about her life, her children and the place she lived. As a result, with the help of her worker, Lillian was able to get other occupants of the apartment building to go with her and to complain to the landlord about the decrepit conditions in his building. The man refused to help, saying he could not afford to do so. Then, Lillian, again with her neighbors' help and the guidance of the center, went to a Legal Aid facility. Through this agency's help, pressure was brought to bear on the landlord and measures were instituted to rid the building of roaches and rats. Finally, Lillian was referred, at her request, to a family planning clinic. Thus, through a call for crisis intervention, the many services of the Community Mental Health Center were brought into play in order to assist two members of the catchment area who were unable to resolve a critical episode without professional support.

SECONDARY PREVENTION

Like primary prevention, secondary prevention again focuses on a population that resides in a catchment area. Within the actual population, there is a *statistical* population, that is, a group that is likely to develop mental illness because of stress which is *probable,* rather than actual. To better understand this, imagine a biostatistician employed in a city public health agency. Such a worker, after studying data of 1971, might conclude that X per cent of diagnosed postpartum psychosis arose in 21 to 24 year old primiparas within a specific geographic area. From these findings, health officials might predict that 1972 would probably show an incidence of XX per cent of postpartum psychoses in the specific age group within the given geographic area. The identification of this *probable* or *statistical* population would alert mental health workers to the need for additional primary prevention techniques and early case finding and the treatment which characterizes secondary prevention.

Secondary prevention reduces prevalence of mental disorders by shortening the duration of illness through early case finding and prompt, effective treatment. Effectiveness of secondary prevention methods is reflected by disability rates in the population at large following a long-term program of this type of prevention.

Target Groups for Secondary Prevention

Community mental health workers in a given area identify the prevailing types of groups and "high-risk" populations within them. This is accomplished by gathering information regarding cultural backgrounds of the community dwellers, family structures and the agencies used for health purposes in the community. Leaders in the area are identified and contacts with them are established. Such people are often priests or ministers, neighborhood midwives, or housewives who act as spokesmen in the occasional meetings attended by the groups. (Parent-Teacher Association meetings provide such an example, as do protest groups.)

In an inner city center located where there is heavy industry, personnel from the center might be interested in studying employed workers within the catchment area. The center personnel might be particularly concerned with that group of workers who are frequently absent, or the group who make numerous visits to the medical office for minor accidents. Again, they might focus on those workers who change jobs frequently. Any of these behaviors may reflect underlying problems which if explored in their early stages could prevent long, disabling and disruptive illnesses. If the center is situated in a small college town, special attention might be given to incoming students, those who were on a warning list for unsatisfactory grades, or that group of students who frequent the infirmary. In a college setting, other groups deserving special attention would be those who sustain significant losses, such as that of a parent, boy or girl friend, or a rejection by a social club. Another group facing potential disability are those known to be using drugs.

Agents of Intervention in Secondary Prevention

As has been discussed, the professional staff of community mental health centers is usually small, and much of the work done with the community is actually conducted by members from the community itself, who are supervised by professional personnel. Thus, a small staff is able to make its effectiveness felt by a large group through the consultation process. In the case of the center situated in an inner city locale, high-risk groups in factories would be appropriately identified and dealt with by foremen, supervisors and the industrial nurse. Occasionally employment personnel might also be utilized. These individuals would be trained and supervised by the community mental health personnel via the consultation process. The therapeutic processes taught them would be utilized for secondary prevention.

In the small college town a community mental health center might look to student health services personnel, faculty, housemothers, and the deans of students for assistance in identifying vulnerable persons and also in treating these people so that their minor problems would not grow and develop into major disabling ones. Again the goal would be secondary prevention.

In the following example, a community mental health nurse was evaluating the characteristics of her catchment area by working with neighborhood assistants in the antipoverty program. Of particular interest to the nurse was the plight of preschoolers who had inadequate play areas and supervision. The isolation of their young mothers was also noted. Consequently this nurse was placed in an observation nursery school, which involved participation by the parents through a discussion group composed of mothers. The nurse became a co-leader of the group. She also interacted and intervened with the children in the play area. The activity was organized to foster healthy socialization experiences for the children and to promote communication and learning among the parent or mother group. The children and adults did not have any diagnosed problems, but as a result of living in an atmosphere of cultural deprivation they were vulnerable to many psychosocial stresses. Thus, they were identified as a "high-risk" population. When one of the children *did* begin to manifest behavior indicative of emotional disturbance, the nurse alerted the mental health team. In the work with this child, secondary prevention techniques were utilized.

> Lisa was three and one half years old. She attended the nursery school on a regular basis with her mother. Lisa was somewhat withdrawn and would not defend her possessions when other children took them. She would play by herself or with one other person, preferably an adult. Lisa avoided small group play. She moved about with head bowed and little shoulders bent. Lisa had a speech problem also, and many people could not understand her. Some shunned her for this reason. Lisa tried to communicate verbally, but she became extremely frustrated at times.
> The nurse observed Lisa's behavior and wished to help, so she met with Lisa and her family. To develop a coordinated treatment plan for the family, it was necessary to arrange a meeting in which representatives from the various agencies involved with the family would assemble to discuss the situation. The goals of this meeting were to establish an avenue of communication, to determine the services to be provided by each of several agencies, and to ascertain the best way for the mental health workers to assist. Frag-

mentation and duplication of services were to be avoided so that a coordinated treatment plan would emerge.

Lisa responded well to the various modalities of therapy used. Family therapy, speech therapy and involvement in enrichment activities at school provided the necessary media for Lisa's growth. She gradually became more spontaneous in play and more aggressive; her peer relationships improved. Before long her speech also was modified. Later Lisa was able to become involved in Head Start, where her behavior continued to improve.

When symptoms indicative of emotional difficulties became overt, therapeutic interventions were introduced which prevented further deterioration of functioning. Lisa was never labeled a "mental health case" and, consequently, her family did not have to deal with that stigma. This was possible because a nurse from the community mental health center was available to identify the early stages of a problem. She then took steps to alter the problem before it became a full-blown illness. In this case, a high risk group was identified and an individual member of that group was treated, utilizing secondary prevention methods.

TERTIARY PREVENTION

The third element of the community mental health program is called tertiary prevention. It includes treatment and rehabilitation services for those persons who have had diagnosed psychiatric illnesses. The main objective of tertiary prevention is to treat and rehabilitate expatients so effectively that their residual disability rate is minimized. Such an objective requires careful follow-up.

Target Groups for Tertiary Prevention

Community mental health centers are, for the most part, connected with state hospitals or psychiatric units of general hospitals. The inpatient unit is characteristically utilized as a "back up" facility to which patients can be admitted as necessary if they are unable to tolerate the stresses of their community. When the hospital is used in this way, it becomes a dynamic, therapeutic element of the total treatment plan, rather than a more traditional, custodially oriented cul-de-sac. The mental hospital, in effect, is one of many agencies that can be employed in the therapeutic program for community members. Patients can be admitted briefly or, if necessary, for more extensive periods.

The center might utilize a state hospital for the acute phase of treatment for alcoholics or drug addicts who need close monitoring of their physiological conditions. Individuals experiencing reactive depressions who demonstrate poor impulse control might be hospitalized briefly until impulsive behavior is no longer a factor in their safety. Schizophrenics who are generally ambulatory but experience transient episodes of serious delusions which threaten the safety of others might need to be committed for varying lengths of time. The postpartum mother who suffers a psychosis after the birth of each of her children would also need the facilities of the hospital briefly after each delivery. Important for all these patients is the presence of a community mental health center from which their aftercare can be supervised and co-ordinated, thus permitting earlier discharge from the confines of the hospital before chronic hospitalization patterns of living emerge as more serious problems than the admitting complaint.

Agents for Intervention in Tertiary Prevention

There are numerous organized groups that meet the needs of ex-patients. The primary function of the community mental health center in utilizing these groups is to make the referral and to check periodically —usually through consultation—to see that the referred client is pro-gressing effectively in the program. Such groups as Alcoholics Anonymous and Synanon (for drug addicts) are examples of organized groups that are effective. Also useful is a more widely organized group for neurotics who have been hospitalized. The center, itself, might institute some type of group activity if such an opportunity does not already exist in the community. Some centers choose to see aftercare patients in groups on a monthly or bimonthly basis; the object is to see that the individual is adjusting satisfactorily to the stresses of living outside the hospital. If this is not the case, personnel from the center explore the situation further via home visits and meetings with the family or those with whom the patient lives; they try to iron out in-cipient problems before they reach such proportions that the patient must be returned to the hospital. In centers that utilize monthly group meetings with expatients, those who are on maintenance doses of drugs are seen briefly by a psychiatrist, and changes or renewals of prescrip-tions are made.

Tertiary prevention is also employed when expatients are rehabili-tated through vocational placement or training. It is sometimes difficult for those who have been ill for protracted lengths of time to find work. The community mental health center is an ideal agency to test the expatient's capabilities and to prepare him for the job interview. The social worker in the center is often the person who can help the former patient to feel more secure as he anticipates his first attempts at selling himself.

For the child or teen-ager who has been severely ill, the center is a coordinating agency and a treatment source. In the former instance, a worker might go into the school to which the child will return and consult with teachers, principal and school nurse, identifying with them the probable sources of stress for the child and the means at their disposal for helping to make the transition from hospital to school and home less traumatic. Periodic therapeutic interviews might be carried on concurrently between the child and a mental health worker.

In this way, the child receives support from two major sources. The parents would also be counselled concurrently by center personnel.

Ethel T., a 37 year old Negro mother of six, was admitted to the aftercare program of the community mental health center after she was discharged from the state mental hospital following her sixth admission to that institution. Mrs. T. had a diagnosis of paranoid schizophrenia. She had become floridly ill after the births of each of her children. During several episodes of psychosis, Mrs. T. had threatened to kill her husband, a day laborer.

Mrs. T. was placed in a mixed group of chronically ill patients who were all receiving medication. The group was conducted by a nurse who, after each monthly session, reported briefly to the psychiatrist about the condition of each patient. The doctor then saw the patients individually, just long enough to renew their medications and see that each of them was in satisfactory physical health.

Mrs. T. did not converse spontaneously, but she did seem to listen to the other group members as they spoke. The nurse visited Mrs. T. in her home also and noted that the patient was caring adequately for her six children. In the fourth month of caring for Mrs. T., the nurse noticed that her patient's abdomen was beginning to protrude suspiciously. She asked Mrs. T. if she were pregnant, but the patient denied the possibility. The nurse looked at Mrs. T. carefully the next month; by now she was certain that the protrusion had grown and that Mrs. T. must be pregnant. After the group meeting, when she reported to the psychiatrist, the nurse mentioned her concern. The psychiatrist saw Mrs. T. and made the same observation, but when he questioned her, he was told that she was "just fat." The psychiatrist referred this patient to the obstetrical clinic but she refused to go. After another four weeks, the nurse and psychiatrist contacted Mr. T. and asked him to come in for a conference. At the meeting between the three, Mr. T. was told of the staff's concern for Mrs. T. The husband promised to get his wife to the obstetrical clinic.

The husband kept his word and a report was sent back to the mental health clinic confirming the nurse's and psychiatrist's suspicion. Mrs. T. steadfastly denied her condition. It was decided to remove this patient from the monthly group and see her individually at weekly intervals. In spite of her intensive therapy, Mrs. T. became progressively worse. As the fetus within her began to move, Mrs. T. explained that this was the devil within her and that she had been raped by Christ.

The nurse who led Mrs. T.'s group and who had followed her closely contacted the nursing staff on the postpartum unit where Mrs. T. would deliver. She explained some of her patient's problems and alerted the staff to the type of behavior that Mrs. T. was likely to display. The nurse left her telephone number, both at the center and at home, so that the floor staff might get in touch with her if Mrs. T. presented problems that they felt unable to handle.

Mrs. T. did eventually go into labor; however, her denial was so strong that she did not indicate that she had any discomfort until she had bulging membranes and was in danger of delivering in the street. Her husband rushed her to the hospital where she delivered a healthy male child in the elevator. Mrs. T.'s first two postpartum days were relatively uneventful. On the third day, however, she awoke threatening to kill the doctor. She addressed persons in the room who were not visible to the nurses and threatened them when they asked to whom she was speaking.

Both the mental health nurse and the psychiatrist were called. Mrs. T. was placed under the special care of the nurse over a 16-hour period, but all efforts of the nurse failed to give Mrs. T. a firmer attachment to reality. The patient was placed on high doses of tranquilizers but to no avail. On the fifth day postpartum Mrs. T. had to be transferred to the state hospital because of her severely psychotic behavior, which posed a threat to her safety and the safety of those around her.

MENTAL HEALTH CONSULTATION

The term "consultation" has run through much of the previous discussion. It is apparent that through the consultative process, the professional personnel of the community mental health center are able to "stretch" themselves so that they, in effect, are treating far more individuals and groups than they would otherwise have time to reach.

Caplan, one of the foremost authorities in the field, has defined mental health consultation as follows: "The interaction between two professional persons—the consultant who is a specialist, and the consultee, who invokes his help in regard to a current work problem with which he is having some difficulty and which he has decided is within the consultant's area of competence."[2] This process places professional responsibility for the client with the consultee. The consultant may offer suggestions and recommendations; however, the consultee is free to accept or reject any part of the help. Thus, an elementary schoolteacher may seek aid as she attempts to help one of her charges. The mental health consultant mentions other appropriate agencies that could augment the teacher's efforts. The teacher may use all the consultant's ideas or she may pick among them and decide what seems feasible to her as she perceives the client (the student) and his family. If the teacher wishes, she is free to reject all advice. In any event, the teacher maintains primary responsibility for her client, the student.

Another aspect of mental health consultation is that the consultant meets with the consultee not only to support him in his current professional work but in order to educate him further so that in future encounters of a similar type, the consultee might be able to proceed effectively without additional help.

ROLES FOR THE NURSE IN COMMUNITY MENTAL HEALTH

There are a variety of positions and roles for the registered nurse who is interested in community mental health. The field is exceedingly flexible, and nurses entering it have many options available to them. A distinct disadvantage to the beginning practitioner is that roles are often indistinct. Actually, there is a remarkable amount of role blurring which makes it difficult for the young nurse to "find a niche" and later to say with any certainty just what her role is.

For the recently graduated, inexperienced nurse, the inpatient service of a community mental health center is likely to be the most appropriate placement. Here the nurse can develop and refine her skills as a therapeutic agent. The more dynamic programs will utilize a therapeutic milieu and will focus on early discharge for its patients. In this type of setting, the nurse can expect to take an active part in the daily living of her patients in the clinical area. She will be expected to speak spontaneously in the ward meetings, to interact therapeutically with patients, and to plan and carry through on measures developed by the treatment team for individual patients and groups.

The nurse must develop an understanding of the culture of the people she serves. This awareness is more than a theoretical grasp of the subject, being a living, usable concept, for the nurse in this setting becomes part of the people with whom she works. She is, in a sense, absorbed into their living patterns and works from the inside out, rather than as a "sometimes visitor." One facet of community mental health is an attempt to bridge the gap between "middle-classism" and the disadvantaged groups usually served in community mental health centers. Only in this way can the health team hope to reach the many who would otherwise remain on the periphery of health attention, untouched by efforts toward health maintenance or the prevention of illness.

Other services of the community mental health center that will shortly be appropriate for the developing psychiatric nurse are the day, night or weekend hospital. These services are likely to be housed in the inpatient area; the difference is that there is a mobile population who come and go according to their own individual needs. The psychiatric nurse functioning in such an area will need some sophistication because the activities she engages in with patients who were hospitalized over a 24-hour period must now be compressed into a shorter time interval; that is to say, the behavioral outcomes of the nurse's therapy must be attained in a briefer interval. Thus, the nurse must have sufficient sophistication to identify her goals in a shorter time and then pick from among her repertoire of plans to find the most effective one for a particular patient in the given time that he will be present on the unit. By definition, then, the psychiatric nurse on the day, night or weekend unit needs some experience behind her so that she has past successful (and unsuccessful) experiences from which to draw.

In addition, the nurse on such a unit must cope with a constantly changing set of stresses to her patients. The individual who leaves the unit intermittently goes out into a community that represents to him the problems which made him ill. In re-experiencing these elements the patient will need varying quantities of support and encouragement to move ahead and grapple with the problems as they present themselves. The nurse in this type of unit needs much flexibility and innovative skill so that she can pace herself according to the ever-changing situations confronting her patients. If this unit is contained within the more traditional setting for continuously hospitalized patients, in addition to the nurse's other responsibilities, she must have the ability to "take a reading" on the ward atmosphere. She must recognize that the incoming and outgoing patients have some effect on the remaining patients and, at times, she must stand ready to modify that effect.

The psychiatric nurse who has attained some skill is now ready to move into the outpatient branch of the program. Contained here is a refreshing and delightful mixture of psychiatric nursing and the public health approach. The nurse will still deal primarily with psychiatric patients, but added to the factors under consideration will be the ambulatory status of the patient and his intramural exchange with family or neighbors. The nurse who treats outpatients will probably spend some time in the field, visiting in homes, evaluating situations and helping to situate patients in new settings. The nurse in this type of work will spend some of her time in an agency close to supervision and instant help, if needed. She will spend part of her time on her own, seeing patients away from the hospital. This is enjoyable work for the psychiatric nurse who has developed some competence and self-confidence.

This nurse focuses on the neighborhood population *in the community,* rather than having them come into the health facility. To accomplish this she may become part of various neighborhood projects. Thus, a nurse might work with the group for better housing conditions; she might march with mothers demonstrating about food stamps; or she might help with a neighborhood clean-up campaign.

For highly sophisticated psychiatric nurses, the emergency services of the community mental health center will prove challenging. Here, crisis intervention techniques are used. The nurse has the opportunity and, indeed, is expected to function at a moment's notice and with a minimum of consultation. Usually the emergency services of a center are attached to one of the previously discussed services. In some settings the 24-hour telephone service is based on the unit where inpatients are housed. With such an arrangement, the community agencies are aware of the telephone number to call for psychiatric help. It is likely that the police would utilize the service frequently when they are called into service on an emergency basis. The nurse receiving a request for aid notifies the team that is on call. Usually a team is composed of a psychiatric nurse and a psychiatrist or a social worker and a psychiatrist. The team accompanies the police, or goes alone if the police are not involved, to the place where the emergency exists. They make an evaluation and disposition based on their observations. In some cases the team is not called. The person answering the phone is expected to evaluate from the phone conversation the emergent nature of the situation and then to handle the problem by phone, if possible, to call in the team, if necessary, or to arrange for therapeutic intervention at a planned time. The psychiatric nurse handling the telephone service must be able to evaluate, and she must know what to do about the situation she has assessed. Sophistication is necessary to assign priorities.

In a typical case the nurse on duty answered a call from the police at 9:30 P.M. The police officer stated he had just taken a 17 year old, married, pregnant woman to the emergency room at one of the local hospitals for treatment of an overdose of sleeping medication. It developed that the young woman was to have a gastric lavage. Afterward she would probably be returned to her home. The officer wanted the crisis team to assess the situation. Consequently a home visit was made at 11:30 P.M. by the nurse and the physician. It was decided that the husband would remain with the patient for the night. An appointment was made for the couple to be interviewed on the following morning at the community mental health center. A treatment plan was developed and follow-up care was provided.

For the most experienced practitioner, the remaining services of the community mental health center provide a challenge. Consultation and education services must be made available to community agencies and professional personnel. The psychiatric nurse who undertakes these functions must be a competent practitioner. In addition, she must acquire knowledge of a wide range of issues—social, economic, political and administrative. These will enable her to plan and to implement programs that focus not only on individual patients but on the community of which they are a part. The psychiatric nurse who assumes this post must, of necessity, know *how* to consult. She must be a proved teacher and clinician. Such an individual is typically the product of an experiential background and an accredited Master's program.

It is seen that there are limitless levels of functioning in a community mental health center. The nurse who wishes to embark on a career in this area will not find herself without challenge.

REFERENCES

1. Berlin, I.: Secondary Prevention. *In* Freedman, A., and Kaplan, H. (eds.) : *Comprehensive Textbook of Psychiatry.* Baltimore, The Williams & Wilkins Co., 1967.
2. Caplan, G.: *Principles of Preventive Psychiatry.* New York, Basic Books, Inc., 1964, pp. 212-213.

3. Caplan, G., and Caplan, R.: Developments of Community Psychiatry Concepts. *In Comprehensive Textbook of Psychiatry,* op. cit.
4. Freedman, A.: Tertiary Prevention. *In Comprehensive Textbook of Psychiatry,* op. cit.
5. Gottesfeld, F.: A Study of the Role of Paraprofessionals in Community Mental Health. *Community Mental Health Journal,* 6:285-288, August, 1970.
6. Greenblatt, M.: Role of Community Mental Health Worker. *In Comprehensive Textbook of Psychiatry,* op. cit.
7. Hargreaves, N., and Richards, H.: Nursing in Response to Social Crisis. *Nurs. Clin. N. Amer.* 6 (No. 4):674, December, 1960.
8. Joint Commission on Mental Illness and Health: *Action for Mental Health.* New York, John Wiley & Sons, Inc., 1961.
9. Leininger, M.: Community Psychiatric Nursing. *Perspectives in Psychiatric Care,* 7 (No. 1):10-20, January-February, 1969.
10. Lowenkopf, E., and Zwerling, I.: Psychiatric Services in a Neighborhood Health Center. *Amer. J. Psychiat.* 77 (No. 7): 917, January, 1971.
11. Ozarin, L., *et al.:* Experience with Community Mental Health Centers. *Amer. J. Psychiat.* 77 (No. 7):912, January, 1971.
12. Stokes, G.: Extending the Role of the Psychiatric-Mental Health Nurse in Community Mental Health—An Overview. *Nurs. Clin. N. Amer.* 5 (No. 4):635, December, 1970.
13. Stubblebine, J. M., and Decker, B.: Are Urban Mental Health Centers Worth It? *Amer. J. Psychiat.* 77 (No. 7):908-910, January, 1971.
14. Visotsky, H.: Primary Prevention. *In Comprehensive Textbook of Psychiatry,* op. cit.
15. Whittington, H.: *Psychiatry in the American Community.* New York, International Universities Press, Inc., 1966.

SUGGESTED READINGS

Adamson, F.: A Mental Health Consultation at Work. *Am. J. Nursing,* 70 (No. 10): 2164-2166, October, 1970.

The reader is again given the opportunity to see the new kinds of roles evolving in the community mental health format.

Anderson, M., Glasser, B., and Manning, M. J.: Nursing and Social Work Roles in Cooperative Home Care and Treatment of the Mentally Ill. *Nursing Outlook,* 11 (No. 2):112-114, February, 1963.

This is a rather exciting discussion of the work done in one outpatient agency. It is rather unusual because the authors focus on collaborative roles primarily, rather than functions of the nurse. It is interesting to read how the authors perceived the differences in their approaches based on their basic preparation.

Arnson, A., and Collins, R.: Treating Low Income Patients in a Neighborhood Center. *Hospital and Community Psychiatry,* 21:111-113, April, 1970.

This is a good article. It is well written and worthy of careful reading because it differentiates middle class orientation from that of low income groups. This is a realistic focus for the serious student of community work.

Barckley, A.: The Nurse in Preventive Psychiatry. *Nursing Outlook,* 8 (No. 4):252-253, May, 1960.

The reader can once more see how another agency is set up and how the nurse evolves her role in that particular setting.

Boone, D., and Brown, B.: The Role of the Mental Health Nurse in a Mental Health Public Health Setting. *Mental Hygiene,* 47:197-198, April, 1963.

The reader should try to locate this article because it is a classic. The authors are well informed in the area of community mental health. Miss Boone is a mental health nurse consultant and senior nurse officer with the public health service (NIMH). Dr. Brown is also connected with the federal service.

Bulbulyan, A.: Nurses in a Community Mental Health Center. *Am. J. Nursing,* 64 (No. 2):328-331, February, 1969.

This is one of the unusually well written, particularly descriptive articles that the reader must not miss. The author goes into great detail to explain how various workers (nurses) in her agency function. This is an extremely valuable addition to the nursing literature.

Eller, F.: A Psychiatric Nurse's Experience in Community Nursing. *Perspectives in Psychiatric Care,* 3:13-28, 1965.

The article describes the work of the author in managing a patient in the community.

LePage, A.: A New Role for the Psychiatric Nurse. *Nursing Outlook,* 7 (No. 12):709-710, December, 1959.

This is an earlier article which, the reader will see, still focuses on the hospital as the basic point of reference. It is also seen, however, that the nurse is beginning to consider moving out of the institution to reach her patients.

Mistr, V.: Community Nursing Service for Psychiatric Patients. *Perspectives in Psychiatric Care,* 6 (No. 1):36-41, January-February, 1968.

This presents a well organized, lucidly written discussion of the nurse's role in outpatient care of psychiatric patients.

chapter 11

OTHER TYPES
OF THERAPY

SOMATIC THERAPIES

CHEMOTHERAPY

During the past 20 years the practice of psychiatry has changed radically. Psychotropic drugs which flooded the market in the fifties and sixties have made possible new techniques in the care of mentally ill patients and in the treatment of their diseases. In keeping with movement away from harsh and brutal management of mental illness, the past 20 years have brought us from the dramatic and sometimes dangerous therapies, such as insulin coma shock therapy, electroshock therapy and psychosurgery, to chemotherapy.

Today, drugs are used liberally. They are not "cure-alls" but are used in conjunction with other appropriate treatment. Through drug therapy, hyperactive patients can be sedated so that they do not become exhausted and face physical deterioration or even death from exhaustion. Isolation or "seclusion" rooms are becoming obsolete; patients need not be removed from the group in order to maintain or regain control. Wet packs, camisoles, other mechanical restraining devices, and deep sleep therapy are used infrequently. Many traditional institutions have borne witness to the efficacy of drug therapy as their doors have been unlocked and patients of long standing have been given the opportunity to move about freely. It has been gratifying to see victims of 20 to 30 years' hospitalization able to leave the confines of the ward and live in the community.

The mental hospital has become, like the general hospital, a treatment center for the curing of disease; it is no longer an establishment occupied with the management of deviant behavior which is intolerable to the community. The mental hospital has become a place of hope for the future rather than an asylum for failures of the past.

Treatment of Psychiatric Disorders with Drugs

The majority of doctors who diagnose mental disease and treat patients with drugs use the drugs as an adjunctive therapy. That is, chemotherapy is utilized along with psychotherapy, social therapies, and intervention in the patient's familial, educational, and vocational life. The large array of drugs available permits the physician to find that specific agent which is most effective for a particular patient. Though a variety of drugs may be generally antipsychotic in their action, antidepressants, or anti-anxiety agents, many drugs within each category have effects which are specific. For instance, some antipsychotic agents calm the patient because of their muscle relaxant properties, whereas others make the patient less anxious because of their sedating effects.

Finding the correct drug for a specific patient does not end the quest. Establishing the effective dosage of that drug is also highly individual. There are great variations in the range of drug tolerance. Some patients can tolerate only 25 mg. of a chemical agent, whereas others may be able to handle 1000 mg. daily.

To find the most effective dosage, a patient's medication is slowly increased from a minimal dose to the point where side effects are unacceptable, and then the dosage is dropped back to the highest dose that preserves optimum improvement with minimum toxicity. This process requires the close attention of the physician during the first month of chemotherapy and the careful observations of the nurse who administers the drug.

The Nurse's Responsibility in Establishing and Maintaining the Drug Regimen

When a drug is ordered, the nurse usually initiates the process that terminates with the prescribed chemical agent's arrival on the ward from the pharmacy. Her work is only begun, however, for the nurse must administer the drug to the patient and then observe for the effects of the drug and report them to the prescribing physician.

Administering psychotropic drugs is sometimes complicated by the patient's feelings about the prescribed medication. Some patients do not want to take drugs because they fear harmful consequences to their physical health and self-esteem. To some, accepting the need for medication is an admission that they are ill. Some fear control by their drug.

Indeed, some fear getting well because they have come to rely on their "sick" roles. When the nurse has secured the patient's cooperation in taking the drug, the second vital part of her task is at hand.

It is important for the psychiatric nurse to be familiar with the drugs she administers. It is necessary for her to understand specific drug action so that effectiveness can be evaluated and untoward responses noted and reported. The nurse must be familiar with usual dosage ranges so that errors can be minimized. Also, some patients for whom drugs are prescribed will be unable to cooperate in reporting day-to-day changes in their physical and psychological sensations which are drug related. Changes described by an observant nurse will help the doctor to ascertain the proper drug level.

> Dennis Y., a middle-aged lathe operator, was admitted to the ward from the emergency room. He had been brought to the hospital in a police cruiser. The officers reported that they had been called to the Y. family's home to settle a domestic quarrel.
>
> Mr. Y. was found in the backyard chasing his grown son with an ax. He was heard screaming as he raced about swinging the ax, "I'm going to kill you. I'm going to kill you when I get you!"
>
> Examination on admission revealed a middle-aged man in essentially good physical health who was able to respond appropriately to the examiner. The patient was highly disturbed, however, and kept insisting that "that fellow" who claimed to be his son was an intruder and the patient felt he had to kill him in order to protect himself and his wife. The patient was admitted to the psychiatric service of the hospital.
>
> Dennis was immediately given 100 mg. of chlorpromazine hydrochloride (Thorazine) intramuscularly. He was put to bed and nurses were assigned to him on a rotating basis. In the next 72 hours, Dennis, who was receiving 100 mg. of Thorazine every 4 hours, became more disturbed. He was found to be developing paranoid delusions about the hospital staff. He told the resident and the nurses that he knew they were all part of a secret society pledged to his destruction. The psychiatrist decided to increase the Thorazine dosage. Dennis was now given 800 mg. over a 24-hour period. The patient became physically more manageable, but his delusions persisted with sporadic episodes of violence. Again the drug dosage was modified. Now he was injected with 250 mg. per dose every 6 hours.
>
> The nurses noted that Dennis slept much of the time on this drug regimen; however, he seemed less frightened of them and was able to cooperate when aroused and given instructions. It was decided to hold Dennis at this level for several days to see if he would build up tolerance to the drug and be able to participate in simple ward activities. Eventually the patient seemed to become more alert. The drug also permitted him to enter into a more trusting relationship with his therapist, so doctor and patient could begin to examine the validity of Dennis' ideas. The patient was soon more rational, and the doctor felt it was appropriate to lower the drug dosage slightly. Dennis was then given 150 mg. of Thorazine every 6 hours. He tolerated the reduction well without showing increased delusional ideas and erratic behavior. At the

same time, he was more alert and the side effects of dehydration and dizziness ceased. Thus, the appropriate level of drug was established for this patient.

The nurse who administers medication communicates the correct expectations for the medication she dispenses. Thus, the nurse giving disulfiram (Antabuse) to an alcoholic who is struggling to overcome his desire to have "just one," or the nurse giving methadone to a drug-addicted patient, needs to convey to the patient that she, too, wants the patient to win his struggle. She needs to convey her confidence in the patient's strength and her conviction that the drugs she administers can and will aid the patient in his battle. The effect of drugs can be influenced by the attitude of those giving them.

Drug Therapy in the Treatment of Thought Disorders

It has been found through extensive research that antipsychotic agents are most useful in treating disorders marked by psychotic disorganization of thought and behavior when psychomotor activity is also altered. These drugs rapidly reduce panic, fear and hostility. Relief of severe emotional tension (excitement, restlessness, aggression, anxiety, agitation, panic) is often followed by the lessening of hallucinatory and delusional phenomena. When the antipsychotic agents become effective, combative, destructive, antisocial and withdrawn behavior decreases, creating an opportunity for hospitalized patients to enter into psychotherapy and adjunctive therapies such as occupational therapy and group therapy.[2] Though other somatic therapies, i.e., electroconvulsive therapy (ECT) and insulin coma, are used in the treatment of schizophrenia, their efficacy has not been clearly established nor have studies shown these somatic therapies to be more effective than drug therapy.[1, 4]

Table 1 lists antipsychotic agents; they are divided into the four major chemical groups: phenothiazines, butyrophenones, thioxanthenes and reserpines.

The antipsychotic agents are used in acute schizophrenia, manic episodes, involutional and senile psychoses, agitated states (associated with toxic confusional syndromes), agitated depression, Parkinson's disease, Huntington's chorea, acting-out phases of psychoses associated with psychopathic personality, chronic psychoses, and the borderline states in which patients present with extremely weak ego strength and fragile adaptation. These drugs are also useful in psychotic disorders occurring after surgery, with myocardial infarctions or ulcerative colitis, and in pre- and postpartum psychosis.

Drug response to the antipsychotic agents. The vast majority of patients with incipient psychosis respond within a six-week period to drug therapy by showing mood stabilization and regularization of their adaptive and sleep patterns. If perplexity, suspiciousness and psycho-

Table 1. *Antipsychotic Agents**

GENERIC NAME	BRAND NAMES	AVERAGE DAILY DOSAGE RANGE† (P.O.)
A. *Phenothiazines*		
Acetophenazine	Tindal	40-80
Butaperazine	Repoise	15-30
Carphenazine	Proketazine	75-400
Chlorpromazine	Thorazine	60-1600
Fluphenazine	Prolixin, Permitil	12.5-100 mg.
Mesoridazine	Serentil	25-200
Perphenazine	Trilafon	16-64
Piperacetazine	Quide	20-40
Prochlorperazine	Compazine	15-200
Promazine	Sparine	25-300
Propiomazine	Largon	10-40
Thiopropazate	Dartal	30-100
Thioridazine	Mellaril	300-800
Trifluoperazine	Stelazine	4-20
Triflupromazine	Vesprin	100-150
B. *Butyrophenones*		
Haloperidol	Haldol, Serenace	2-15
C. *Thioxanthenes*		
Chlorprothixene	Taractan, Solatran	30-600
Thiothixene	Navane	6-10
D. *Reserpines*		
Deserpidine	Harmonyl	0.1
Reserpine	Serpasil	0.5-5

* These drugs are also known as "major tranquilizers," "ataractics" or "neuroleptics."

† Dosage in milligrams unless otherwise noted.

motor retardation have been characteristic of the illness, the patient may require longer to show progress.

In the paranoid patient, antipsychotic drugs cause a suppression of suspiciousness and thinking disorders; there is also a decrease of communication, decreased spontaneity and limited socialization. In these patients, slight to moderate improvement may be expected from medication.

The excited, panicky patient requires very large doses of phenothiazines. (When giving medication by the intramuscular route, the injection should be deep into the buttocks. Intramuscular chlorpromazine is an irritant and will produce a marked inflammation when used repeatedly.) In schizo-affective patients, the phenothiazines promote a reduction of angry agitation, a decrease in anger, the disappearance of delusional material and flights of ideas. Social participation may then increase. The response of the retarded schizo-affective is less dramatic than the response of other types of schizophrenic patients; there is gradual restoration of normal activity, with loss of suspiciousness and perplexity.

Side effects of the antipsychotic drugs

Central Nervous System Effects

PARKINSON'S SYNDROME. This side effect is characterized by loss of motor control, muscular rigidity, alterations of posture, tremor and autonomic symptoms. Also seen, though less frequently, are mask-like facies, shuffling gait, loss of associated movements, hypersalivation and drooling.

DYSTONIA. There are uncoordinated spasmodic movements of the body and limbs, or coordinated, involuntary, stereotyped rhythmic movements, known as dyskinesis.

INVOLUNTARY MOTOR RESTLESSNESS. This side effect consists of constant pacing and inability to sit still, fidgeting, chewing and lip movements, and finger and leg movements.

All these side effects develop within the first 40 days of phenothiazine therapy. In general, antiparkinsonism medication is effective in their treatment. (Approximately one fourth of the patients treated with antipsychotic agents never develop drug-induced parkinsonism.)[11]

DROWSINESS. This effect occurs in the first few days of treatment and usually lasts one or two weeks, terminating when patients develop tolerance.

CONVULSIONS. Convulsions may occur when high doses of phenothiazines are used, but this is a rare side effect.

Autonomic Nervous System Effects. These side effects include dizziness, faintness, weakness, dry mouth, throat and eyes, nasal congestion, nausea, vomiting, constipation, diarrhea, urinary disturbances, blurred vision and hypostatic hypotension. Inhibition of ejaculation occurs, as do menstrual irregularities. For women, weight gain may be a problem. Galactorrhea is also seen. Nausea and vomiting have been noted upon withdrawal of chlorpromazine, thioridazine and chlorprothixene, generally within the first 48 hours.[11]

Skin and Eye Effects. Pigmentary skin changes have often been noted. They usually consist of a blue-gray metallic discoloration over areas exposed to sunlight. The skin changes often start with a tan or golden brown color and progress to slate gray, metallic blue or purple. Eye changes have been observed after long-term high dosage of chlorpromazine. Corneal opacities are seen, and in some patients the conjunctivae are discolored by a brown pigment. Research indicates that eye changes are associated with skin reaction. In the cases of eye changes, lens changes are associated with corneal changes. These side effects seem to be dose related, with an appreciably greater incidence at high doses.

Rare Side Effects

JAUNDICE. Jaundice occurs within the first month of treatment. It is preceded by prodromal fever, malaise and gastrointestinal symptoms, followed by liver enlargement, tenderness, pruritus and a slight lessening of the malaise at the onset of jaundice. The jaundice is usually self-limited. It is thought that this condition is probably due to a hypersensitivity reaction which causes small bile duct obstructions.[11] Most patients recover spontaneously within a few weeks of the discontinuation of medication.

AGRANULOCYTOSIS. Agranulocytosis occurs in the first six weeks of treatment. It develops in a few hours and is accompanied by sore throat, ulcerations and high temperatures. If the drug is discontinued and the initial phase is not fatal, the white blood cell count returns to normal within seven to ten days and recovery is rapid.

Because of these complications it is wise to see that appropriate blood and liver studies are done every week during the first month of treatment, every two weeks in the second month, and monthly until the sixth month. If symptoms of side effects have not developed by that time, it is likely that they will not appear.

Drug Therapy in the Treatment of the Affective Disorders

The treatment of the affective disorders was greatly enhanced by the discovery of the imipramine-like drugs and the monoamine oxidase inhibitors in the late 1950's. All these drugs are effective in mood elevation. In addition, psychostimulants have found a valued place in the treatment of depressed patients. Table 2 lists the mood active drugs. They are divided into the tricyclics (or imipramine-like drugs), the monoamine oxidase inhibitors (MAO inhibitors) and the stimulants.

Table 2. Mood Active Drugs

GENERIC NAME	BRAND NAME	AVERAGE DAILY DOSE*
A. *Tricyclics*		
Amitriptyline	Elavil	75-150
Desipramine	Pertofrane, Norpramin	50-100
Imipramine	Tofranil	100-150
Nortriptyline	Aventyl	20-100
Protriptyline	Vivactil	10-60
B. *MAO Inhibitors*		
Furazolidone	Furoxone	400
Isocarboxazid	Marplan	10-30
Nialamide	Niamide	75-200
Pargyline	Eutonyl	10-25
Phenelzine	Nardil	30-75
Tranylcypromine	Parnate	20-60
C. *Stimulants*		
Amphetamine	Benzedrine	5-30
Dextroamphetamine	Dexedrine	5-30
Deanol	Deaner	100-300
Methamphetamine	Amphedroxyn, Desoxyn	5-15
Methylphenidate	Ritalin	20-30

* In milligrams unless otherwise noted.

Drug response to the mood active agents. Agitated depressions respond quickly to the phenothiazines used in conjunction with anti-parkinsonism medication. Beneficial effects upon agitation and insomnia take place within the first few days after treatment begins. When the appropriate drug levels are reached, the depressed patient's complaints lose vigor. Usually after two to three weeks the complaints lessen and may disappear. In some cases, however, patients do better on a combination of phenothiazines and imipramine. For a few, no psychotropic drug seems to alleviate their symptoms.

Some neurotic patients with chronic, persistent type of depressions do not benefit from the major antidepressants; some show marked benefit from either an imipramine-like drug or an MAO inhibitor. When an antidepressant drug is effective with these patients, the change may be so subtle that the patient is not aware of it. In patients who are helped, personality changes include a more self-assertive, outgoing, extraverted manner. The patient's increased self-assertiveness may lead to difficulties with employers, colleagues, therapists and relatives who are used to dealing with the patient as a passive, compliant person. Such patients become problems for nurses when they refuse medication, saying the drugs do not treat their main problem.

The imipramine-type antidepressants. It is important that patients started on these drugs be kept on them for at least four weeks, since improvement may not be seen sooner.

Side Effects. Many somatic complaints associated with antidepressant drugs are commonly associated with depression. Thus, it is necessary to evaluate the patient's complaints in terms of their being associated with the drug or with the disease.

CENTRAL NERVOUS SYSTEM EFFECTS. Imipramine and amitriptyline may cause a persistent, fine, rapid tremor, usually in the upper extremities and very occasionally in the tongue. Twitching, convulsions, paresthesias, peroneal palsies, sudden falls and ataxia may rarely occur. In some instances insomnia is present, though there is often a sleep regularization effect by the drugs. Both imipramine and amitriptyline occasionally bring about angry states, as well as manic and schizophrenic excitement. Visual hallucinations of a mescaline type have been reported on daily doses of imipramine approximating 300 mg.[11]

AUTONOMIC SIDE EFFECTS. Dry mouth, palpitations, tachycardia, loss of visual accommodation, postural hypotension, faintness, dizziness, vomiting, profuse sweating, urinary bladder atonia, constipation and aggravation of glaucoma occur. Tricyclic antidepressants and drugs such as the phenothiazines and antiparkinsonism drugs potentiate each other. Such drug action may result in urinary retention and paralytic ileus.

Sweating about the head and neck occur with imipramine. In predisposed patients, the tricyclic drugs may cause acute congestive glaucoma. To prevent this complication, patients should be asked if they have attacks of blurred vision accompanied by ache or pain in or around the eyes or if colored rainbows are seen around lights at night. Occasional galactorrhea has been reported from use of imipramine.

CARDIOVASCULAR EFFECTS. Some changes may be seen on the electrocardiogram (EKG). Postural hypotension occurs in the elderly, as do coronary thrombosis, congestive heart failure and pulmonary emboli.

ALLERGENIC AND HYPERSENSITIVITY EFFECTS. These side effects are usually noted early in treatment, and they subside with a decrease in dosage. Rarely are photosensitivity and jaundice seen. Also seen infrequently are agranulocytosis and other blood dyscrasias. Because of the danger of these side effects, however, *it is important to assume responsibility for knowing that appropriate blood studies are ordered routinely.*

WITHDRAWAL EFFECTS. In patients for whom imipramine dosages above 150 mg. daily have been used, sudden withdrawal may cause nausea, headache, malaise, vomiting, dizziness, chills, cold sweat, abdominal cramps, diarrhea, insomnia, anxiety, restlessness and irritability.

The monoamine oxidase (MAO) inhibitors

Side Effects

CENTRAL NERVOUS SYSTEM EFFECTS. The MAO inhibitors can convert retarded depression into an agitated or anxious depression and may precipitate hypomania or an acute schizophrenic psychosis. The drugs may also cause acute confusions, with disorientation, mental clouding and illusions.

AUTONOMIC SIDE EFFECTS. Dizziness, orthostatic hypotension, epigastric distress, delayed micturition and ejaculation, constipation, dry mouth, impotence and paroxysmal hypertension occur. A syndrome consisting of headache, hypertensive crisis and, rarely, intracranial hemorrhage may also be seen.

THE "CHEESE" REACTION. Hypertensive crisis and headaches occur after the patient has been on MAO inhibitors for long periods. The headaches have a sudden onset and may be associated with high blood pressure, sweating, pallor, chills, painful stiff neck, nausea and vomiting, fright, restlessness and muscle twitching. These attacks, though frightening and often painful, usually disappear within a few hours. Another, more serious syndrome includes sudden onset of severe hypertension, profuse sweating, palpitations, chest pains, apprehension, pallor, headache and collapse. Still a third syndrome includes chest pains, palpitations, sweating, headaches, high blood pressure, pallor and intracranial bleeding. This syndrome may prove fatal. Through research it has been established that these three syndromes (which are actually one syndrome with progressive stages of intensity) are related to diet and drug consumption. Headaches and hypertension crises have occurred within two to 20 hours of ingestion of cheese, particularly cheddar or other cheeses containing large amounts of *tyramine,* which is a pressor amine normally destroyed by MAO. Other foods that contain tyramine are beer, Chianti wine, chicken livers, yeast products, creamy pickled products such as herring, and chocolate. Strong mature cheeses usually have a higher tyramine content than the more bland varieties. Because of this incompatibility, patients on MAO inhibitors should be educated regarding the potential danger of consuming cheese and other foods containing large amounts of tyramine.

It is likely that the doctor ordering antidepressant drugs will have done a thorough work-up of the patient first so that pre-existing conditions that would contraindicate their use will be known. Nonetheless, it is important that the nurse be aware of the inherent dangers of the drugs she administers so that she can observe for early symptoms of adverse reactions. With the antidepressant drugs it is a real problem to distinguish side effects of drugs from symptoms which the patient reports that reflect his depressive condition. Impotence, for instance, is a side effect of the imipramine group. This symptom is also seen in depression, and it is not easy to differentiate the cause of the symptom; however, it is comforting to the anxious patient if he can be told that certain symptoms were expected from the drug's use. Such remarks should be timed judiciously. They should not be made before the symptom appears, because the patient may never have the problem; however, if the situation does arise, it is helpful to the patient to know that it has been anticipated and that the condition is not a new problem with unknown etiology.

The psychomotor stimulants. These agents act directly on the nervous system, and their effects are felt almost immediately, but wear off rapidly. The drugs are used as mood elevators, as appetite depressants and to combat the effects of fatigue and sedation. The psychomotor stimulants are legitimately prescribed for such reasons as mild psychic depression and hyperactivity syndrome in children, as an anorexic agent in obesity and for narcolepsy.

While the drugs are being metabolized, they cause increased motor activity and an upsurge of energy. These feelings are quickly lost, however, when the drug's effects have ceased. In patients with more severe depression, when the drug has worn off the patient is sometimes left with a worse feeling of "let down" than before the medication was used.

Zealous but lazy dieters should be warned that the injudicious use of these types of drugs can be habit-forming. While at first the drug's effects help to curb appetite, if their use is continued too long, the patient can unwittingly become addicted. Removing the medication will leave such an individual so tired and lethargic that activity is not possible. Students studying for examinations and cramming during exam week, truckers using these drugs to stay awake on the highways, and adolescents seeking "thrills" are all vulnerable to the same problem when they have used psychomotor stimulants too long and then, unwittingly, try abruptly to stop using them.

Side effects of the psychomotor stimulants are agitation, cardio-vascular effects, insomnia and mental disorganization leading to psychotic states. These agents should be used with caution and under the care of a physician.

In the following all too typical case, a nursing student discovered one of the dangerous side effects of drug abuse.

> Jill, a vivacious 20 year old junior nursing student at State University, had elected a two-week tour of night duty in Obstetrics. She loved the experience, and after the second night looked forward to returning to the unit each evening. She had classes scheduled in the late afternoon, which caused her some consternation because she could not get into the habit of going to sleep at 8 A.M. Consequently when she did finally fall asleep close to lunchtime, it was all too soon time to arise for class. Jill had connections in the hospital, and one of her friends soon found her a handy supply of amphetamine, "Bennies." This solution was perfect. When Jill awoke after three hours of sleep, she simply popped a pill and went on her way. Jill knew she needed more rest but she didn't have time. In fact, she felt so good that she didn't really even care. During the second week of her night duty experience Jill noticed that she was unduly short with the patients and their new babies. She also realized that she felt a constant fine tremor, and she often caught herself close to tears. Jill was sure that her condition would be remediable as soon as she came off the night tour and stopped taking drugs.
>
> The day after Jill's last night tour, she got up for classes. She reached automatically for her pill and remembered that she was not going to take any more. Slowly she pulled back her outstretched fingers. She could hardly wake up. After sitting on the edge of the bed for a while Jill forced herself to get up and to wash. The cold washcloth felt a million miles away. Jill dressed, feeling as if 20 tons were upon her shoulders. She left her room and made her way to class. During the lecture Jill fought to keep her chin off her chest; she tried to listen to the lecturer but could not concentrate. After class she returned to her room and slept until midnight.
>
> The nursing student awoke feeling refreshed. She dressed and went to the night cafeteria for a sandwich. Soon Jill felt again that she could not keep her head up, so she returned to bed. In the morning, Jill again got out of bed, assuming that she would feel better. However, when she had washed and dressed, Jill realized that she did not feel better. She had to take a "Bennie."
>
> Jill was a smart student and she knew that she was in trouble. She went to the student health clinic and with some embarrassment explained her plight. A programmed regimen was planned and implemented to gradually wean Jill from the drug that her body had come to need physiologically.

Lithium and the treatment of mania. Mania is experienced in the manic-depressive psychosis or in response to antidepressant therapy or ECT. Management of the manic episode requires large doses of phenothiazines, chlorpromazine being preferred because of its soporific effects. (Manic insomnia does not respond well to barbiturate sedation.)[11] Also used are ECT, sedation, wet packs and isolation. Many studies, however, indicate that lithium is the drug of choice in treatment of mania. It is not clear whether the drug shares the antipsychotic properties of the major tranquilizers, but its action is antimanic without the production of sedation. The lithium-treated patient feels appropriate happiness, joy or excitement without manic elation or loss of control.[11]

Lithium, the third element in the periodic table, was demonstrated to be of use in this disorder during the 1960's. Though the drug is considered dangerous by many clinicians, with increase in knowledge concerning its mechanism of action, properties and side effects and with proper clinical and biochemical monitoring, lithium is a reasonably safe drug.[11]

Side Effects. Diarrhea, vomiting and nausea are common during the first few days of therapy. Symptoms of severe toxicity are drowsiness, tinnitus, blurred vision, fatigue, thirst, vertigo, uncertain gait, dry mouth, slight confusion, coarse tremor and muscle twitching. Occasionally reversible EKG changes are noted. An advanced state of lithium intoxication is marked by excessive thirst with accompanying spontaneous increase in fluid intake and urinary output, ataxia, giddiness, tremor, confusion, persistent diarrhea and vomiting, nystagmus and seizures.

Food and salt intake must be maintained despite the patient's nausea. Patients who do not maintain their sodium intake may quickly become toxic. Lithium use requires continual supervision and should not be given to patients with renal or cardiac failure. Such side effects as diarrhea, nausea and vomiting, tremor, thirst, ataxia and giddiness, if ignored, can progress to toxicity, coma and anuria. The first two weeks of treatment should be carefully supervised. Since it takes six to ten days for the drug to become effective, other drugs such as the phenothiazines may be necessary in the initial stages of therapy. Other somatic treatments used successfully are the butyrophenones such as haloperidol and trifluperodil. ECT is also of benefit; however, relapse rates are high and frequently occurring within two or three weeks of the treatment's termination.

Drug Therapy of the Neuroses and Personality Disorders

Sedatives and anti-anxiety agents (minor tranquilizers or non-neuroleptics) are sometimes used to bring about more comfortable states in patients with neuroses or personality disorders. Tables 3 and 4 list nonbarbiturate anti-anxiety agents, sedatives, and nonbarbiturate hypnotics.

Drug response to the anti-anxiety agents. This group of drugs is used to suppress the less severe manifestations of anxiety and tension.

Table 3. *Nonbarbiturate Anti-anxiety Agents and Sedatives*

GENERIC NAME	BRAND NAME	AVERAGE DAILY DOSE*
Buclizine	Softran, Vibozine	50-300
Chlordiazepoxide	Librium	10-100
Chlormethazanone	Trancopal	300-800
Diazepam	Valium	4-40
Doxepin hydrochloride	Sinequan	25-300
Hydroxyphenamate	Listica	600-800
Hydroxyzine	Vistaril, Atarax	75-400
Mephenoxalone	Trepidone	1600
Meprobamate	Miltown, Equanil	600-1200
Oxanamide	Quiactin	1600
Oxazepam	Serax	30-120
Phenaglycodol	Ultran	1200
Tybamate	Solacen	800-3000

* In milligrams unless otherwise noted.

Table 4. *Nonbarbiturate Hypnotics*

GENERIC NAME	BRAND NAME	AVERAGE DAILY DOSE*
Ethchlorvynol	Placidyl	500-1000
Ethinamate	Valmid	0.5 mg.-1 gm.
Glutethimide	Doriden	0.25 mg-1 gm.
Methaqualone	Quaalude	150-300
Methprylon	Noludar	200-400

* In milligrams unless otherwise noted.

Formerly called the "minor tranquilizers," these drugs effect changes that are far different from those of the erstwhile "major tranquilizer" category (now termed antipsychotic agents). The anti-anxiety drugs help to control mild to moderate degrees of emotional upset in patients with neuroses and in normal individuals under unusual stress. Additionally, some of the anti-anxiety agents help to decrease hyperexcitability in such patients as alcoholics in delirium tremens. The anti-anxiety agents have a central depressant action; however, they do not usually bring about soporific effects. Unlike sedatives they do not affect the state of consciousness or psychomotor performance. Some of these agents act as muscle relaxants. Some have antihistaminic or anticonvulsant effects as well. Some are useful in patients in whom depression is a component of the anxiety. It is safe to say that the many types of anti-anxiety agents act in a variety of ways.

Side Effects of the Anti-anxiety Agents. The anti-anxiety agents are relatively safe so long as they are taken as prescribed and are not used along with other drugs which potentiate their effect. A prevalent side effect of these drugs is sedation. This property is potentiated by alcohol and other central nervous system depressants. *Patients should be warned of these effects and cautioned against even mild indulgence in alcohol or the use of other sedative agents while on the prescribed medication.* Other central nervous system effects include blurred vision, diplopia, slurred speech, tremor and hypotension.

Addiction potentialities and paradoxical reactions are also adverse effects of these drugs. To protect the patient against addiction he is cautioned to take his medication only as prescribed, i.e., time and amount. Paradoxical reactions are seen when the patient becomes stimulated or hyperactive or demonstrates an angry outburst or depersonalization. Also reported in this category are difficulty in concentration and thought blocking.

CONVULSIVE THERAPIES

The convulsive therapies have been used since the 16th century when Paracelsus utilized camphor to produce "magnetic" changes in the brain.[12] It was not until 1935, however, that camphor was again used in conjunction with the treatment of mental illness. Since that time, other agents such as pentylenetetrazol (Metrazol), electricity, insulin, and flurothyl (Indoklon) have replaced the first agent, camphor.

Though the agents used seem to affect patients' symptoms, the reasons for these effects are, for the most part, unknown. Studies indicate that the convulsive therapies, while modifying symptoms of mental illness at the time they are utilized, do not create a long-term, stable improvement.

Electroconvulsive Therapy (ECT)

This form of therapy was first introduced by an Italian physician Cerletti and his associate Bini in 1937. Until the advent of psychotropic drugs in the 1950's, it was the treatment of choice in many conditions. Today ECT is used only to treat severely depressed patients. It is found to be most useful for those patients whose symptoms have accumulated rapidly and are of an acute nature. ECT has also been particularly helpful in the treatment of suicidal patients and those who are so profoundly depressed that they are immobile. The latter symptoms tend to decline rapidly when treatment is instituted.

ECT can be administered in the hospital, clinic or doctor's office. The outpatient should be instructed not to eat or drink for at least four hours prior to therapy. Before the patient is placed on the treatment table, the bladder should be emptied. It is the nurse's responsibility to see that this has been done, as well as to check to see that dentures are removed. (If the patient has a partial denture, it is probably better to leave it in so that he does not have an uneven line of teeth that could do him harm while convulsing.)

The patient is placed on a well padded treatment table. In private practice he is usually given a quick-acting anesthetic, like sodium pentothal or methohexital sodium (Brevital). A muscle relaxant is also given to decrease the severity of the clonic movements, and as soon as the latter has been administered, the shock is delivered through tongs applied to the skull. Assistants place a well padded tongue depressor in the mouth to prevent the tongue's being bitten or swallowed. They also gently restrain the limbs to prevent fractures. The patient is only briefly unconscious; however, when he awakens he is usually hazy and may show some confusion about past events. For this reason the patient should be observed for at least one hour after treatment.

Patients receiving ECT are usually frightened of their first treatment. The idea of an electric shock and subsequent convulsion is unpleasant, and for some, barbaric.* Patients discover during the initial treatment that there is no pain associated with it. Nonetheless, many continue to be afraid, and their fears multiply as the course of therapy continues. Some patients have described feelings of dread in which they feel a sense of impending doom. Additionally, patients tend to lose parts of their memory as treatment continues. This may last for one to several weeks after therapy ends, but it does decrease and finally disappear. (Amnesia for the actual treatment procedure continues.) A typical course is eight to 20 treatments, with sessions three times per week.

There is little that the nurse does as an adjunct to the therapy itself other than to provide physical care; she can play an actively supportive role, however, by making herself available to talk to patients, for it gives some a sense of relief to be able to discuss their feelings about ECT. Also, it may be of comfort to them when the nurse explains that any memory impairment is only temporary.

Insulin Shock

This type of therapy requires a competent team of physician and nurses and should be administered only in a hospital employing such a group.[10] Complex monitoring of the patient is requisite in this therapy, which can become dangerous even when physical signs and symptoms are closely observed.

Only a small number of patients can safely be managed at one time; it is advisable to have no more than 12 patients monitored by a single team of one doctor and at least three or four nurses. "The im-

---

* *The Bell Jar* (Sylvia Plath, 1971) offers a particularly poignant description of a patient's fears regarding ECT.

portance of having trained key personnel cannot be overstressed. In hospitals with teaching and training functions, complications frequently arise when a new resident takes over or when key nurses go on vacation. One or two experienced nurses should always be on duty."[10]

Insulin shock therapy is used very infrequently today, but when it is prescribed, it is used in the treatment of the schizophrenic patient. When it was first administered, it was given to increase weight and to inhibit excitement. It was a fortuitous accident to find that the therapy did indeed help the schizophrenic patient in other ways. In 1940 insulin was first utilized in the formal treatment of the schizophrenic. Since that time, the procedure has changed little.

Typically, the NPO patient begins treatment early in the morning with an injection of insulin. Approximately one hour after injection, the patient manifests the first signs of hypoglycemia. Symptoms include perspiration and feelings of tiredness and somnolence. *The attending nurse needs to be completely familiar with the signs and symptoms that she is dealing with, for it is only through knowledgeable observation that she will know where the patient is in terms of the depth of his coma.*

During the second hour the patient's sensorium becomes clouded and he falls asleep. Some patients may be restless, toss about and yell. Others are disoriented or show hallucinatory behavior. Speech becomes incoherent. Motor activity during the second hour consists of automatic movements—forced grasping, myoclonic twitchings and various dystonic manifestations. Sometimes patients will convulse during the second hour of hypoglycemia. (These convulsions are considered by some to be of value; however, when they occur during later hours of hypoglycemia, they are considered a danger sign and require immediate termination of the treatment.)

In the third hour the patient can go into true coma. Deepest coma is reached when the patient no longer responds to painful stimuli.

Generally patients are not left in coma for more than one hour. To terminate treatment, the hormone glucagon is administered intravenously or intramuscularly. The patient should awaken 10 to 20 minutes after the medication is given; if this does not occur, more glucagon is injected.

A typical course of treatment is 50 to 60 comas, with a coma being induced only five days in any one week.

Of particular concern to the nurse should be the possibility of a second hypoglycemic coma which might occur several hours after the termination of treatment. The patient again may perspire, feel tired and lie down "for a nap after lunch." *Such a patient must be carefully watched because sleep may turn into coma.* To guard against this, the patient should have sugar with him and be told eat some of it at the first sign of uneasiness. He should be warned against sleeping during the afternoon of treatment. It is expedient for the nurse to encourage insulin patients to stay with the other patients in the afternoons and to participate in group activities. If this is done, the patient can be kept under surveillance without its being so obvious.

Indoklon (Hexafluorodiethyl Ether)

This is a relatively recent addition to the pharmacological repertoire. Although used originally for other purposes, the drug was found to induce convulsions. It is given as an inhalant by means of a mask and vaporizer. The patient loses consciousness rapidly before the onset of tremors and clonic movements. Nursing measures surrounding its use are similar to those in other convulsive therapies.

Psychosurgery

In 1890 a Swiss psychiatrist named Burkhardt removed portions of the brain cortex to rid patients of their fixed hallucinations. Surgery had been performed prior to this time, to alter mental disease. One method utilized was trephining to "let out evil spirits." This primitive precursor of psychosurgery was employed by the Greek and Roman physician-priests. The technique reappeared in medieval times.

In 1935 a surgical technique was once more utilized. This time it was a prefrontal leukotomy or lobotomy. It entailed surgical separation of the frontal lobes, which are responsible for thought, from the thalamus, which is the seat of emotion. The procedure was used extensively in the forties and fifties. A variation on the basic procedure was the transorbital lobotomy. In both procedures the nerve tracts between the frontal cortex and the thalamus are severed. This involves the drilling of small holes on the side or top of the skull. A sharp instrument is inserted and rotated in a 35-degree arc anterior to the frontal lobes. The transorbital technique utilizes a cutting instrument inserted into the thin, bony structure separating the eye and the brain. The latter technique is considered simpler and tends to have fewer postoperative complications.[12]

Though research on effects of the surgical procedures does not yield conclusive findings, most studies indicate that in the psychological sphere there is a decrease in the intensity of the patient's affect. In the physical sphere it is observed that immediately after surgery patients seem sluggish and unmotivated, but over an extended convalescence the former pace of activity is resumed. [In a recent discussion, Dr. Frank Ayd, Jr., said that psychosurgery is once more becoming an important mode of treatment.[3] He reports that not only severe behavioral problems are so treated, but also some incapacitating neuroses that do not respond to drugs. Dr. Ayd said that the lobotomy procedure has been modified to the degree that little brain tissue is destroyed. In fact, some psychosurgery is done on an outpatient basis, and the postoperative patient may return to work within days of the surgery.]

GROUP THERAPIES

It is natural for human beings to gather in groups. Nations consist of groups of people with a common language and purposes; cities and towns are composed of groups, as are community organizations and families. The latter are the individual's primary group.* Within the group, the individual acts and reacts. His anxiety increases or decreases, depending on the group's emotional behavior toward him. It is often advantageous to treat the patient in a group, because his problems involve his feelings and behavior toward others as well as their feelings and behavior toward him. This process of action and reaction occurs because the individual has developed a set of attitudes and behaviors toward others based on his perceptions of people in his primary group. As the individual matures and joins secondary groups, the roles that he perceived in his family (or primary group) are perceived by him again in the individuals he encounters in secondary groups. (This is similar to the psychoanalytic situation in which the analyst is cast by the patient in the roles of significant persons in the patient's past.) Group therapy effectively utilizes the individual's potential for transference of roles from the primary to secondary groups.

Group therapy traditionally refers to the treatment of psychiatric patients in a group with a therapist-leader. The group, which is a formal one, i.e., planned and structured and with some predetermined goals (s), meets in a specified place for a specified period of time. For the psychiatric nurse, group therapy is a practical mode of treatment because it permits the nurse to care for several patients at once. (Research in the technique indicates that the more effective groups contain no more than six to eight patients.)

Within the group the nurse may observe several patients as they relate to one another, utilizing functional and faulty mechanisms for socialization. The nurse has an opportunity to evaluate patients' levels of behavior and their potential for growth.

Through group process the nurse leader can see that certain of the group members' needs, such as recognition, acceptance and a sense of belonging, are met. The leader fosters trust and closeness in the

---

* The original family is the patient's primary group. Secondary groups are school classes, work groups at the place of employment, and the patient group on the ward.

group, so that the members can have their needs met by one another. In this way the group becomes more like secondary groups found in the community, and rehabilitation is enhanced.

SELECTION OF GROUP PATIENTS

There is little agreement among group therapists as to *how* to select patients for group therapy. Some advocate choosing patients with the same problem; others recommend a random selection. For the nursing student who will work with a group for only a short time, it is probably best to select a group of patients for whom there is a common goal, i.e., to be more verbal in expressing their feelings, to talk about discharge, or perhaps to learn to act in a group through planned activities.*

When the therapeutic goal (s) has been identified, patients can be selected. The main criterion becomes not one of diagnostic label, but who will benefit from the planned objective. It is likely that external factors such as sex of patients in the group, age, and location of patients will be determined from the ward (s) available to the nurse. For re-socialization groups (see Chapter 9, p. 178) it is valuable to use a group of both men and women. It is probably useful to select a group of patients from the same or nearby wards, because the experiences of learning to relate can then be carried over into the hours spent on the ward. If patients are being selected from the acute services, and the patients are verbal and ready to work intensively, then a mixture of patients from varying wards might be indicated. Such a group would come together only to work therapeutically, but then would separate until the next session. When intensive work is being done, this is more acceptable because it decreases the possibility that members might get together extracurricularly to work out group problems that should rightfully be handled in the group setting with the therapist.

PHYSICAL ARRANGEMENTS

The meeting place should be one where the group can be comfortable, where privacy is possible and where disruptive noise can be minimized. Ventilation is important. (A tiny room without windows becomes agonizingly hot when eight people are tense, perspiring and smoking.) Basic necessities are chairs and ash trays. Comfortable chairs are more conducive to group work than straight-backed, armless ones.

---

* Such would be an activity group; it is more appropriate for chronically ill, regressed patients who cannot handle verbal skills.

They should be placed in a loose circle, i.e., facing into the center, but not so close together that the group members feel imprisoned.

THERAPEUTIC CONTRACTS

The group therapist establishes her group by meeting with each of the potential members and explaining the purpose of the therapy and the patient's role in it. The patient needs to know: (1) why he has been selected, i.e., the therapeutic goals he can hope to obtain; (2) where the meetings will be held and when, i.e., how often; and (3) how he is to respond, i.e., that he will be expected to talk or to behave in some certain manner.

The following conversation between a nursing student and a schizophrenic patient on a chronic female unit will help to demonstrate the initial contact between therapist and patient.

Patient: (Looks up but says nothing.)

Student: As part of your care you are going to be starting group therapy twice a week. The doctor [the student must clear all patient choices with the medical staff] and the nursing staff feel that we can offer you more through this kind of treatment. What do you think about it?

Patient: I don't think I want any therapy, thank you.

Student: We want you to give this a try, Mrs. S. We think you can expect to feel more comfortable in your life on the ward after you have been in the group for a while. We know that it is frightening, at first, to try anything new, but this therapy is going to be worth the effort you put into it.

Patient: What do I have to do?

Student: You and I and five other patients are going to meet in the dayroom each Monday and Thursday from 2 to 3 P.M. We shall talk about how things go on the ward and what the various members of the group are thinking. If any member wants to bring up something in particular, the group will be a good place to talk about it.

Patient: I don't like to talk to a bunch of strangers. . . .

Student: I don't think you'll feel the group members are strangers after you've been with them a few times. You'll probably feel that they are your friends. They will be telling you things, and you will tell them what you wish, and everyone will speak only in the group about matters that come up in the group.

Patient: Well, I don't know. . . .

Student: I shall be looking forward to seeing you in the group for the first meeting next Monday. In fact, I shall come by to pick you up about 1:45. You may bring a pack of cigarettes with you if you like to smoke.

Patient: (With an evident lack of enthusiasm.) Okay, . . . I'll be here.

TASKS OF THE THERAPIST IN THE GROUP

The tasks of the therapist vary with the therapist's philosophy of group therapy and the type of group that is formed. The majority of groups provide an arena for the learning of greater interpersonal effectiveness. This occurs as a result of the relationships that are established between group members and the process of working through difficulties encountered in those relationships.

The therapist creates and convenes the group. In the beginning he is the group's primary unifying force. To him falls the task of developing the group's rules of behavior, or "group norms." Such behavior includes free interaction among the group members, self-disclosure, high levels of involvement, nonjudgmental acceptance, acceptance of patient role, and communication of conflict and affection.[20]

Some philosophies of group therapy indicate that the therapist is an expert in the technical aspects of group life. When a given therapist feels this way, he and the group will expect solutions to the group's problems to emanate from the leader via interpretations on his part. Other philosophies conceive of the therapist as simply another group member. As such he tries to focus responsibility for conflict resolution back on the group when members attempt to cast him in the role of expert. Through this process the group learns to take responsibility for its own growth. The therapist is seen as one of the individuals who is part of the search. He does not have a solution which he holds in abeyance. The problem is part of the life of the particular group, and a solution does not exist until the group formulates it.

Some psychoanalytically oriented groups proceed under certain assumptions that center the group's activities around the therapist. In such groups the goal is not to develop greater interpersonal effectiveness through group interaction, but it is often to resolve the transference that is permitted to develop between each of the group members and the therapist. In these groups the therapist does not allow himself to be cast simply as a group member. He is often seen as a benevolent authority. He is less active in the group process but subtly manipulates the group so that transference phenomena develop. In groups of this type the therapist is apt to offer interpretations concerning the unconscious meanings of members' statements and behavior. There is less attention to the "here and now" than is seen in groups in which leadership responsibility is shared by the entire group.

Thus, it is seen that the therapist's tasks will be determined by his philosophy of therapy. This is a highly controversial area, and the nurse who wishes to practice in this modality will have to identify her own preferences. If she becomes a private practitioner this choice will come from extensive reading and training. If she is connected with an agency or has a co-therapist, her views will likely reflect compromise with her co-workers.

PATIENT ROLES IN THE GROUP

It will be noted that as the group becomes solidified, each member begins to act in a characteristic manner within the group setting. Some of the behaviors will contribute to building relationships and cohesiveness among the members; others will be destructive of the group's cohesiveness. A major part of the therapist's work will be to encourage the constructive behaviors and to modify the destructive ones.

Some of the constructive behaviors are as follows:

Harmonizing or mediating. This is the ability to clarify points of disagreement and attempts to reconcile disagreements.

Gate-keeping. The effort to keep communications open.

Supporting. Letting others in the group know that they are understood, or at least heard and held in esteem.

Relieving tension. Draining off negative feeling by bringing a topic to a close or diverting attention, or jesting.

Initiating. Bringing up topics for discussion.

Some of the destructive behaviors are:

Silence. The patient who will not participate causes tension and lack of cohesion. If the group therapist has chosen a non-verbal member on purpose, it is wise to select not more than one such person for the small group.

Acting out. The use of nonverbal behavior to express a message that might otherwise be transmitted through verbal means. Such behavior should be interpreted and questioned by the leader or, hopefully, by group members themselves.

Monopolizing. The means by which an individual patient takes over the group and talks continuously, not allowing others to participate. Such behavior is usually defensive in nature and is a means to cope with overwhelming anxiety. It is more useful to the patient if he can be limited without being punished. Thus, the therapist who can say, "Mr. R., that is a very interesting point. Now let's see what Mr. S. has to say about it," is being supportive of the first patient. If she cannot limit the patient, it is possible that the patient group will tell him to limit himself in a far less gentle manner. (If the group has been working together over a long period and is well integrated, patient intervention is ideal; however, in the typical student-led group which is limited in time, it is unlikely that a group would reach that point in its working relationships.)

DEVELOPMENTAL PHASES OF THE GROUP

Formative phase. Any new group must determine the reason for its formation, that is, its primary goal, and a means of attaining that goal. In the therapy group this phase is often observed in the members' questioning of the group's worth: "Why am I here?" "I can't see how this is going to help me!"

Members size up one another and search for role models for themselves. They are very insecure and are constantly seeking sure, stable, unwavering *truth*. This is why the therapist can be so successful in introducing group norms. Members will turn to anyone in the group who is willing to offer models of behavior. Because the therapist offers them, the group observes hungrily and usually incorporates them.

The content and communication style of the formative phase of the group is somewhat stereotyped and restricted. Patterns of socially acceptable behavior that have been useful in the past are brought into the therapy situation. There is an abundance of etiquette, group support and tranquility. Giving and seeking advice is a time-consuming activity of the early phases. Though the advice is of questionable value, it provides a means by which members can communicate interest and caring.

Working phase. One may recognize when the group emerges from the formative phase because the social niceties no longer dominate the group's interaction. Instead of preoccupation with acceptance, approval, commitment to the group, definitions of accepted behavior and the search for orientation, structure and meaning, the group is now immersed in a sea of negative embattlement. A struggle for dominance, control, and power ensues.[20] In this phase of the group's development, conflict may be between group members and the leader, or between group members. Out of this struggle, a group hierarchy is established. It is during this process that individual's roles from other kinds of groups become more evident. Also reflected in these struggles are members' maladaptive ways of problem-solving. It is during this process that the therapist will be most tempted to set limits on behavior, while at the same time encouraging confrontation. In this stage of development there are few oases of serenity. The group is usually in flux, and themes are generally negative.

Out of these struggles emerges true group cohesiveness. This phase is recognized through the presence of group spirit, cooperation and freedom of communication. The group is concerned with closeness. The formation of a viable state for working through its problems is near, provided the group does not choke off further access to negative feelings that must be expressed from time to time in the group's life. The remainder of the group's work may then proceed until the goals of the group are met, or the group must terminate because of a time limit, or other extra-group factors determine a premature closure.

Termination phase. As in individual therapy, termination is not pleasurable. The group has derived comfort and gratification from the members' affiliations with one another; the cohesiveness that has grown out of the sharing of pain and strife will not be duplicated. The group members must be helped to face the pain that loss of the group means. They will require support as they disclose their feelings about separation. The phase of termination is one in which the members recognize the need to end the group, and go about bringing the experience to closure in an orderly, meaningful way.

MILIEU THERAPY

Milieu therapy is a treatment of the patient that utilizes the environment in which the patient finds himself. It is perhaps misleading to discuss milieu therapy under the general heading of group therapies, because in this type of therapy the members of the group include all patients and staff in a particular designated location. Thus, selection and assignment are not the issues that they are in other group therapies.

In the residential treatment center, the patient is typically seen by the therapist for an hour several days a week. Why then is the patient kept in the hospital the other 23 hours per day? In a well developed therapeutic program, the patient's milieu is considered part of the treatment regimen. His existence in the environment, his thoughts and his behavior, and the corresponding thoughts and behavior of those living with the patient can be significant in altering the pathological aspects of the patient's living style. In an untherapeutic milieu, the maladaptive patterns of the patient may be reinforced. In a truly therapeutic milieu, the learning of new patterns of behavior which are more effective in the patient's life is a goal.

It is felt that the social role of the patient should be structured and modified in milieu therapy. How is this done? The staff who admit a new patient to the unit observe the patient and acquaint themselves with the types of behavior that the patient exhibits. They identify those patterns that are useful to the patient and those which seem maladaptive. When study of the patient has been completed, staff members confer about their observations. The outcomes of such meetings will present the staff group with several questions: What does the patient need in order to develop more efficient responses? How can we, as individuals, help him to learn these behavioral responses? The answers to the first question will be agreed on by the total group. The second inquiry must, of necessity, be more individualized. Perhaps the patient needs to learn to express his anger. Perhaps he needs to learn control of his impulsive behavior. A patient may need to learn to experience himself as a more aggressive, decision-making individual. How each of the staff helps the patient to learn these responses will depend partially on the temperament of the particular staff member. One person may be able to point out areas in which the patient can be more decisive; another may be comfortable in waiting until the patient comes to a decision no matter what the question. Still a third staff member may need to help the patient by pointing out all the alternatives. Nonetheless, each staff member will try to interpret the approach decided on by the group in terms of his own personality and his normal modes of behavior.

It is felt that milieu therapy when properly planned can improve behavior because the environment provides relationships which satisfy emotional needs; it reduces psychological conflict and deprivation, and it strengthens impaired ego functions.[25] The staff who observe the newly admitted patient and draw from their conclusions ideas about the needs of the patient will provide an environment in which the patient can acquire a social role which he can enact and experience during his stay in the hospital community. Through his acquired role, he can learn behavioral responses which are, at the time of illness, deficient in his life style. Basically the staff must agree upon the needs of the patient and they must be consistent in their approaches. The staff members who feel committed to the value of milieu therapy will continue to observe the patient's behavior. Efforts must be made to reflect to the patient what his behavior communicates to others. Staff must react in such a way that the patient understands that his behavior does affect others. This is not to say that staff should be punitive, but they should be feeling and responsive. It is the staff's responsibility to provide a stable, lucid environment. Every attempt should be made to reduce ambiguity by explaining to the patient whenever there is a question about his comprehension of reality. Also, the staff and other patients can be utilized to strengthen the patient's confidence in the predictability of the behavior of others in his environment. Thus, the patient who is subtly aggressive and acts in ways to irritate others can be told "Look, I think you are going out of your way to be annoying. I am wondering if you may be angry at me and, if you are, why you can't just come out and say so instead of acting this way?"

Other ways in which the staff can reinforce new behavioral modes are to provide opportunities for the individual to utilize them. Thus, if a patient needs to be more decisive, the attendant might suggest that in the morning the patient choose between one dress or another. When an outing is planned, the patient can be asked to make a choice between one destination and another. When the patient demonstrates a more effective response, the staff commend the patient for it.

PSYCHODRAMA

Psychodrama is a form of group therapy. It involves a structured, directed and dramatized acting out of a patient's personal and emotional problem, or the problem of a group. This technique was first introduced in the United States in 1925 by Moreno.[26] Psychodrama is not acting in the theatrical sense that is familiar to the reader; rather, it is a spontaneous dramatization of a problem (or theme) that is decided on by the central patient and patient group just prior to the acting out of the drama. The goal is self-realization. It is based on the principle that action and dramatic psychotherapy give the opportunity for greater depth of awareness than is possible through verbalization alone. The technique includes catharsis,* abreaction,* free association in acting, and an "encounter" between various members of the drama team.

In psychodrama the major goal is spontaneity, total perception of unhealthy responses, a more accurate perception of reality, involvement with other persons and learning through experience.[27] Elements of the psychodrama that are used to obtain the goals are the group, that is, the audience and the participants; the protagonist, that is, the acting subject; and the auxiliary egos, that is, other persons in the group who act out roles assigned to them by the director, who is the therapist.

The protagonist is an individual patient who presents his own personal problem, or takes the main character in a drama depicting a group problem. The auxiliary egos help him to bring "personal and collective drama to life and to correct it. It is important that the theme, whether private or collective, be a truly experienced problem of the participants (real/symbolic)."[26]

It is not likely that the nursing student will observe a psychiatric nurse acting as director in a psychodrama, for that task is a highly complex one requiring special training. To help one become such a therapist, there are courses and workshops available; however, the therapy itself is extremely interesting to watch. Should the student have an opportunity to observe any session of a group that is led by a competent therapist, the experience is highly recommended.

THE ENCOUNTER GROUP

Again a technique is presented, not because the nurse will find herself in a position to use it, but because it is interesting and, in this

---

* See Glossary.

case, relatively new and becoming popular. The encounter group is a product of the sixties and early seventies. It is a type of group activity that is consonant with the trend of social life in the United States in which social and interpersonal relationships are of a temporary nature.

Because of the mobility and transient character of social relationships in this age of technology, social deprivation and mass alienation occur.[21] The encounter group has grown out of this trend and is a reaction to it. The encounter movement attempts to put individuals in touch with themselves again and in touch with one another by reawakening their awareness of their own feelings and the feelings of others. The encounter group experience is sought by many who do not label themselves as "mentally ill" specifically, but who do feel the need to become more in touch with themselves and others. The experience is one that many in the psychiatric field have been interested in, not so much from the *treating* perspective, but from that of the *treated*. Many have reported gratifying results from this type of experience.

The most important aspect of the encounter is feeling. Emphasis is placed on the immediate experience, on the here and now. An ongoing battle is waged between getting in touch with feelings versus intellectualization of behavior.[23]

In the traditional group, the orientation is basically historical, that is, the "whys" and "where froms" are necessary for the functioning of the group; in the encounter situation, "subjective truths are shared, irrational and ineffectual behavior appears incongruent, to be dropped in favor of new, more intimate and competent behavioral patterns."[23] Thus, the new technique is fundamentally "ahistorical" and emphasis is placed on the "what" and "how now" instead of the "whys" and "where froms." Group members are asked to come to terms with their immediate experiences in the here and now. They are encouraged not to postpone, or evade, or hide. Each member of the group is required to share with the others his feelings now, not what they were yesterday or may be tomorrow.

While encounter groups are gaining popularity and many people are deriving benefit from them, there is a segment of the population to whom their advent is a disservice. Borderline and psychotic individuals should not go into encounter experiences. For these people the experiences can be sufficiently traumatizing that they develop overt mental illness and require formal psychiatric care, so the encounter group is contraindicated.

Well qualified leaders for encounter groups can be found. Some are in residence at the larger centers for "growth experiences," such as Esalen, California;* The National Training Laboratory, Bethel, Maine; the Western Behavioral Sciences Institute, LaJolla, California;

---

* "The Esalen Institute at Big Sur, California, is named for an Indian tribe that once roamed the area. It is staffed by such diverse sorts as dancers, theologians, businessmen, practicing psychologists, social workers, and medically trained persons."[21]

and the American Institute of Humanistic Psychology, San Francisco, California. Some leaders travel circuits and hold encounter groups in multiple locations. Among the best known leaders (or trainers) are such people as George Bach, Carl Rogers and Virginia Satir. There are many more, however, who are also extremely talented and competent. To be able to identify them, the encounter group enthusiast must investigate the background of the trainer in terms of his training and objectives. Reputable trainers are people who have worked with competent teachers. Generally they have had experience in therapy and may themselves have been analyzed. They are knowledgeable about dealing with countertransference phenomena and are prepared to support the group in constructive ways.

If there is a role for the psychiatric nurse in the encounter movement, it is probably to be a teacher, to disseminate information about the new group therapies and to discourage those persons from attending who are obviously poorly integrated and emotionally unstable. For the better integrated, the encounter group seems to provide an experience by which individuals can once more get back in touch with themselves through sharing their subjective lives with others.

The nurse may be asked if there are differences between encounter groups, sensitivity training and T groups.† At this time, the differences are becoming less pronounced. The term "sensitivity training" was coined in 1954[22] and refers to programs which are oriented to making people working in industry, such as managers and executives, better able to function in a humanistic rather than authoritarian manner. These programs are characteristic of the National Training Laboratory in Bethel, Maine. They have been regarded as quite conservative compared to the approaches and objectives of the encounter, or human potential movement, in the West, which is characterized by Esalen, in California. Encounter and growth potential seem to be terms indicative of the Western approaches to this type of training. Sensitivity training and T groups are terms that usually indicate the more conservative East Coast orientation.

FAMILY THERAPY

As has been discussed, the primary group of any individual is his family. This group is composed of father and mother, the architects of the primary group, and the children they raise. Sometimes father and mother are referred to as the original dyad. Family therapists claim that treatment of the individual is not so effective as treatment of the whole family, because the sick individual only reflects a group (the family) in pain. They feel that the symptomatic individual, usually a child, who comes to the attention of teachers, school nurse or other interested resource people is not "the sick one," "the different one,"

---

† Training groups.

or "the one to blame," but that he is the individual family member who reflects a lack of homeostasis in the family.[24] The therapist regards this individual's symptoms as an "SOS" about the parental relationship which is causing family imbalance.

Advocates of family therapy believe that to treat the individual member creates a hardship for that person because he is unjustly labeled "sick." They feel that the family malfunction remains even though the individual patient is trying desperately through his therapy to bring about change in all the members. Therefore, the patient suffers blows additional to his symptoms. First, he takes the blame for a larger problem than he is responsible for and, secondly, he puts great effort into making the family well, which again is not his responsibility.

Family therapy attempts to improve all interactional behavior within the primary group. The therapist is a resource person whom the family can trust. He acts as an observer of communication processes in the family and is able to report to them impartially on what he sees and hears.[24] The therapist acts as a teacher, helping his clients to check on their tacit assumptions, to question one another, and to request sufficient feedback from each that all concerned in the family know what each member is saying, doing and meaning. Like the more traditional group therapist, the family therapist supports one member or another when the necessity arises. All maneuvers are utilized, however, to help the total family mature by developing more functional means of communicating with one another.

REFERENCES

Somatic Therapies

1. Ackner, B., and Oldham, A.: Insulin Treatment of Schizophrenia. *Lancet,* 1: 504-506, 1962.
2. A.M.A. Council on Drugs: A.M.A. Drug Evaluations, 1971. Chicago, American Medical Association, 1971, p. 231.
3. Ayd, F., Jr.: Personal communication, 1971.
4. Baker, A., Game, J., and Thorpe, J.: Physical Treatment of Schizophrenia. *J. Med. Sci.* 104:860-864, 1958.
5. Freedman, A. M., and Kaplan, H. I.: *Comprehensive Textbook of Psychiatry.* Baltimore, The Williams & Wilkins Company, 1967.
6. Freyhan, F. A.: Neuroleptic Effects: Fact and Fiction. *In* Sawer-Foner (ed.): *The Dynamics of Psychiatric Drug Therapy.* Springfield, Ill., Charles C Thomas, 1958.
7. Gordon: *The New Chemotherapy in Mental Illness.* New York, Philosophical Library, 1958.
8. Himwich, H.: Biochemical and Neurophysiological Action of Psychoactive Drugs. *Science,* 127:59-72, 1958.
9. Hock, P.: Drug Therapy. *In* Arieti, S. (ed.): *American Handbook of Psychiatry.* Vol. 2. New York, Basic Books, Inc., 1959.
10. Horwitz, W.: Insulin Shock Therapy. *In* Arieti, S. (ed.): *American Handbook of Psychiatry.* New York, Basic Books, Inc., 1959, p. 1486.
11. Klein, D., and Davis, J.: *Diagnosis and Drug Treatment of Psychiatric Disorders.* Baltimore, The Williams & Wilkins Company, 1969.
12. Millon, T.: *Modern Psychopathology.* Philadelphia, W. B. Saunders Company, 1970.

13. Musser, M., and Shubkagel, B.: *Pharmacology and Therapeutics.* 3rd ed. New York, The Macmillan Company, 1965.
14. RN Magazine: Drug Interactions. Oradell, New Jersey, 1970.

Group Therapy

16. Armstrong, S., and Rouslin, S.: *Group Therapy and Nursing Practice.* New York, The Macmillan Company, 1963.
17. Berne, E.: *Principles of Group Treatment.* New York, Oxford University Press, 1966.
18. Holmes, M., and Werner, J.: *Psychiatric Nursing in a Therapeutic Community.* New York, The Macmillan Company, 1966.
19. Johnson, J.: *Group Therapy: A Practical Approach.* New York, McGraw-Hill Book Co., Inc., 1963.
20. Yalom, I.: *The Theory and Practice of Group Psychotherapy.* New York, Basic Books, Inc., 1970.

New Group Therapies

21. Goldberg, C.: *Encounter: Group Sensitivity Training Experience.* New York, Science House, Inc., 1970.
22. Howard, J.: *Please Touch.* New York, McGraw-Hill Book Co., 1970.
23. Ruitenbeek, H.: *The New Group Therapies.* New York, Avon Books, 1970.
24. Satir, V.: *Conjoint Family Therapy.* Palo Alto, California, Science and Behavior Books, Inc., 1967.

Milieu

25. Stainbrook, E.: The Hospital as a Therapeutic Community. *In* Freedman, A. M., and Kaplan, H. I.: *Comprehensive Textbook of Psychiatry.* Baltimore, The Williams & Wilkins Company, 1967.

Psychodrama

26. Moreno, J.: Psychodrama. *In* Arieti, S. (ed.): *American Handbook of Psychiatry.* New York, Basic Books, Inc., 1959.
27. Rubin, J.: Psychodrama. *In* Freedman, A. M., and Kaplan, H. I.: *Comprehensive Textbook of Psychiatry.* Baltimore, The Williams & Wilkins Company, 1967.

SUGGESTED READINGS

It is recognized that the undergraduate student's exposure to group therapy techniques is typically minute. Nonetheless, more and more training programs are beginning to look at the possibility of introducing group, rather than individual methods of nursing intervention. For students who might be in such programs, the four texts listed under Group Therapy references are highly recommended. Though it is unrealistic to suggest all four, I offer them as possible choices. The Holmes and Werner is interesting and well written. Because it is discussed from the point of view of nurses, it is particularly valuable. For a comprehensive text (more so than the basic student would need) I recommend Johnson without any reservations. It is a delightfully readable book and includes a wealth of information about group work.

Ayd, F.: Chemical Assault on Mental Illness: The Major Tranquilizers. *Am. J. Nursing,* 65:70-78, April, 1965.

Ayd, F.: The Minor Tranquilizers. *Am. J. Nursing*, 65:89-94, May, 1965.

Ayd, F.: The Antidepressants. *Am. J. Nursing*, 65:78-84, June, 1965.

This series is well written and highly informative. The nursing student would do well to study the above series carefully prior to administering drugs in the clinical area of the hospital.

Bueker, K.: Group Psychotherapy in a New Setting. *Am. J. Nursing*, 57:1581-1588, December, 1957.

This article combines a discussion of work with patients receiving concurrent insulin shock therapy and group therapy. The group is led by a doctor and a nurse, which provides for an additional look at co-therapy. Parts of the group dialogue are reproduced, making the article well worth the reader's time.

Goodson, M.: Group Therapy with Regressed Patients. *Perspectives in Psychiatric Care*, 2 (No. 4):23-31, 1964.

The paper is a good presentation of group work with chronically ill male patients.

Kirshenbaum, E.: Group Work Method in Psychiatric Nursing Practice. *Am. J. Nursing*, 64:128-132, October, 1964.

A report of an experimental project with schizophrenic patients who were engaged in activity groups by the nursing staff.

Lego, S.: Five Functions of the Group Therapist, 20 Sessions Later. *Am. J. Nursing*, 66:795-797, April, 1966.

A concise and lucid discussion of the functions of the group therapist after the group has moved into the working relationship phase. The article is a good review of basic techniques and responsibilities as well as more advanced considerations.

Rogers, C.: Facilitating Encounter Groups. *Am. J. Nursing*, 71:275-279, February, 1971.

The well known and widely respected author describes his own style of activity in leading encounter groups.

Swanson, M.: A Checklist for Group Leaders. *Perspectives in Psychiatric Care*, 7:120-126, 1969.

This paper will be very helpful for persons trying to examine their group work in an organized, meaningful way.

chapter 12

THE PATIENT WHO
ABUSES ALCOHOL
OR DRUGS

Drug abuse in the United States and in other parts of the world has become a pervasive public health and legal problem. From the college campuses to the ghettos, from the world of business to the world of play, from private parties to Woodstock, one hears of, or has personal experience with, individuals who consume drugs indiscriminately. Such agents as LSD, peyote, alcohol, mescaline, barbiturates, marihuana, nutmeg, glue and even banana skins have been described as the keys to bliss, contentment, inner self and nirvana. Health and legal authorities are increasingly concerned with a generation of people who have apparently opted to "cop out." Today's scene is one of drugs. The "skid row" alcoholic is no longer the interest of a concerned few; the occasional opium user no longer exists. Drug abuse is a problem of massive proportions. The world is crying for answers as scientists, parents, doctors, nurses, teachers, social workers and industrialists ponder the nature of drug abuse—a deadly route taken by so many which renders them as unproductive as they are broken on the rack of toxicity and dependence. They become cirrhotic, infected with abscesses and psychotic; they contract syphilis and other venereal diseases; they have acute and chronic brain syndromes; they hemorrhage from bleeding varices. A growing number of drug users who are not incapacitated by poor health are rendered unproductive because they are in jails, prosecuted for illegal activities connected with their drug abuses and addictions.

ALCOHOLISM

One of the oldest and most abused chemical agents is alcohol. Its uncontrolled use leads to alcoholism, a condition which has been variously described as a "sin, a scourge, a sign of weakness." It is only in recent years that many people, indeed, the majority of workers in health fields, have become sufficiently accepting of the alcoholic to identify him as being sick. Some investigators who are sociologically oriented perceive alcoholism as a disease which develops as a result of the growing child's observation of patterns of alcohol usage in the family setting. They believe that alcoholism results from conflicts in the culture (as reflected in the family) over drinking behavior. If drinking is accepted, it is not a stressful factor. If there is conflict over whether drinking is acceptable, the individual never knows when he may drink and when he should not.

Another group of investigators who are physiologically oriented theorize that alcoholism is the result of a metabolic defect which renders the alcoholic incapable of using foodstuffs from his normal diet. They believe that inordinately large needs for such dietary essentials as vitamins cause cravings for alcohol.

Some psychoanalytically oriented theorists consider alcoholism to be the result of fixation of personality development with superimposed conflict and stress. Wexberg writes, "There is some evidence in the dynamics of alcoholic patients that they were less able to 'take it' than the average person, a long time before they started drinking to excess."[9]

Another writer reports that the chronic alcoholic is an individual who from earliest childhood on has lived in a state of insecurity. The character of the alcoholic involves a chronically tense person with the tendency to give in passively to assumed pressure or to react with over-compensation. Alcohol reverses the process. It gives security and acceptance as long as the intoxication lasts. With the wearing off of the effects of the alcohol, the underlying tensions and terrors reappear in increased form and create the demand for renewed drinking.[8]

In short, the "cause" of alcoholism has not been identified. Proponents of a unitary disease theory, that is, that alcoholism is one specific disease entity, insist that the differences in the presenting picture and the differences in psychological and behavioral manifestations accompanying alcoholism are irrelevant. *The* disease, they say, is the uncontrollable, addictive drinking; all else is secondary.[7]

Critics of the unitary disease theory say that compulsive or uncontrollable drinking is not a disease of and by itself, but rather a symptom or syndrome or disease condition found in association with many different personality disorders. It is apparent that drinking represents a tension-reducing device. The strength of the habit depends on the degree of anxiety which prompts it and the individual's tolerance of frustration.

Definition

Alcoholism may be regarded as a chronic disorder in which the individual is unable, for psychological or physical reasons, or both, to refrain from the frequent consumption of alcohol in quantities sufficient to produce intoxication and, ultimately, injury to health and effective functioning.[7]

Alcohol is an effective tension reducer because it is a depressant. Used in sufficient quantities, it narcotizes the individual so that feelings of anxiety are obliterated. The effects of alcohol advance along a path from the uppermost portions of the brain extending to the caudal region.[3] Functions of the brain utilizing the cortical area seem most susceptible to the effects of alcohol. Thus, memory, judgment and reasoning are adversely influenced before simple reflexes are involved.

THE DEVELOPMENT OF AN ADDICTED DRINKER

The Pre-alcoholic Symptomatic Phase

All drinking starts with social motivation. The child observes adults around him drinking. He sees them enjoying it, reacting to it or being reacted to negatively. Later in life the prospective alcoholic finds himself feeling relief from stress when he drinks. The relief is greater for this individual than for the ordinary social drinker because the social drinker either has less tension than the potential alcoholic or he handles his tensions differently. In the early history of the disease there is occasional drinking for relief. The amount of alcohol needed to promote relief grows steadily, but drunkenness is not yet observed.

The Prodromal Phase

In this phase blackouts, i.e., amnesia for single events or episodes, become evident. These occur without intoxication or loss of consciousness.[7] This phase may last for a few months or it can extend over several years. The accompanying behavior and feelings of the addicted individual indicate that drinking is no longer a source of relief or idle pleasure, but now alcohol is sought as a drug which the individual needs. Typical behaviors include: surreptitious drinking, preoccupation with the supply of alcohol and gulping of drinks when alone or with a social group. The individual feels enormous guilt and avoids reference to alcohol. Usually any tendency to heavy drinking is categorically denied. This is the terribly painful period when the alcoholic arises in the morning and must have a drink to "steady" his nerves so he can make it to work. Lunchtime becomes a progressively longer period which is used to have "a few" to keep the tremors down. By late afternoon such an individual has left the office to stop at the neighborhood tavern to "have a short one" on the way home. Once home, several drinks usher in the evening's relaxation. This is the period when the addict drinks two while he mixes one for his guest. This is the period when a noticeable tremor, if questioned, is rationalized as "a little weakness in my hands from the bout with a virus last week." The alcoholic is not simply a liar; he is an individual who feels himself trapped in a quandary. He feels unable, rather than unwilling, to break away from his habit. He feels increasingly worthless as he recognizes his downhill course and is extremely sensitive to the regard of those around him. In this phase there is occasional loss of control. It is at this point that the crucial phase of alcohol addiction begins.

The Crucial Phase

"Loss of control is the inability, consistently, to choose whether to drink or not."[7] Once started, a drinking binge does not stop until the individual is too drunk or too sick to consume more. Episodes may last from a few hours to several weeks. The alcoholic describes these periods as nightmares of sickness, filth, degradation, loss of consciousness and animal-like existence. Those who live through them are frightened and disgusted. They resolve to stop drinking forever, . . . or at least to stop their intemperate drinking. For the lucky, the resolves are followed by brief periods of controlled drinking until the next crisis prevails. In this phase, grandiose behavior, isolation from surroundings, marked aggression, a decrease in outside interests, frigidity, impotence and nutritional impairment become evident. Addicted drinkers in this stage of illness are very sick. By this time most gainfully employed alcoholics have lost their jobs; all have lost their self-respect; and many have lost their families.

The Chronic Phase

In this final stage of the disease, the individual shows extensive emotional disorganization. He is drunk in the morning and during the work week, and he remains inebriated for days on end. Prolonged bouts of inebriety are termed "benders." The addicted individual manifests a marked loss of sense of ethics, an impairment of reality testing, profound regression, grandiosity and resentment. He is profoundly self-pitying and helpless. The addicted drinker who reaches this point in the progression of his illness is truly on "the bottom." He has reached the point of psychological deterioration that ushers in psychosis. Physically such an individual is on the brink of, if not actually struggling with, diseases of the central and peripheral nervous systems, the liver and the vascular system.

Medical Treatment

When the medical team is confronted with an addicted drinker who is as ill as the individual in the chronic phase, his care is first and foremost medical. Such an individual must have *tranquilizers* to control his symptoms of acute brain syndrome, i.e., confusion, dulling of senses and psychomotor agitation. He must have *polyvitamin therapy* with a concentration of vitamin B, *intravenous and oral fluids,* maintenance of his *electrolytes,* and a *high protein, high carbohydrate diet.*

Psychotherapy

For the student of alcoholism who believes that uncontrolled drinking is the core of the disease, the treatment would be the abolition of alcohol. Needless to say, this is not a practical solution; but just for instance, let us fantasy about it. Suppose that the production and distribution of alcoholic beverages could be controlled and, in this situation, obliterated. Would this cure the disease? Many think not.[5, 8, 9]

They feel that any comprehensive treatment must take into consideration the fact that alcoholism does not exist by itself, but is part of the total personality malformation which exists at the time. Whether the alcoholic can be successfully treated will depend on his motivation, his insight and his potential for change. Those for whom the treatment outlook is most hopeful are those people with a high degree of emotional development, i.e., development not fixated at the more primitive levels, for instance, the oral or anal. Though such alcoholics are extremely anxious and vulnerable to conditions created by stress, they are better integrated than the severely regressed. The addicted drinkers who have the potential for greatest gain in therapy have a high degree of social and economic involvement and responsibility and are capable of utilizing assistance and responding to pressures from family, doctor, clergy and friends.[7] In short, representatives of the middle classes and above are considered better treatment candidates. Such is discouraging information when nurses consider the numbers of alcoholics coming to their attention who are not verbally facile, are not employed, do not have understanding families and do not have good work histories; this group is found in our ghettos, in our emergency rooms, and on our state hospital wards.

No matter what the social class of the addicted drinker, no matter who the therapist, it is crucial to realize that:

1. The addicted drinker uses alcohol for relief of tension and insecurity.

2. The addicted drinker has a greater need for tension relief and relief of insecurity than others. The ways that he has become more tense and more insecure are numerous. Some have passive-aggressive personalities, repressed Oedipal urges or unmet dependency needs. Some are homosexual, depressed or basically schizoid. The reasons are numerous, and because of this treatment must aim at different goals for different patients.

3. A good treatment plan for the alcoholic must be individualized.

According to Chambers, who has achieved excellent results in the treatment of addicted drinkers, it is necessary that the patient gain the insight that he must give up alcohol. He must see that *he* has a hold on it, not that *it* (alcohol) has a hold on him.[12] The therapist with whom the alcoholic will gain this necessary insight must be a person who is tolerant, trustworthy and patient. The alcoholic will need time to develop a relationship with his therapist in which he can look candidly at his addiction to alcohol and his underlying problems that influence his addiction. The therapist must be prepared for exacerbations as reflected in the patient's temporary return to drinking. Many patients, when severely frightened by blackouts or delirium tremens, resolve "never to touch the stuff again," but these moments are usually forgotten with the next major stress. Backsliding will occur. It is necessary to acknowledge that drinking has resumed in a matter-of-fact way. For some alcoholics, a period of hospitalization may be necessary to start the patient on the road to sobriety. With help some may be able to stay away from alcohol long enough for the therapy to get underway. Treatment will strengthen the patient so that he can gain sufficient insight to recognize the role of stress in his drinking and to face basic issues without his crutch.

The therapist does not promise or expect a "cure." He does not hold out to the addicted drinker the possibility of being able to drink again in moderation. For the alcoholic controlled consumption of alcohol is so rare as to be considered a fallacy. For him, alcoholism might become a problem 20 years after successful treatment if he chooses to drink again. The goal of therapy, then, is to enable the addicted drinker to stop using alcohol as a tension reliever by identifying the underlying causes of his stress and by building in him different means for coping with it.

COMPLICATIONS OF ALCOHOLISM

Delirium Tremens

The most frequent psychosis seen in chronic alcoholics who have been drinking for a period of a decade or more is delirium tremens or "d.t.'s." This psychosis is the result of accumulated toxins. It is often brought on by abrupt cessation of drinking, though this is not always the case. Delirium tremens is differentiated from other underlying psychoses because in typical d.t.'s, hospitalization, drugs, fluids and diet usually quell the accompanying hallucinations within several days. If the symptoms continue beyond this interval, an underlying psychosis must be considered.

The patient with incipient d.t.'s is usually well-oriented but highly agitated and frenzied as he begins to experience auditory hallucinations. The full blown episode is characterized by extreme agitation and great fear as the patient has auditory and, occasionally, visual hallucinations. In this stage there is a clouding of consciousness and disorientation, and comprehension is poor. Thought processes are frequently illogical, and persecutory delusions are common. The patient shows mistrust, suspicion and uncertainty. Evident is a coarse tremor of the hands, tongue and face, especially around the mouth. The symptoms are usually worse at night and upon awakening from sleep. Moderate fever, sweats, leukocytosis and tachycardia are common. The syndrome usually runs its course in three to four days unless complicated by other factors such as pneumonia.

Needless to say, the appearance of d.t.'s creates a critical situation for the patient as well as the nursing staff. A particularly difficult situation is one in which the patient has been admitted to the hospital for reasons other than delirium tremens. Typically, such a patient comes to the unit for surgery, orthopedic therapy or a medical problem. There is no mention of alcoholism in the admitting history. Characteristically the patient begins to show signs of increased agitation after 24 to 36 hours in the hospital, since he has been withdrawn from alcohol for this period of time. The nurses are unaware of an impending problem unless they have seen such a situation before. Within another six to 12 hours the patient is acting as if in a full blown psychosis. There is disorientation to time, place and person. The patient may be seen running as if for his life. When stopped and restrained he screams that "they" are about to attack him or kill him, or some other theme of a persecutory nature. It is difficult to reassure such a patient.

The patient is sedated. He must be watched closely, for such persons are likely to commit suicide unintentionally in their frenzied efforts to "get away" from whatever it is that they are hallucinating. If the patient is in a room with a window, it should be adequately covered by bars or reinforced screening. The patient should not be left unattended. Bright light in the room is preferable to light that creates shadows, with a possibility of illusions. If at all possible, it is more humane not to restrain the patient. To understand the patient's dilemma, the reader need only imagine being restrained in bed while watching snakes, bugs or other odious crawling creatures move slowly up the sheets toward her body.

When it is necessary to administer medicine or treatment to the uncooperative patient, it is best to take enough staff members into the patient's room initially to properly restrain him. It is frightening enough for the patient to be handled and given medication that he fears, but it is worse when the patient is put in a position where he struggles unsuccessfully. The most humane approach is to have sufficient staff members present to administer whatever is prescribed without undue stress on anyone's part.

People, places and the time should be identified whenever appropriate. If the patient describes the nightmarish phenomenon that he is experiencing, the listening nurse should acknowledge her awareness of his fright, but state that she does not see or hear that which is evident to the patient. She can also indicate that the experience that the patient is undergoing is part of his illness and will disappear as he recovers from it.

The following complications occur only after years of heavy drinking. They may appear even though the alcoholic is sober.

Korsakoff's Syndrome

This disease occurs in chronic alcoholics. It is manifested by impairment of thought processes, confusion, loss of sense of time and place, and the tendency to recreate memories from fantasy rather than reality.

Wernicke's Syndrome

This syndrome, again seen in chronic alcoholism, is manifested by disturbed functioning of vision, memory loss, confusion, wandering of the mind, stupor and, sometimes, coma.

Polyneuropathy

Involvement of sensory and motor nerve endings is seen, producing irritability, pain, itching and loss of control of the limbs.

Korsakoff's and Wernicke's syndromes are much less common than polyneuropathy. Other complications frequently found in association with acute intoxication are cardiac strain, gastritis, hemorrhage of the esophagus, liver damage, pancreatitis, emphysema, diabetes and pneumonia.

Special Therapies

Antabuse. In 1948, disulfiram (Antabuse) was introduced. It is inert in the body until alcohol is consumed. It then produces intense throbbing headache, severe flushing, extreme nausea and vomiting, palpitations, hypotension, labored breathing and blurred vision. The drug is effective for several days after its administration. Knowing the effects of the drug reinforces the patient's resolve not to drink. The obvious drawback to the therapy is that the patient must take the drug. Thus, the patient who decides to drink need only stop the drug to resume the drinking habit. Results with Antabuse are poor without concurrent psychotherapy—individual, group or family.

Conditioned reflex or aversion therapy. The patient is subjected to revulsion-producing or pain-inducing stimuli at the same time he takes a drink. This process establishes a whiskey-pain or whiskey-revulsion association. Proponents of this type of therapy claim that periodic repetition of the conditioning process produces automatic, unconscious and lasting rejection of whiskey.

LSD-25. Much research is in progress utilizing this hallucinogenic agent to treat the alcoholic. Some workers report success ranging as high as 75 per cent. The exact mechanism in LSD-25 that is therapeutic has not been established, though some workers think that the drug induces insight-producing experiences. All agree that further research is indicated.

Alcoholics anonymous. "A.A." is responsible for the sobriety of more alcoholics than any other therapy—social, religious or medical.[7]

A.A. is a loosely organized, voluntary group of alcoholics who gather together for the purpose of helping themselves and each other to get sober and to stay sober. The membership is composed solely of addicted drinkers. The only condition of membership is that the individual be an alcoholic who wants to stop drinking. A.A. is not involved in any movement to combat or restrict the use of alcohol in general. It does not support any causes, even those designed to help alcoholics. It does not sponsor or support hospitals, nursing homes or sanitariums for alcoholics.[7]

A.A. instructs and supports the addicted drinker in his effort to stay sober for one day at a time. It helps the drinker to give up denial, rationalization and the other defense mechanisms that have characterized his thinking. The alcoholic is confronted with the seriousness of his problem. He must make realistic assessments of himself and move to correct these problems through concrete acts. A.A. provides fellowship and acceptance and support. In A.A. group meetings and individual encounters many psychological needs of the alcoholic are met.

Nursing Care

In the general hospital. The nurse is likely to have to develop nursing care plans for the alcoholic in two areas: the first, the emergency room, at which this patient arrives in acute illness; the second, the medical, surgical or orthopedic unit to which the patient is admitted and finds himself going into d.t.'s from withdrawal. In the emergency room the addicted drinker is typically treated punitively. He is usually known to the staff from numerous previous appearances. The alcoholic has a peculiar way of turning up on Saturday nights when the emergency room is literally overflowing with patients, many of whom are in grave distress and needing immediate attention. Nurses, doctors and attendants tend to push the alcoholic off in a corner, and each time he bobs up again, to shove him down more punitively, telling him to sit down, be quiet and stop bothering them. This is not helpful to the alcoholic.

Probably the emergency room is unable to do better under the pressure of the workload; however, if this poor wretch can be turned over to an alcoholism counselor or another designated person who is assigned the care of alcoholics, this is preferable. The alcoholic most likely needs medication, fluids and the support of some individual who is understanding, tolerant and patient.* He needs firmness. The alcoholic needs to know that the person in attendance knows what is going on. He does not need a lecture about the error of his ways. If he could control his consumption, he doubtlessly would. Hearing about his "weakness of character," and so forth, does nothing useful for him. The patient may offer a fantastic story about the reasons for his latest debacle. He does not need an appreciative audience. Indeed, what he does need to hear is that he has had too much; it's made him ill and it's time to sober up and hopefully look at some of the things that make him uncomfortable enough to get in this condition.

If the patient indicates willingness to follow through he can be referred to on-going treatment. A.A. is one source. Other possibilities are state mental hospitals, if they have alcoholism units, general hospitals, day or night hospitals and alcoholism clinics. Ideally such agencies should provide orientation lectures; medical treatment, including drugs, counseling and psychotherapy; programmed activities; resocialization measures; access to A.A.; diagnostic services; family casework and treatment; and information and referral services. Other agencies to which such a patient can be referred are recovery houses and halfway houses.

It would be folly to permit the nursing student to think that all these facilities are available in every large city. In fact, they are not; however, most communities of any size have some kind of program available for the addicted drinker. The emergency room nurse should keep a current list of these facilities and the people in them to be con-

---

* It is well to be sure the individual with alcohol on his breath, who appears stuporous and uncoordinated, is not suffering from diabetes, minor stroke or other metabolic diseases or encephalopathy.

tacted so that alcoholics coming into the emergency room are not simply discharged. Not to refer the alcoholic creates the "revolving door" situation in which the patient comes in, is treated, goes out, and comes in again the following night. A percentage of alcoholics will end up this way no matter how they are handled, but each should be given the opportunity of being moved into an active treatment program.

Industry. The nurse employed by industry is likely to meet alcoholics on the job. It is important to recognize the employee who is losing his battle with alcohol. Such a person has a record of spotty attendance. He may have reddened eyes, tremors of his hands or numerous complaints of gastritis. He may become noticeably withdrawn, irritable or, at least, changed in personality. His record may reflect increasing numbers of accidents. The industrial nurse needs to be on the lookout, because an addicted employee is a sick employee. He needs understanding help. Many firms such as DuPont, Eastman Kodak, and Allis-Chalmers have initiated educational programs on alcoholism.

The National Council on Alcoholism has made efforts to develop such programs for industries requesting them. The industrial nurse can keep track of absenteeism and decreased effectiveness in alcoholic employees. With her statistics she is in a position to sell management on the worth of requesting help from the National Council on Alcoholism in working out procedures for care of the alcoholic employee. Such programs ultimately increase output, which supports the industry.

It has been found that the alcoholic is characteristically able to manipulate employers to give him leeway, to "tolerate" his problems. If the alcoholic is going to be helped, he must find out that: (1) the employer recognizes his alcoholism as an illness; (2) the employer expects him to seek and stay in treatment; and (3) the employer expects to see improvement, and if not, the employee will be fired.[7]

In the community. The public health nurse is likely to deal with the problems of the alcoholic's family, for the addicted drinker who is not in crisis is not likely to seek medical attention. He does not hurt, and so he does not perceive himself as ill. For his family, it is another story. The alcoholic can create untold havoc in a household. The people there tend to protect him, to hide his problems from the neighbors. For them life is often a nightmare as their lives become more and more enmeshed with that of the drinking member. Families of alcoholics need the support of the public health nurse who is willing to drop in simply to chat. Her acknowledgment that there is a problem and her repeated visits offer some reassurance to the family members that someone will accept them. The visiting nurse can suggest appropriate referral for family members, whether or not the addicted drinker is in therapy. A.A. has separate groups for spouses of alcoholics and for adolescent offspring. In addition, there are church-sponsored groups in some communities to which the family can go for guidance as they try to make acceptable lives for themselves.

The nurse can also keep an eye on the alcoholic to see that his physical condition is maintained as long as possible. She can suggest those foods that offer the most amounts of necessary vitamins in the least amounts of food needed, since the alcoholic is a notoriously poor eater. Above all, the nurse remains in contact with the addicted drinker, letting him know that she knows, that she accepts, and that she understands his inability to control his alcoholic consumption. She communicates her willingness to stand by and to make the appropriate referral when the patient is ready to try to let go of his destructive habit.

DRUGS

Any discussion of drugs being abused currently is bound to be outdated by the time of publication, for each new day brings with it reports of some heretofore innocuous chemical agent which suddenly receives great notoriety because of its effects on the user. Whatever the agent, the effects can be broadly described as contentment-inducing, hallucinogenic or tension-reducing. Some of the drugs, like marihuana, do not seem to induce grave physiological damage; others create physical dependence that makes them impossible for the user to give up without special medical treatment.

The indiscriminate use of drugs, known as "drug abuse," is a behavior pattern by which people try to cope with the stress of overwhelming and uncontrollable change in or disruption of their lives. According to Yolles, "The hopeless despair of chronic poverty and the frustrating alienation of an increasingly mechanized society send the ghetto-dweller, as well as the economically affluent, to the same drugs. Poverty and alienation breed a common compulsion to 'cop out' or 'turn off' through drugs, from the surburbs to the slums."[12]

DRUG ADDICTION

One cannot write with authenticity about the "characteristics" of drug addicts. They include both men and women, educated and uneducated, poverty-stricken and financially secure. They all have become drug dependent because they believed that the drug they took would magically supply their needs. Thus the ghetto dweller may have believed that he could be "important," that his life would have significance and that he would be of some consequence and would be heard. The college student who had not found himself, or who felt inadequate to compete with his peer group, may have felt that with the introduction of heroin into his veins he would be competent to deal with his problems. The harassed housewife who without drugs felt tense and unable to assume her daily responsibilities felt immediately calm and serene when she maintained her blood level of barbiturates. Most of these people, no matter what they sought, no matter which drug they sought it from, had one thing in common: They were not existing in the real world; they were not in touch with their real selves. The problems resulting from their drug dependence catapulted them into a world that was unlike that of other humans.

Drug addicts create an external world for themselves which must be as problematic as the internal or external worlds they have sought to escape. They are constantly driven by internal forces to seek satisfaction through ever-increasing drug consumption. Drugs require money. Users are always concerned with getting money and acquiring drugs. Pretenses must be kept up. Reality must be bent so that the addict himself does not face the awful truth about the existence that he has shaped. Those who come in contact with the addict, such as family and friends, must not know about the secret life. Though jewelry, small appliances and other valued objects are taken from the home to pawn or sell, the addict tries to keep from his unaddicted friends and relatives the meaning of their losses.

When other means of revenue have been exhausted, when the spiraling cost of the habit gets beyond job potential, the addict must stop work or take time off to hustle. He must find other means of supporting his habit. He may borrow for a while, but eventually friends and family grow wary. Then the user turns to illegal means. Women become shoplifters or prostitutes who "turn tricks." Men burglarize, shoplift, pick pockets and forge signatures. Sometimes when the addict is feeling sick because his last fix has worn off, he will steal an item and take it directly to the pusher. When he is feeling sicker and more pressured he may in desperation hold up a victim at knife or gun point. Fiddle notes that addicts under this stress go to the pusher with their wares, such as tape recorders that would legally sell for $50 to $100, and they will gladly trade them for a few bags of drugs which would normally cost three to four dollars each.[4]

The drug addict's life is not tranquil. He is continuously looking for means to buy his fix, to find connections, to avoid the police. The addict is always hunting; he is always hunted. Added to the misery that he creates for himself is the constant risk of overdose and of hepatitis. He accepts all this for the *"nod."* This is "the culmination of the shot and represents the narcotization and apparent stimulation which the addict craves. It represents the end of striving, the cessation in varying degrees of all troubled reflection as well as the abandonment of all other projects except that of the quest for apparent euphoria or homeostasis."[4]

Yet even in the reward is the punishment. Illegal drugs are usually cut to provide the pusher a greater profit. The addict who may be used to a large dose in order to create the high he seeks may be sold a fix of uncut drugs; when he injects the fix, he dies from overdose. Should the addict be fortunate enough to escape this fate, he is still constantly hounded by the taste and smell of vomit that surrounds him. It decreases as tolerance for the drug increases, but a run-down condition or lack of food heralds its return. Thus, death, disease, disgust, ceaseless toil and the constant threat of arrest are continuous reminders to the drug addict of his miserable plight.

TYPES OF DRUGS

The types of drugs most commonly abused are: (1) sedatives, (2) stimulants, (3) tranquilizers, (4) hallucinogens, and (5) narcotics.

Sedatives

These drugs are usually barbiturates. They are commonly referred to as "goof balls." The barbiturate addict develops irritability, he often talks loudly, changes mood rapidly or becomes quarrelsome. In time such a person cannot concentrate. His intelligence is compromised and his judgment impaired. The barbiturate addict may develop slurred speech, tremor or staggering gait. Mental depression and suicide occur. If drugs are not available, withdrawal symptoms, i.e., restlessness, anxiety, increased irritability, nausea, vague pains or delirium may be reported. In severe cases, coma and death occur.

Stimulants

Stimulants are primarily amphetamines.[8] (See Chapter 11, p. 222.) Initially the stimulant addict may appear alert, describe a sense of well-being and have the ability to think quickly and to concentrate. However, with continued usage he becomes loud, irritable, agitated, unable to sleep and tremulous. Delusions of persecution and psychosis are seen in individuals addicted to these drugs. Interestingly enough, the adolescent group who are particularly prone to addiction to this type of drug have picked up or developed a language to go along with their drug culture. One of their terms is "paranoid." When they use it, they mean that the individual has developed delusions of persecution.

Tranquilizers

The same symptoms that are seen in those addicted to barbiturates are seen in users of tranquilizers.

Addiction often starts from the continued use of prescriptions that were probably written for a specific short-term problem or for others in the family. Other influences are dares, friendly persuasion that boasts of "kicks" and the fear of peer group rejection. For the adolescent it is not "cool" to be different. Thus, what the peer group does is likely to influence the behavior of any individual within that group. It is not difficult to find tranquilizers. In some school systems, disruptive children, termed "hyperactive," are treated with them; harried executives "pop" them to ease pressures; worried housewives depend on these drugs to calm their fears and tensions. The enterprising potential addict need not look far for his supply.

Hallucinogens

These are the chemical agents which induce altered states of consciousness. Some, like marihuana (also called pot, grass, and Mary Jane), produce relaxation and sometimes euphoria. Others, such as peyote, LSD and STP, induce visual hallucinations, alterations in tactile sensation, and expansion of feelings, usually described as feelings of omnipotence. These latter drugs are felt to be particularly dangerous because the users may have "bad trips." These are experiences of frightening proportions in which the "tripper" may be terrorized enough to commit suicide if not restrained. If not intentionally, he may commit suicide accidentally because of perceptual impairment or a loss of judgment. The trip itself can be fraught with danger; however, equally prevalent is the problem of "flashbacks" in which the person who is supposedly free of the drug's influence suddenly has a recrudescence of his symptoms, days, weeks, or months after the drug's ingestion. This may occur anytime and any place. One can imagine the effect if a drug user suddenly begins to hallucinate in the middle of a heavily traveled, high-speed highway! "Trippers" who need help are seen in neighborhood counseling centers, emergency rooms and college infirmaries. If they are unable to be calmed through verbal intervention, the drug of choice is usually Thorazine in large enough doses to sedate them until the effects of the hallucinogen have worn off. Of course, close supervision is essential.

The hallucinogens are not addicting. Individuals using them may feel the psychological need for them, but physiologically they are not imperative. It should also be said about these agents that, used under medical supervision for bona fide reasons, they sometimes yield useful results. Such is the case with LSD (lysergic acid diethylamide) in the treatment of alcoholics (see page 252) and the terminally ill. As with all drugs, use by rational authority is not drug abuse.

Narcotics

Though the statistics are changing rapidly and drug users are getting younger,* the "hard core narcotic user" is not typically an adolescent.

---
* Drug use is reported in the elementary schools, and death from overdose has been recorded for a 12 year old.

He is more often a school dropout, older than the high school age group. He is likely to come from worse social and economic straits than the users of other drugs. The student takes drugs for kicks, or because of dares, or to be like the others in the gang, but the narcotics user takes them to escape. His life is hard, his hopes are slim and, like the addicted drinker, he has found something that makes him feel good. Before much time has elapsed, such a drug abuser is "hooked." He finds he cannot stop taking his drug even if he wishes. Such a person will usually report an initiation by a "friend" who has described the good feeling associated with the drug's use. (Heroin, known as "H" or "horse," morphine and Demerol are used.) The addict characteristically starts by "snorting," or inhaling, the drug. Then he turns to "skin popping" or injecting it subcutaneously. Finally, he graduates to "mainlining" or injecting it directly into the vein for the heightened and more quickly obtained effect. Hard core narcotics addicts come to the attention of the nurse when they are admitted to the wards for treatment of their abscesses or hepatitis. Occasionally they are admitted for other types of medical problems, and the admission physical examination reveals typical puncture marks and the collapsed veins of the addict. Such individuals are usually given methadone while hospitalized, if they claim drug dependence.

TREATMENT

The treatment of the drug abuser addicted to narcotics is similar to that of the alcoholic in that the addicted individual must first tolerate separation from his drug (unless he is treated with methadone); then he must begin the exploration of his feelings in order to find out why he turned to drugs for comfort and how to protect himself against the necessity for them in the future. Unlike the alcoholic, it is almost impossible to treat the narcotics user on an outpatient basis. This is so primarily because of the emotional meaning of "the street" to the addict. Where alcoholism is an isolated process, i.e., the alcoholic buys his drink, consumes it and sleeps it off, the narcotic addict is hounded by the many people who prey on him. In his neighborhood are junkmen, pushers who know him and want him to continue to use drugs because his habit creates revenue for them. Thus, the narcotics addict is not only vulnerable because his own body craves the drug, but people around him are ever ready to help him get hooked again. A "fix" is as handy as the nearest pusher looking for a sale.

When treatment for addiction first gained popular interest, stress was put upon *detoxification* and rehabilitation in hospitals and community facilities. *Dechemicalization,* which is at once chemical, physiological, psychological and social, was not widely attempted. These programs have been succeeded by the current interest in a variety of treatments oriented around halfway houses and comparable group structures.

Studies show that the exaddict faces a multitude of problems: He is alienated from both addicts and nonaddicts. Family members are wary and unwilling to trust him again. Friends no longer acknowledge his presence. They identify the exaddict as a "junkie." Other addicts also represent a threat to the exaddict, who fears joining them socially. Loneliness is, therefore, a major problem of the exaddict.

Added to this is the ambiguity he is likely to face in family roles. Because he has been a drug addict he has become the sick, the dependent, the unreliable member of the family. His functions as a provider and supporter, or as a contributing member of the group, have been usurped. Often by the time he has been rehabilitated, his role has been taken over by a more adequate family member. This means that when he returns to the family he must once more win his place. Until this happens, his role is an ambiguous one. Still another problem the exaddict faces is failure in job adaptation. It is tough to tolerate the discipline of a nine to five job, the direction of a rigid or uninterested foreman, the requirement to produce steadily. It is tough to handle the questions pertaining to absences in the past. It is even tough to stand by and hear one's fellow workers talk about "junkies" and the hopelessness of addiction and express their disfavor of that group. All these factors make the exaddict's reintegration into society a hazardous undertaking.

At present these are basically two types of programs for the treatment of drug addicts. One utilizes readdiction by methadone. This type of program is controversial, though its results are promising. The chemical is distributed under federal control and there are restrictions on its use. Because readdiction is implicit in the treatment, a usually stated criterion for admission into such a program is that the addict must show evidence of addiction over a stated period (it varies from two to five years) and must have failed at other methods of withdrawal. Limitations are placed to insure as much as possible that an individual who might be able to come off drugs entirely is not unnecessarily readdicted; on the other hand, the limitations impose harsh conditions on addicts who really want the treatment, but who have not been addicted long enough or who have not been exposed to other types of programs.

The other basic means of treatment is withdrawal. It may be gradual, with decreasing amounts of narcotics used over a long period and support from other types of medication given in an inpatient setting. It may be abrupt withdrawal, known as "cold turkey."

Methadone

This is a synthetic drug which was created by German chemists during World War II.[2] It appeases the desire for opiates without producing the euphoria of narcotics. The drug blocks the action of other narcotics, such as the "high," and at the same time it prevents the addict from feeling "sick." "Sick" is the symptom complex associated with drug letdown, or withdrawal. Once the maintenance dose of methadone is reached, increases in dosage are not required, as with other narcotics, to produce the individual's good feelings associated with the drug. Methadone is given by mouth. Even if the addict has had a large habit, the dosage is small initially and is gradually increased over a period of six to eight weeks. It is prepared daily in fresh or artificial fruit juice to disguise the taste. One milligram of the drug is mixed with 1 ml. of liquid. The medication is prepared daily because the fruit juice is unstable after 48 hours, and preservatives interfere with monitoring done by urinalysis.

In 1970 there were approximately 30 methadone programs in the United States serving about 4000 people. One such program is found in St. Louis. The St. Louis State Hospital became a center for a methadone clinic in 1968. It was funded under the 1966 Narcotic Addict Rehabilitation Act. The program is operated jointly by the St. Louis Division of the Department of Psychiatry of the University of Missouri School of Medicine and by the Missouri Division of Mental Health. A year after its inception the clinic moved to a storefront building in an area where there was heavy use of drugs. This clinic distributes methadone to approximately 230 patients, maintains necessary surveillance through urinalysis and attempts social rehabilitation. The clinic serves also as a point of entry into a total program for addicts. After evaluation, addicts are referred for further withdrawal (preferably as inpatients in the program's 20-bed unit at the state hospital), to a therapeutic community operated for 50 addicts at a former hotel or for methadone maintenance.[6]

The staff of the clinic are a registered nurse who is the director, a receptionist, a chief counselor and one other counselor who are both exaddicts, and a psychiatrist who comes half a day per week. A social worker, a rehabilitation counselor and additional exaddict counselors come by appointment. The clinic also receives the services of a pathologist, laboratory technicians, a pharmacist and an epidemiologist.

When an addict comes to the clinic, he is likely to be asked for a urine specimen, which will be tested for the presence of drugs other than methadone. (Patients in most clinics are not asked for a specimen every time because, anticipating such a test, they could then falsify the results by bringing specimens that they did not excrete.) The test takes six and a half hours to complete. Methadone is given on the day the sample is submitted. The results of the urine analysis are returned the following day. If the results show the presence of drugs, the patient is questioned about this on his return visit.

This treatment has been found to be safe and effective.[7] Through methadone the addict is protected from the discomforts of being without drugs; he is able to remain out of prison, and normal social roles are attainable. Though the drug is the main feature of treatment, doctors, nurses, vocational counselors, exaddicts and legal advisers are needed in the total rehabilitation program. Initially they help to combat the "street problems" which hound the addict and make his social rehabilitation difficult. Eventually they support the addict as he identifies and explores his basic problems. Finally, they counsel him during his search for and efforts to forge a new life.

Withdrawal as a Treatment

Informal types of groups such as Synanon and Phoenix Houses, Exodus House, and Daytop Lodge are springing up all over the country, designed to reach out to the drug addict and to help him to kick his habit. The programs usually consist of groups of addicts with counselors or leaders, many of whom are former addicts, who live together for a prescribed period of time. The leaders and older members of the group have successfully withdrawn from their dependence on drugs. They oversee the novitiate's withdrawal. It is generally felt that the former addict is well equipped to help the newer patient because he knows more precisely what is happening both physiologically and psychologically to the withdrawing patient.

Synanon is an organization which has had remarkable success with rehabilitation of the drug addict, or drug "fiend" as members of that organization prefer to call themselves. The organization was founded by an exalcoholic and corporate executive named Chuck Dederich. This man has been described as a genius in understanding and solving human problems. He began Synanon on an unemployment check and a charismatic personality which was able to attract people who needed help. Today this same organization has grown to the point where it is all but self-sufficient.

Synanon is a voluntary treatment facility. The addict presents himself at one of the five houses located in Santa Monica, San Francisco or San Diego, California; Reno, Nevada; or Westport, Connecticut. There he is interviewed by staff members who are exaddicts, and if he is accepted by them, the addict is told the conditions of his admission. He will work at jobs to which he is assigned by others; he will attend the functions of the House; and he will not use drugs or physical violence. If the addict accepts the conditions, he becomes a member. When an addict comes in "loaded," he is taken to the living room and shown to a couch where he can come off his drugs "cold turkey." The addict is given no medicine. Twenty-four hours a day sympathy is available, as are massage, egg nog and observation. The drug stock of the house consists of vitamins and aspirin.[11] While the addict goes through "kicking the habit," which is likely to mean several days when he is intensely uncomfortable and weak, the new member is supported and kept company by older members. After this period of withdrawal the person, as he is called at Synanon (no one is called "patient"), is assigned to a job. Everyone in the organization works for the group. There is no "we" and "they."

Rehabilitation is accomplished through an active program oriented around group process. There are "synanons," which are group discussions, several times a week. New groups are formed from the house members for each synanon so that permanent membership does not breed "agreements," such as "You don't bring up my problem and I won't bring up yours." There are also unscheduled "haircuts," which are sessions attended by relatively new patients and four or five of the older members of the organization. In these sessions the new member is "taken apart" and his performance to date is pointed out to him, both constructively and destructively, together with suggestions for his future behavior. Haircuts are seen as brutal verbal attacks, but persons in the organization seem to improve as a result of them and they do not shrink from them. In Synanon, words are important, but actions are more highly valued. Pure insight is scorned and openly ridiculed. As was explained by a Synanon member: "You (professionals) are all involved with drug addiction. You want to know how an addict uses it, how much, and all that crap. Around here we are interested in helping exdope fiends grow up by talking about living clean."[11]

The synanon gets people to interact on an intense personal level. They grow by imitating the role models provided by older members. They are encouraged to be upwardly mobile, and this is a reality in the organization because there is stratification in the groups through job differentiation. Thus, a variety of jobs are available involving real needs of the organization. Food must be procured and cooked; there are office tasks, maintenance and service crews, automotive and operations crews and a coordinating staff. The new member starts in a menial job. As he grows and remains longer in the group, he stands a good chance of promotion to jobs which involve direction of Synanon. (All directors are exaddicts.)

Synanon is a large and growing organization. It transfers addicts from the East Coast to the West and vice versa in order to break old and pathological ties. Indefinite stays are prescribed. Indeed, many of the members elect to live permanently with their families in Synanon. It is possible to live without contacts in the outside community; Synanon is becoming more self-sufficient each year. Economic and social resources become stronger and stronger. "Synanon Industries" has several warehouses and factories. It accepts industrial contracts for manufacturing machine tool parts and has shown a profit. Looking ahead, the residents of Synanon hope to create a city where members can live and bring their families. At this time there have been marriages among the group members, and a nursery is available to care for their children.

Synanon hopes that "through group process a man will become less alienated from himself, less stupid, less absurd, less concerned with his own problems and more concerned with becoming a functioning member of society."[4]

Regrettably there is little systematic research done in the area of treatment of the narcotic addict, unless he is treated in a place such as the federally run hospital in Lexington, Kentucky, or other institutions administered primarily on the medical model. It is known that both gradual and abrupt withdrawal are notable for relapses of treated patients. Methadone helps; it seems to permit a better social adjustment. Programs such as Synanon look promising. Considering all, it is recognized that new treatment methods are needed.

Nursing

The nurse is appropriately assigned in the care of an addict with hepatitis or abscess. Her clinical practice is well outlined in medical and surgical nursing texts; aside from these situations, however, it is difficult to say explicitly what the nurse's role is. In the clinic she gives methadone. In the community she may refer an addict for medical attention. The question still remains, what can the nurse do for the addict? At this point in time there does not seem to be a specific role for the nurse in the actual treatment of addiction. The few studies available indicate that addicts are best treated in groups. They are helped by the pressure of the group they live with when they are told to fight it out, to give up the drug, to sit down and talk about their problems. The nurse is an ancillary person in such a setting. She offers herself as an understanding listener and as an enthusiastic supporter of the addict's progress. The nurse should act toward the drug addict's family as she does toward the family of the alcoholic by counseling, making appropriate referrals and keeping in contact. If necessary, the nurse may have to provide emotional support to the family as they turn over their loved one, the addict, to the law.

The nurse and the drug-habituated adolescent. The nurse who cares for the adolescent coming "down" from drugs, or withdrawing, must be prepared for a hostile, negativistic person. She is dealing with someone who is at best ambivalent about the therapy, and at worst completely against it. There will be recriminations, accusations, tears and frustrations. Such a patient needs understanding and tolerance. As with the alcoholic, an understanding, nonpunitive attendant is necessary. It is distressing to give up that which the mind and body have come to require in order to function. It is equally distressing to begin the exploration of issues that created the potential in an individual for drug abuse. The outlook for the individual who has been taking sedatives, stimulants, hallucinogens or tranquilizers, however, is far more optimistic than that for the narcotics user.

The nurse who works in a school is quite likely to encounter the adolescent on drugs. She may recognize his problem from his emotional instability, his sluggishness or tremulousness. The school nurse who moves about in her working environment may become aware that drug traffic is heavy in the bathrooms. "Joints" (marihuana) are smoked here and pills are popped. It is here, in the cafeteria and in the locker rooms that drugs are consumed and traded. It is in these places that the school nurse must begin to work with her vulnerable population. It is not recommended that the nurse begin by telling the students about the evils of drug abuse. Rather, the potentially helpful nurse must become known as being understanding and "with it." She is a person to whom the students can go to discuss other matters, i.e., family conflicts, feared pregnancies, felt inadequacies. As in helping the alcoholic, being an understanding listener is a prerequisite. No progress can be made until the drug user feels a permanent bond with the nurse so that he or she is willing to consider the possible distress that withdrawal will entail.

When the drug-using student indicates his readiness to seek definitive treatment, the school nurse may help him to contact a private or clinic source for therapy. Finally, if the nurse has earned a reputation for fairness and honesty, she will be sought out for "the facts" about drugs. If she is lucky, the information she disseminates may influence some students not to experiment.

REFERENCES

Alcoholism

1. Blum, E.: Psychoanalytic Views of Alcoholism. *Quart. J. Studies on Alcoholism,* 27:259-299, 1966.
2. Chambers, F.: *The Drinker's Addiction: Its Nature and Practical Treatment.* Springfield, Illinois, Charles C Thomas, 1968.
3. Himwich, H.: Views on the Etiology of Alcoholism. *In* Kruse, D. (ed.): *Alcoholism as a Medical Problem.* New York, Hoeber Division, Harper & Bros., 1956, p. 34.
4. Jellinek, E.: *The Disease Concept of Alcoholism.* New Haven, Conn., College and University Press, 1960.
5. Kaufman, F.: *In* Kruse, D. (ed.): *Alcoholism as a Medical Problem.* New York, Hoeber Division, Harper & Bros., 1956.
6. Kruse, D. (ed.): *Alcoholism as a Medical Problem.* New York, Hoeber Division, Harper & Bros., 1956.
7. Milt, H.: *Basic Handbook of Alcoholism.* Maplewood, New Jersey, Scientific Aids Publications, 1969.
8. Schilder, P.: Psychogenesis of Alcoholism. *Quart. J. Studies on Alcoholism,* 2: 272-292, 1941.
9. Wexberg, I.: Alcoholism as a Sickness. *Quart. J. Studies on Alcoholism,* 22:217-230, 1951.
10. Zwerling, I., and Rosenbaum, M.: Alcoholic Addiction and Personality. *In* Arieti, S. (ed.): *American Handbook of Psychiatry.* New York, Basic Books, Inc., 1959.

SUGGESTED READING

Anonymous: Alcoholism, Addiction, Depression: A Nurse's Story. *Nursing Outlook,* 3: November, 1965.

This very real, very touching account of a nurse's struggles with her feelings and alcohol may help the reader to see the addicted drinker as a person, more human, more troubled than otherwise. The article is highly readable and graphically portrays the hellish existence of the uncontrolled drinker.

Gelperin, E., and Gelperin, A.: The Inebriate in the Emergency Room. *Am. J. Nursing,* 70:1494-1497, July, 1970.

This timely, medically oriented discussion on the alcoholic who presents in the emergency room warns the nurse not to be lulled into a false diagnosis of simple drunkenness when the patient presents with alcohol on the breath. There are other more virulent conditions which may be influencing the patient's seemingly stuporous condition.

McNatt, J., and Sahler, S.: Caring for the Alcoholic on a Medical Unit. *Am. J. Nursing,* 65:114-116, March, 1965.

The article presents a lucid and very handy guide to the sometimes anxiety-provoking care of the acutely ill alcoholic on a medical unit.

Moore, M.: An Account of a Nurse's Role and Functions in an Alcoholic Treatment Program. *J. Psychiatric Nursing,* 8:21-27, May-June, 1970.

This is another interesting account of how the work is planned and implemented in one particular setting. It permits the reader to look at how a workable plan functions. This may not be the right set-up for every agency, but it offers one functional scheme.

Parry, A.: Alcoholism. *Am. J. Nursing,* 65:111-115, March, 1965.

Alcoholism is presented as a medical disease requiring the care of a medical team, replete with nursing care, special dietetics, drug therapy and psychotherapy. The article provides a good, thorough look at the broad considerations.

Quiros, A.: Adjusting Nursing Techniques to the Treatment of Alcoholic Patients. *Nursing Outlook,* 5 (No. 5):276-279, 1957.

This is an excellent article which explores the use of nurses in the treatment of alcoholics. The author says so much more than the nurse "should be a good listener." One has the impression the writer has truly wrestled with the problem of nursing care for the alcoholic and she has constructive suggestions to make.

Randall, T.: *The Twelfth Step.* New York, Charles Scribner's Sons, 1957.

I cannot recommend this book highly enough. It is old and thick and the print is not large; however, for the persevering reader the pages of this story will yield information about the life of the alcoholic that can come from no textbook account. The reader who peruses the pages of Randall's book will know the morass that is the drinker's life as if she had been there.

Drugs

1. Byrd, O. (ed.) : *Medical Readings on Drug Abuse.* Reading, Mass., Addison-Wesley Publishing Co., Inc., 1970.
2. Carlova, J.: Methadone: Growing Hope or Grim Illusion? *Medical Economics,* (special issue), April 20, 1970, p. 83.
3. Dole, V. P., Nyswander, M. E., and Kreek, M. J.: Narcotic Blockade. *Arch. Intern. Med.,* 118:304-309, October, 1966.
4. Fiddle, S.: *Portraits from a Shooting Gallery.* New York, Harper and Row, 1967, p. 36.
5. Hekimian, L. J., and Gershon, S.: Characteristics of Drug Abusers Admitted to a Psychiatric Hospital. *J.A.M.A.,* 205:125-130, July, 1968.
6. Knowles, R. R., and Anderson, G.: Setting up a Methadone Maintenance Program. *Hospital and Community Psychiatry,* 22: February, 1971.
7. Nyswander, M., and Dole, V.: The Present Status of Methadone Blockade Therapy. *Am. J. Psychiat.,* 123:1441-1442, May, 1967.

8. Osbourne, R.: Drug Abuse and Abusers. *In* Byrd, O.: *Medical Readings on Drug Abuse.* Reading, Mass., Addison-Wesley Publishing Co., Inc., 1970.
9. Robinson, L.: Marihuana Use in High School Girls: A Psycho-social Case Study. Unpublished doctoral dissertation. University of Maryland, College Park, 1970.
10. Weech, A.: The Narcotic Addict and the Street. *Arch Gen. Psychiat.,* 14: March, 1966.
11. Yablonsky, L.: *The Tunnel Back, Synanon.* New York, The Macmillan Co., 1965.
12. Yolles, S.: The Drug Scene. *Nursing Outlook,* 8: July, 1970.

SUGGESTED READING

Caskey, K., Blaylock, E., and Wauson, B.: The School Nurse and Drug Abusers. *Nursing Outlook,* 18 (No. 12):27-30, 1970.

The author presents a highly readable, most valuable account of the school nurse's potential role in the prevention, counseling and treatment of the drug user.

Childress, G.: The Role of the Nurse with the Drug Abuser and Addict. *J. Psychiat. Nursing,* 8 (No. 2):21-26, March-April, 1970.

The article presents a lucid account of the problem and the nurse's position in relation to it.

Fiddle, S.: *Portraits from a Shooting Gallery.* New York, Harper & Row, 1967.

This interesting and well written book shows intimate knowledge of the lives of addicts.

Osnos, R.: A Community Counseling Center for Addicts. *Nursing Outlook,* 3 (No. 11):38-40, 1965.

This is another well written account of one agency's method of delivery of health services. It seems to be a good plan.

Poplar, J.: Characteristics of Nurse Addicts. *Am. J. Nursing,* 69:117-119, January, 1969.

This is a particularly useful article because it reminds the reader that "drug addicts" are people we know, not clinical specimens.

Rodewald, R.: Speed Kills: The Adolescent Methedrine Addict. *Perspectives in Psychiatric Care,* 8 (No. 4):160-168, 1970.

The author has written a particularly good overview of the whole problem of adolescent drug abuse. She has utilized many resources which the reader will appreciate as she reads this article. Additionally, the reader is treated to short anecdotal accounts of the author's work with this particular population. Overall, this is a most useful article for the nursing student to study.

Russaw, E.: Nursing in a Narcotic-Detoxification Unit. *Am. J. Nursing,* 70:1720-1723, August, 1970.

An inpatient treatment program is described. The author, as a result of her observations, concludes that the nurse's role is a supportive one. She perceives the exaddict in a more functional capacity vis-à-vis the hospitalized addict. This article is especially interesting because it is written by a nurse who sees other than nursing personnel in key roles. She very much reflects the team approach to the drug addict's care.

Taylor, S.: Addicts as Patients. *Nursing Outlook,* 12:41-44, November, 1965.

The author writes from the viewpoint of a public health nurse. She sees different things and draws conclusions that reflect her orientation, which is slightly different from those already presented.

Yablonsky, L.: *The Tunnel Back, Synanon.* New York, The Macmillan Co., 1965.

Yablonsky, a sociologist, has produced a fine account of Synanon. He has lived with the groups and discusses many interesting facts about them which serve to create a living image of Synanon for the reader.

chapter 13

PATIENTS WHO MANIFEST SYMPTOMS OF PSYCHIATRIC ILLNESS FROM ORGANIC CAUSES

There are a wide variety of organic problems which arise in the central nervous system and cause behavioral disturbances. Some of them are reversible; many are not.* Organic brain syndrome, the complex of symptoms which results from the majority of central nervous system diseases, includes impairment of orientation, memory and intellectual functioning, i.e., comprehension, calculation, knowledge, learning and judgment; lability of emotion; and shallowness of affect. In acute brain syndrome (abs) the symptoms are reversible; in chronic brain syndrome (cbs) they are not. To complicate the picture, some disorders which seem to be reversible initially can ultimately leave permanent damage.

Diseases of the central nervous system can be divided into brain syndromes associated with: (1) intracranial infectious disorders, such as encephalitis and meningitis; (2) systemic infections; (3) drug or poison intoxication, such as lead poisoning and barbiturate overdose; (4) trauma, such as automobile accidents in which victims sustain concussions or skull fracture, which sometimes leaves residual disturbances such as epilepsy; (5) circulatory disturbances, such as cerebrovascular accidents; (6) cerebral arteriosclerosis; (7) neoplasms; (8) syphilis; and (9) diseases of unknown origin, such as multiple sclerosis, Huntington's

---
* Aging is included in this category, but will be discussed separately.

chorea and Alzheimer's disease. Medical and neurological considerations differ with the various disorders; however, the psychiatric nursing problems and interventions are, for the most part, similar.

Several of the disorders will be discussed in order to show the basic commonalities of nursing care, or to identify for the nursing student specific details pertinent to particular disorders.

BRAIN SYNDROME ASSOCIATED WITH CEREBRAL OR SYSTEMIC INFECTION

DELIRIUM

There are several paths by which the physical condition of a patient can lead to that syndrome known as delirium. One of these is alcoholism, and the type of delirium observed is called delirium tremens. (See Chapter 12.) A similar syndrome may result from systemic infections such pneumonia, typhoid fever and various others, including the genitourinary group, which produce high fevers. In these illnesses the organism causing the infection produces toxins which irritate the brain.

A third manner in which delirium is caused is through actual invasion of the brain by the infecting organism. Intracranial infections are usually localized in the subarachnoid space (meningitis) or are spread diffusely within the brain (encephalitis), or are seen in encapsulated regions within the brain or meninges (abscess).[10]

Delirium may be mild or severe. In its mild form, symptoms such as irritability, insomnia and restlessness appear. If the infection is overcome rapidly, the symptoms tend to subside. With increasing severity of infection, there are increasing symptoms of delirium. They may include combativeness, visual hallucinations, impairment of memory and altered states of consciousness such as lethargy, drowsiness, stupor and coma. Though these symptoms subside when the causative organism is controlled, changes of personality and intellect may persist.

The patient suffering from delirium is highly anxious. He is aware of his poor state of health and fears this as well as the feelings he experiences as a result of decreased awareness. The environment should be familiar. If possible, nurses who are known to the patient should be assigned to him. Family members should be encouraged to remain with the patient. This is not to suggest a large group, but one or two close relatives. The patient should not be left alone. Every effort must be made to assist the patient in maintaining his grasp on reality. Such things as mirrors, calendars, newspapers, orienting (i.e., information giving), conversations and familiar faces have this effect. Also important in decreasing disorientation is the use of light that does not cast shadows that might stimulate illusory perceptions.

Sedation and analgesia should be requested from the attending physician if the nurse observes the need for them; however, it is important for the nurse to remember the depressant effect such medications have on cerebral function. The patient must be well hydrated, kept from undue exposure and generally supported by good bedside nursing.

ENCEPHALITIS

Encephalitis is a term for several types of infections that are spread diffusely in the brain. Encephalitis may produce sequelae, including postencephalitic parkinsonism and certain enduring behavior disorders. Psychiatric symptomatology may range from severe organic states to paranoid or catatonic schizophrenic disorders and manic-depressive symptoms. Some patients have tendencies to obsessive behavior. Impulsive, aggressive behavior is not unusual. In children, mental retardation and extremely asocial, aggressive and abnormal sexual behavior have been reported.[6] Postencephalitic changes vary from mild behavior syndromes, including poor impulse control, to severe psychoses. The nursing care of patients with acute encephalitic phenomena is basically like that of patients in delirium. In postencephalitic sequelae, care is oriented around the patient's psychological needs. Though etiological factors may vary, the patient's feelings are like the feelings of others with similar behavior patterns who have already been discussed.

BRAIN SYNDROME ASSOCIATED WITH CEREBRAL ARTERIOSCLEROSIS

This disorder is usually associated with advancing age. It is not inevitable, but it is seen in most elderly people. The disease process involves hardening and thickening of the artery walls, which produces narrowing of the lumina of the vessels. Circulation is impaired, and the cells of the brain do not receive the oxygen necessary to survival and optimal functioning. Thus, there is destruction of brain tissue.

Individuals with this problem may become easily tired. They tend to be forgetful, emotionally labile and irritable. In the early stages such individuals can usually be maintained outside of hospitals if families are willing to give the extra supervision needed. Later symptoms may include marked disorientation, incoherence and even delusions. Sleep disturbances with reversal of day and night patterns are not unusual. If the symptoms progress to this degree, the patient may require hospitalization during which bed rest, diet and medication are utilized in treatment.

BRAIN SYNDROME ASSOCIATED WITH CIRCULATORY DISTURBANCES

This disorder is related to cerebral arteriosclerosis because much of the circulatory disturbance seen is the result of arteriosclerosis, particularly in the elderly. The brain syndrome occurs in patients suffering from several other types of vascular disorders as well. They include emboli, arterial hypertension, cardiorenal disease and cardiac decompensation. The neurological and psychic symptoms observed depend upon the size and location of the occluded vessels.

One of the more frequently occurring problems is catastrophic cerebral hemorrhage. Patients who are seen in the emergency rooms and intensive care units fall into two large groups: the younger patients present with subarachnoid hemorrhage, and the older patients with intracerebral hemorrhage.[4]

The patient who presents with a cerebrovascular accident (CVA) may die in the first few hours after hemorrhage or he may stabilize and improve, depending on the location and size of the vascular lesion. Cerebrovascular accidents consist of cerebral infarction or hemorrhage. Ongoing arteriosclerotic processes result in reduction of blood supply to the brain. When occlusions occur, the ensuing symptoms manifest themselves in a syndrome called CVA or "stroke." The term has little descriptive meaning because, depending on the location of the circulatory disruption, one patient may present with loss of a sensory or motor function while another might demonstrate impairment of intellectual functioning. In widespread disruption of physiological functioning in the brain, there may be vast changes in the patient's thinking and behavior. In such situations, emotional responses may be sudden, inappropriate and disproportionate to the stimulus.[3]

If the patient stabilizes and it is apparent that he will improve, his progress will be, in large part, influenced by nursing care. The keystone of that care is nursing assessment. The patient must be seen in his totality, his disease being a part of his person rather than the reverse. In some progressive neurological units, medical, nursing, psychological, social work, occupational therapy and speech therapy specialists all plan together for the patient's care, based upon their individual assessments. A baseline is established for the patient by identifying his level of functioning and his permanent disabilities (as identified in each specialist's area). To this assessment are added the goals that are desired by the patient and that seem realistic to the staff in view of the patient's potential. His treatment plan is built around this assessment.

Of particular interest to the nursing student with special focus on psychiatric nursing are the patient's emotional needs and the problems of supporting him over what is likely to be an extended convalescence. The "stroke" patient regains consciousness (if he has lost it) with many questions. Some questions he feels he can verbalize to his family or attending staff; some he chooses to keep to himself. It is these latter questions and speculations which tend to produce special problems for the patient. For anyone who has not experienced unexpected hospitalization, sudden loss of consciousness, the effort to reconstruct time lost and the assimilation of all new input, it is difficult to understand the patient's emotional situation. The patient becomes aware of the brain inside *his* head. Most individuals do not focus on parts of their bodies. Thus, the heart beats without rest, the brain is constantly vital and the lungs expand and contract, but the individual does not actually focus on any of these parts of himself, because they *are* part of his functioning whole. Suddenly, when one of these vital areas becomes dysfunctional, the individual, in a sense, stops, looks and listens. Psychologically he places the organ at arm's length and inspects it. He wonders how his self is contained in the part and how its dysfunction will ultimately affect that total self which is, in part, the organ that he is attempting to scrutinize. It is in these very private speculations that the nurse may be supportive to the patient if she is intuitively aware. Her therapeutic value lies in her willingness to listen and, if she can, to communicate her acceptance of the patient as a human being like herself. If she can communicate to the patient that she recognizes him as a whole person, perhaps with temporary impairment, rather than a strange specimen with some part of his mysterious brain gone, the patient may then begin to view himself as his actual self, the person with whom he is familiar.

When the initial adjustments are made, the patient will need support during his and the staff's efforts to rehabilitate him. To learn to speak again, to walk, to dress, to lift a cup—all these activities that were once taken for granted are frustrating to relearn. Sometimes, the weeks and months of work required become overwhelming. The nurse in the hospital or caring for the patient in the community is helpful if she can judge when to listen, when to comfort and when to discourage his tears and demand a greater effort from the patient.

BRAIN SYNDROME ASSOCIATED WITH SYPHILIS

In a society that is moving toward increased impermanence, in which there is a marked increase in drug abuse, in which there seems to be a decrease in the importance of familial relationships and an increase in temporary bonds, there is a marked increase in sexual promiscuity. There is a parallel increase in the incidence of venereal diseases. Syphilis is caused by the organism *Treponema pallidum*. It is transmitted through contact between infected and noninfected mucous membranes. Occasionally it may be transmitted through superficial wounds. The only other means by which it is contracted without direct contact is in the newborn, who receives the disease in utero. Some who contract syphilis do not realize it, for when the classic chancre, which indicates the point of entry of the spirochete, disappears, there are no other clinical problems for some time. The disease progresses very slowly and may not be evident in the central nervous system (CNS) for 20 years.

Victims of CNS syphilis manifest exaggerated characteristics of their basic personalities. There is increased irritability, fatigue, lack of concentration, confusion, depression, superficial or absent emotional response and marked carelessness with lack of interest in activities. Social behavior deteriorates rapidly. In later phases there are confabulation, poor judgment and marked displays of delusions, usually of a grandiose nature. These patients can be quite unpredictable in their behavior, and sexual as well as combative activities provide a chronic source of problems to staff members.

Physically the syphilitic patient with CNS disease has pronounced difficulties in speech and writing. An ataxic gait is seen. There is progressive weakness and incoordination of all muscles. Pathological reflexes are seen as well as loss of sphincter control. At this point the patient is critically ill. In the terminal phase the physical nursing needs far outweigh the psychological. Until the terminal phase, however, the psychological needs of the patient such as recognition and acceptance require great ingenuity from the psychiatric nurse. A very basic problem is to prevent staff members from withdrawing from the patient and to continue to approach him as a sensate human being.

BRAIN SYNDROME ASSOCIATED WITH DISEASES OF UNKNOWN CAUSES

MULTIPLE SCLEROSIS

This degenerative disease of the central nervous system is a progressive chronic ailment which is manifested by remissions and exacerbations. In the early phases, when there are few plaques (areas of demyelinization) on the nerves, the patient has minimal symptoms of dysfunction. With increased plaques, the patient shows blurred vision, weakness of the lower extremities, incoordination, parathesias and sphincter disturbances. Unilateral retrobulbar neuritis is often seen, as are nystagmus and coarse tremor. The patient in an exacerbation is often emotionally labile, laughing and crying easily and inappropriately. At times a marked euphoria is seen.

The cause of multiple sclerosis is not known. At this writing, treatment is confined to the administration of steroids to limit the severity of exacerbations, a good balance of rest and activity, nursing care and the prevention of invalidism through rehabilitative efforts.

One of the striking characteristics of this disease is its predilection for young adults. The first episode may be in adolescence or between the early 20's and 40. The disease may run a swift downhill course, or it may be characterized by periods of incapacity followed by remission of symptoms. The average total duration from the time of diagnosis is 15 to 20 years.[16] In later stages the patient is bedridden, febrile and in great pain from muscular spasms.

The outstanding need for the multiple sclerosis patient is his need for emotional support in the light of a diagnosis that is prognostically bleak. This patient must come to terms with the knowledge that he is going to become progressively more handicapped until he can no longer care for himself. Possible loss of sight, loss of mobility and consequent loss of independence are predictable. The patient never knows when the next exacerbation will occur, nor how it will present. It is no wonder that suicide is not uncommon.

To adequately nurse the patient with multiple sclerosis is to care enough to listen, to share the human agony, and to respond. For one nurse this may be sitting and listening, for another it may be talking and occasionally touching the patient. For all it means being with him, not only to give the physical care which becomes an increasing requirement, but also being with him in order to prevent his isolation. Social ostracism is often the fate of the patient for whom we cannot alter the outcome.

HUNTINGTON'S CHOREA

This degenerative disease is known to be hereditary. In the disorder certain cells in the brain which regulate muscle movement die early and are not replaced. The patient, who is usually diagnosed between the ages of 30 and 45 years, manifests involuntary, irregular, jerky movements associated with the upper extremities, neck and face. The movements spread to the trunk and lower extremities. Although they are continuous in periods of wakefulness, in sleep the movements cease.

Severe mental changes appear in the majority of patients, usually after the onset of neurological symptoms. Speech becomes incomprehensible, and patients tend to become paranoid and severely depressed. The patient deteriorates and usually dies in a five to ten year period after diagnosis.

The course of Huntington's chorea is similar to CNS syphilis in that in the final stages the patient presents in the mental hospital with severe organic as well as psychic illness. The patient who has reached the point of institutionalization for his mental deterioration is apt to have difficulty in locomotion and swallowing. He is chronically fatigued from his inability to stop moving. This is the end product. What, though, of the offspring who have watched a parent die of this hereditary disease? What are their feelings, their fears, their fantasies each time they experience a symptom of unknown etiology? What nightmarish terror do they experience each time they await a doctor's diagnosis? How, indeed, do they tolerate the terrible news when the doctor tells them that their "tremor" is due to Huntington's chorea? What possible succor is there for a patient who has watched his own parent die a miserable death from this devastating disease and then must face the eventuality of his own death in the same manner? Equally agonizing must be wondering if one has passed the disease on to one's children.

Whatever is done for such a patient in the early stages of his disease does not fit under the confining rubric of "nursing," but should probably be seen as the acts of one responsive human being to another. The first necessity is to help the patient over the appalling shock that comes with the diagnosis. (For the majority this will not be completely unexpected, for one parent will have died of the disease and, if it was properly diagnosed, the family will know that it was hereditary and that a 50 per cent possibility existed for its transmission.) Nonetheless, it *is* appalling for any reason to be told that one's life is soon to be snuffed out. It is worse, if possible, for victims of this disease, who are destined to deteriorate in such a cruel and painful way.

Nursing personnel working with such a patient can do little physically for the patient other than to make him as comfortable as possible. This is a rather vain effort, because drugs are not yet known that can stop the patient's uncontrollable movements and the pain that accompanies them. Psychological care can help. The patient is alive and aware as long as he can communicate in some form. One of the worst and commonest tragedies that befall the hopelessly ill patient is that he is prematurely abandoned. It is a wonderful thing when staff members do not permit this to happen. Deliberate and honest introspection is required to prevent withdrawal, but abandonment will lead to isolation of the patient, which is comparable to psychic death.

BRAIN SYNDROME ASSOCIATED WITH INTRACRANIAL NEOPLASM

"Brain tumor" is a term used to designate a growth in any part of the brain. The brain consists of a variety of tissues governing an equally wide range of functions. The symptoms of such tumors depend on the type and rapidity of growth, the location of the tumor and its tendency to increase intracranial pressure. Brain tumors may be either malignant or benign, but the latter tumor, if located in an area that is not operable, may have as poor a prognosis as a malignant neoplasm.

A wide range of symptoms may herald the presence of a cerebral lesion. Some symptoms depend to a great extent on the basic personality of the individual. (This is true in the majority of organic diseases that manifest themselves in behavioral change.) Thus, the basically depressive individual may show marked depression. The introverted person may become particularly withdrawn. The expansive extravert may become hypermanic in his euphoria. The psychiatric nurse will most often encounter such patients when their tumors are inoperable and personality changes require institutionalization.

BRAIN SYNDROME ASSOCIATED WITH DRUG AND POISON INTOXICATION

LEAD POISONING

The human consumption of lead occurs in two basic situations: in the child, lead poisoning occurs because young children who are left unsupervised or without adequate activity will sometimes chew on windowsills and other painted surfaces on which leaded paints have been used; in adults, lead poisoning occurs from contact with industrial products such as solvents. The lead may be inhaled or absorbed through the skin. After several weeks of exposure to toxic doses patients develop headaches, nausea and mood changes. Both manic and depressive syndromes, excitement and delirium are observed. Adult patients with lead-induced psychoses have a good prognosis. Once they have been removed from the source of poison, the lead levels usually decrease rapidly. In some cases drugs such as Versene are used to hasten this process.

BRAIN SYNDROME ASSOCIATED WITH TRAUMA

EPILEPSY

There are several forms of epilepsy involving motor or sensory symptoms associated with seizures. The causes of these disorders are multiple. In some cases heredity is indicated. Complications of pregnancy, fetal diseases, malformations, birth injuries and infectious diseases are all considered causes of seizures in infants and children. Epilepsy has been diagnosed as a sequelae of trauma to the brain.[6]

Epilepsy can be a rather easily controlled disease causing little handicap to the patient. For a shrinking minority who have frequent seizures, it may cause psychosis, mental deficiency and deterioration.[6] The latter symptoms are rare, however, since aggressive treatment with anticonvulsant drugs usually controls the symptoms. If seizure activity is found to originate in accessible areas of the brain, surgery may be performed to explore for and remove the focal point.

When seizures are first experienced by the patient, he is often frightened or embarrassed. Such a patient needs repeated assurances that he is not peculiar or outlandishly different from others. Additionally he needs information about the drugs that will be prescribed to control his symptoms. Finally, the epileptic patient should be helped to adjust his activities so that they do not present a danger should he lose consciousness unexpectedly.

AGING

When one considers aging as a normal part of the developmental cycle, it seems more acceptable, more a natural part of life. (See Chapter 5.) In many ways birth and death, childhood and senility, adolescence and elderliness have mutual characteristics. Birth and death signify the beginning and the end. For those who do not believe in a life after death, the state of nothingness is the antecedent of birth and the condition after death. A complete cycle is etched in a lifetime. Childhood represents the era when problem-solving skills develop; senility robs the individual of them. The adolescent struggles with a recrudescence of the exaggerated personality characteristics of the oedipal period. They represent erstwhile interpersonal conflicts that re-emerge; their final resolution is observed in the psychologically stronger personality with which the young adult leaves adolescence. In the era of aging these same personality characteristics appear once again. Thus, one sees recurring patterns in the life cycle. The beginning and the end share similarities.

Lidz divides old age into three phases: elderly—the period when retirement and adjustment to a nonworking life style occur and independence is still possible; senescence—the period when the aged person deteriorates physically and is forced to become dependent on others; senility—the period when the brain ceases to function as an organ of adaptation.[8] These periods may overlap and some may not occur at all.[8] Such productive persons as Chief Justice Holmes, Sir Winston Churchill, Bertrand Russell and Albert Einstein are representative of some in whom all these phases did not occur.

ELDERLY

The first stage of becoming old may be the most traumatic phase of aging. It begins for most at approximately 65 years when the employed individual decides to retire or is forced by company policy to do so. For the male this step is fraught with psychological danger. If his identity has been oriented around an occupation, he must then re-identify himself. For some this is not possible, and the remainder of life is insignificant and without meaning.

For the woman these years may also be distressing. The possibility of child bearing is long over. Physical appearance is no longer at its best, and the years are upon her when she is likely to lose her spouse. If not widowed, she is faced with the constant presence of her husband who no longer works. The daily routines that have become her way of life and which provided a major portion of her security are interrupted. She, too, faces a realignment of her life style imposed by the change in the life of her spouse. This may be difficult after 40 or more years of particular living patterns.

During these years the aging individual recognizes the inevitable approach of physical deterioration. He wishes to continue to make meaningful contributions and he dreads becoming a burden on his family. This wish is illustrated in the comment of E. S., a 62 year old mother, who said to her married daughter: "I hope we can take a house in Italy for the summer while we are all still healthy and can enjoy it. Daddy and I will keep the kids while you and Tom travel. . . . Italy is so beautiful."

SENESCENCE

In this phase, which is often anticipated with dread, physical deterioration progresses, forcing dependence on others. Loss of sight and hearing are common. Teeth fall out and benign prostatic hypertrophy occurs. Though the majority of these conditions can be modified, i.e., by cataract surgery, hearing aids, dentures and urological surgery, the senescent person is failing physically. Medical science has made fantastic strides which prolong life; however, the physical body eventually tires and wears out. Parts cannot be replaced without end. In this phase are the heartbreaking scenes when old people are placed in mental hospitals and nursing homes because there is no one able or willing to assume their care. Such placements are often a reflection of others' solutions to the problems of the aged individual. The solutions are often expensive and inhumane. It is in this phase that the worst fears of the individual are realized. He lives to see himself become dependent, and lose his autonomy. For some who are given shelter by their children, tyrannical practices which were used upon the latter during their youth are now practiced by them upon the aged parent. The tables are turned. For some elderly women who must share cramped quarters with their married daughters or daughters-in-law, the presence of two homemakers will prove disastrous unless the elder woman can restrain herself from competing with the younger one. Senescence is not easy for either the elderly or their families.

SENILITY

In this last phase of aging, the brain ceases to function as an organ of adaptation. Brain cells have been diminishing for some time,* but

---
* Intellectual functioning begins to diminish in the mid thirties.

now there is gross malfunctioning which results in apparent psychotic behavior. In senility the aged individual has little or no recall for the recent past, and he lives more and more in the remote past.

> T. I., a 97 year old man, was approached by the nurse and asked if he wished to be pushed out on the sun porch with the others. He replied that he did not think so because his mother would soon be home to take him to the store.

The senile person is likely to misidentify those in his present life as persons in his past. He may even feel that he is himself a child again. This situation accounts for the often described "second childhood." Some workers feel that senility is not an inevitable phase of the body's deterioration but rather that it represents an emotional breakdown in the elderly caused by anxiety which overtaxes the individual's ability to function.[11] They feel that senility should be regarded as a treatable psychosis in which the precipitating cause and, if possible, the antecedents should be identified and resolved. They propose treatment in groups as soon as the person is in contact with reality. Oberleder writes that predisposing factors in senility are unresolved conflicts of the middle years such as repressed anger, fear, love, need and guilt. She further cites unfulfilled ambition, insecurity, failure, feelings of rejection and sexual repression as problems of a lifetime which finally culminate in the psychosis termed senility.

The aging process is as difficult as was the maturational process of childhood. Stresses impose great anxiety and handicaps; however, all is not bleak. In the twilight years pleasure comes from experiencing the rewards of fulfillment and the successes of children or institutions that the aging person has helped to create. There are contentment and relief from strivings and struggles. Until physical deterioration, through loss of sight or hearing, and the discomfort of arthritis and other chronic diseases occur, there is time to enjoy longed-for pursuits that have not been possible earlier.[8]

"The person who reaches 65 still has a life expectancy of over 12 years. If a person survives to reach 80, he will still have an expectation of another 10 years. With advancing age, the body's decline seems to slow down."[8] Medical science is adding years to the lives of our citizens; these years, however, bring multiple physical, psychological and social problems. What can the nurse do to alleviate some of these problems?

First, families need to be taught how to prevent mental deterioration by providing healthy environments and plentiful opportunities for the elderly to develop satisfactory roles and good self-attitudes. Their living quarters should be bright and cheery, with cherished memorabilia surrounding them. If necessary, measures must be taken to decrease noxious odors. If confinement to a wheel chair or bed is necessary, the family or caretaking staff need to recognize that the size of the individual's environment shrinks. Self-respect can be increased even in these diminished environments by allowing the bedridden or chair-bound to do all that he can, such as feeding himself and moving his own body. Shaking hands with the infirm may be important, for it gives an opportunity for warm contact and helps the individual to feel more respected and significant.

The nurse may be able to teach others the importance of recognizing that with aging comes a diminution of problem-solving skills and the ability to think in abstract terms. As a result, there is increased rigidity. Added to this unpleasant potential is the proclivity for exaggeration of basic personality traits. Thus, bitterness, aggression and being demanding or envy and spitefulness may return without the ameliorative effects of compensatory behavior seen in the middle years. The family of such an elderly person will need support and counsel as they develop means of living with their relative and providing him with security and self-respect without sacrificing their own lives. It is tragic to see the elderly treated like children, either patronized or tyrannized, but equally sad is the family that relinquishes all activities and interests to strength-sapping care for the aging individual.

Social security, medicare and third party payment health insurance are bringing about brighter vistas for the aged. There are a growing number of nursing homes. Some are inferior, whereas others provide congenial and healthful environments. If families are considering such placements, the nurse may be of help by indicating the criteria of good facilities. Ratio of staff to patients, staff preparation and leadership should be questioned. The philosophy of the institution is important, as well as the means by which it is carried out in the care of residents. Is an attending physician identified? The kinds of life-supporting equipment that are available should be noted. Prevailing attitudes of care-taking personnel are especially important. Are residents addressed as Mr. X and Mrs. Y or are they referred to as "Grandma over there" or "Grandpa?" The cleanliness of the institution is of paramount importance. Is the smell of urine present? What are the food preparation facilities like? Important also are the presence of qualified physical and occupational therapists. Finally, the cost of the care facility must be taken into consideration. Can the family afford to keep a relative there? All these factors are significant.

The nurse may be of assistance to the family who is considering such a placement by indicating to them the importance of having the aged person take part in the decision making. The inevitable separation anxieties must be recognized and dealt with. Once the actual placement is made, the aged person must not be abandoned. Visiting is crucial, as is taking the person who is able out of the facility for holidays and special treats.

SUMMARY

There are a multiplicity of disorders involving the brain and spinal cord. Some are acute processes which will resolve; some are acute processes that will move quickly to terminal situations. Many neurological diseases are of a chronic nature and characteristically do not improve. The vast majority of disorders in this area tend to grow worse, causing gradual degeneration, increasing handicap and ultimate death. It is no wonder that those working in neurology and neurosurgery are often thought of as particularly "cool" toward their patients and "academically" or "scientifically" oriented. When it is not possible to help such a large segment of one's patients, it is sometimes necessary to withdraw to the less painful area of interest in the disease process or study of the cerebral area damaged as manifested by the signs and symptoms.

What, though, of the person who harbors the signs and symptoms? What of this individual who must learn of the disease that afflicts him? What of the person who must acknowledge the presence in himself of a disease process from which he will die? The psychological needs of the patient are great. The nurse must come to terms with herself and her feelings if she is to create anything of value for and with her patient. It is characteristic to avoid thoughts which are painful. Death is painful, as are progressive deterioration and loss of mental functioning.

The nurse who is in daily contact with these phenomena among her patients sometimes needs to withdraw her feelings and her investment in her patients in order to survive the psychic onslaught of pain when she responds to those around her. This is understandable; however, for the patient from whom she withdraws it means isolation and abandonment. No one knows how it feels to be dead; therefore, death is not feared. It is the *process of dying* that is dreaded. It is the fear of loss and of isolation. Thus, when the nurse withdraws from the patient, she validates that which he dreads—abandonment, or dying as he perceives it. If this concept is accepted, then the paramount feature in nursing the terminally ill patient is to make sure that he is not isolated. It is the major responsibility of nurses and nursing care plans to provide someone who can be near him. If a given nurse must withdraw, as all must from time to time for emotional renewal, then that person must be replaced by another. The dying or deteriorating patient must not be permitted to feel alone. When nursing personnel are provided, what do they do? It has been observed and reported by many that conversation need not center on dying, living, weather, pain or any other topic.[7, 12–14] The imperative feature is another person's presence. When an individual has spent considerable time with another and there have been honesty and acceptance, words become secondary. Closeness, a feeling of oneness, is created. All that is necessary can be communicated in a look or a touch.

When nurses and doctors can accept death as a property of life, when they can relinquish the need to save lives and can value assisting human beings to die with grace and dignity, then the patient may be unafraid. He will be neither left in pain nor abandoned.

REFERENCES

1. Bibring, G.: Old Age. *In* Lowenstein, R., Newman, L., Schur, M., and Solnit, A. (eds.) : *Psychoanalysis: A General Psychology*. New York, International Universities Press, Inc., 1966.
2. Burnside, L.: Loss: A Constant Theme in Group Work with the Aged. *Hospital and Community Psychiatry*, 21:173-177, June, 1970.
3. Busse, E.: Brain Syndrome Associated with Circulatory Disturbances. *In* Freedman, A., and Kaplan, H. (eds.): *Comprehensive Textbook of Psychiatry*. Baltimore, The Williams & Wilkins Co., 1967, p. 720.
4. Clipper, M.: Nursing Care of the Patients in a Neurological Intensive Care Unit. *Nurs. Clin. N. Amer.*, 4:218, June, 1969.
5. Comstock, R., Mayers, R., and Folsom, J.: Simple Physical Activities for the Elderly. *Hospital and Community Psychiatry*, 20:377-380, December, 1969.
6. Freedman, A., and Redlich, R.: *The Theory and Practice of Psychiatry*. New York, Basic Books, Inc., 1966.
7. Kubler-Ross, E.: *On Death and Dying*. New York, The Macmillan Co., 1970.
8. Lidz, T.: *The Person*. New York, Basic Books, Inc., 1968, p. 478.
9. Markson, E., Kwah, A., Cummings, J., and Cummings, E.: Alternatives to Hospitalization for Psychiatrically Ill Geriatric Patients. *Amer. J. Psychiat.*, 127: 1055-1062, February, 1971.
10. Mulder, D., and Allan, D.: Brain Syndromes Associated with Infections. *In* Freedman, A., and Kaplan, H. (eds.) : *Comprehensive Textbook of Psychiatry*. Baltimore, The Williams & Wilkins Co., 1967.
11. Oberleder, M.: Emotional Breakdowns in Elderly People. *Hospital and Community Psychiatry*, 20:191, July, 1969.
12. Robinson, L.: *Psychological Aspects of the Care of Hospitalized Patients*. Philadelphia, F. A. Davis Company, 1968.
13. Saunders, C.: *Care of the Dying*. London, The Macmillan Co., 1959.
14. Verwoerdt, A.: *Communication with the Fatally Ill*. Springfield, Illinois, Charles C Thomas, 1966.
15. Waggoner, R.: Brain Syndromes Associated with Intracranial Neoplasm. *In* Freedman, A., and Kaplan, H. (eds.) : *Comprehensive Textbook of Psychiatry*. Baltimore, The Williams & Wilkins Co., 1967.
16. Walton, J.: Demyelinating Diseases. *In* Harrison, T. R., et al. (eds.): *Principles of Internal Medicine*. New York, McGraw-Hill Book Co., 1958, p. 1647.

SUGGESTED READING

Anonymous: Death in the First Person. *Am. J. Nursing*, 70:336, February, 1970.

This is a particularly poignant plea written by a dying nursing student. She pleads not to be treated like a piece of baggage on an assembly line. The writer cites that she is dying and that she has never had this experience before, even if those caring for her have. She begs for warmth and compassion because she is afraid. One cannot read this article without reacting.

Anonymous: A Way of Dying. *In* Skipper, J., and Leonard R. (eds.): *Social Interaction and Patient Care*. Philadelphia, J. B. Lippincott Co., 1965.

The writer is a widow who presents dying from another point of view. It is one that is not often recognized by the health professions that are dedicated to prolonging life.

Gunther, J.: *Death Be Not Proud*. New York, Harper & Brothers, 1949.

John Gunther has presented a living memorial to his deceased son in this small chronicle about the boy in his losing battle with a brain tumor. Again the reader is afforded a view of the dying patient and his family that is not always evident in the hospital situation.

Hall, B.: The Mental Health of Senior Citizens. *Nursing Outlook*, 4:206-208, April, 1956.

Here is a particularly warm and readable account of the problems of the geriatric patient and the responsibilities of health workers around him. Though the article does not focus on neurological deficits per se, organic brain syndrome is implicit.

Moser, D.: An Understanding Approach to the Aphasic Patient. *Am. J. Nursing*, 61: 52-55, April, 1961.

This is a useful article for the nurse who is working with a patient who has had a stroke or tumor that has caused him to be unable to communicate by speech. The author gives simple, helpful clues as to ways that the nurse might approach this patient and his problem.

Nursing Clinics of North America, June, 1969, 1: Neurologic and Neurosurgical Nursing.

The nine articles included are interesting and especially useful to the nursing student studying in this area. Of particular worth are the sections on care of patients in an intensive care unit by Clipper, and nursing care assessment by Hamilton et al.

chapter 14

EMOTIONAL AND MENTAL ILLNESS IN CHILDREN

by Leona Weiner, R.N., Ed. D.*

Reliable surveys on the incidence of emotional and mental illnesses in children are unavailable. An increase in the number of residential and outpatient treatment facilities in recent years, with long waiting lists of children needing therapy, would indicate that the problem is becoming more acute, or that the public is becoming more aware of the need for help. Of the children of school age who are receiving psychiatric services, there are indications that boys outnumber girls by as much as three to one. This ratio begins to reverse itself after adolescence.

CLASSIFICATION AND DIAGNOSIS

There is very little agreement among child therapists as to a functional classification of childhood mental and emotional disturbances. In the "Diagnostic and Statistical Manual of Mental Disorders," published by the American Psychiatric Association, most of the childhood disorders are not listed separately from the adult classifications.[4] Only

---

* Associate Professor, Department of Nursing, Long Island University, Brooklyn, New York.

two categories of disorders pertain specifically to children: "transient situational disturbances," and "behavior disorders of childhood and adolescence." In general, these categories fail to take into account the developmental factors and dependency needs of children. Under the category of "unsocialized aggressive reactions," for example, are listed such items as temper tantrums, stealing and lying—characteristics that may be normal during certain stages of growth and development.

In general, most mental and emotional disorders in children fall into three broad categories: disturbances that are of a temporary nature, behavior and neurotic disturbances, and psychotic disturbances.

Disturbances that are of a *temporary* nature include behavior responses that are part of normal growth and development such as temper tantrums. They also include behavior that follows a crisis situation such as a hospital admission. If handled properly, the behavior need not result in any repeated or prolonged disturbance.

A *neurotic* or *behavior disorder* results when temporary upsets are not handled properly or when the child has had a painful or frightening experience, particularly if separation has been involved and he has not been able to verbalize his experience. The child will manifest behavior that is not in keeping with his age expectations, such as the six year old who continues to have temper tantrums. He may regress to an earlier level of behavior, as in the case of the enuretic child who has been previously toilet trained and does not return to his former achievement. Sometimes he exhibits bizarre behavior such as facial grimaces. The neurotic child is aware of and responds to reality, although not always in a socially acceptable way. Disorders that can be included under the broad classification of neurosis are phobias, tics, behavior disorders, personality disorders, and so forth.

The *psychotic* child appears to be out of touch with reality. He exhibits bizarre behavior most of the time and does not follow normal growth and development patterns. He fails to communicate with others in a meaningful way, if at all. Examples of psychosis that fit into this category are infantile autism and childhood schizophrenia.

The causes of mental illness in children are multiple and complex. Studies carried out at the James Jackson Putnam Children's Center have shown that the components present in the history of atypical children were those of a disturbed mother-child relationship, a detached father, and trauma to the child before the age of two, resulting in a separation of the child from the parents for a period of time. There was usually a history of physical illness in the child before the age of two.[8]

Often there is a physical component that either precipitates the disturbance or results from it and it is difficult to separate the two. The child with mild brain damage, for example, will exhibit out-of-control and bizarre behavior. The autistic child will often fail to develop speech or have weird physical manifestations.

Diagnosis of mental illness in children is usually made after an extensive study of the child and interviews with the parents or other significant adults.

The child should undergo a complete physical examination. If neurological signs are present, a neurological work-up, including an electroencephalographic study of the brain waves, is done. The child is also given a battery of psychological tests, depending on his age. The most popular tests include an IQ determination, a modified version of the thematic apperception test, the Rorschach test and perceptual tests. The thematic apperception test is a series of pictures showing a child and an adult interacting. The child's story about what he sees in the interaction often gives a clue to the child's thought processes and personal experiences. The Rorschach test is a series of ten standardized inkblots at which the child can look and describe what he sees. He tells his thoughts, impressions and associations and identifies shapes that he sees in the blots as animals, people or objects. The scoring is standardized, being based on the inkblots used, the nature of the objects seen, and the colors and the forms that the child has responded to.

The psychotherapist generally sees the child for one or two play sessions. If the child is of preschool age he may be observed, together with his mother or father, in a nursery setting with several other families. The observers can be psychotherapists, nurses, social workers, teachers or any other person on the therapeutic team.

A history is taken from the family, both through a written application form and through interview. Usually it is the social worker who does the intake interview, although the nurse may also have this role in some agencies. Items that are looked for in doing an intake interview include (1) the problem as seen by the parent, (2) what the parent feels that the agency can do for the child (3) the developmental history of the child, (4) the education and work goals of the parents, and (5) the relationships between family members.

The intake interview is also used to explain agency policies, to clear up misconceptions and to answer questions. The following excerpts from an interview with Mr. T., father of a disturbed five year old girl, will illustrate some of these points.

> When I had Mr. T. begin by asking him what the problem was, he seemed surprised. He said that the pediatrician thought there was a problem and that he referred him to Dr. P. He continued that Dr. P. feels that the child has "a personality defect, has many irrational fears and is both very shy and very bold." Also that they (the parents) had started her in nursery school in September and she had to be withdrawn two months later because she had a "negative attitude." She would bite and hit the other children. He added that the teacher told him and his wife that their child was very good, would listen and that it was only outdoors that she showed this "negative" attitude. He went on to say that perhaps

"they" didn't have enough teachers and that "my little girl" was the youngest in the class. . . .

When I asked, he said that frankly he and his wife didn't see any problem with the child. (Mr. T. never once used his child's name). He agreed that she was different, but that she was not abnormal. . . .

He asked a great many questions about the actual treatment here and when I noted that the children are not necessarily taken for treatment at the center following the diagnostic procedures, he showed a change in his previous attitude. He emphasized that Dr. P. felt that it was important and that he should make sure to mention his name to us; that he felt that treatment here was what the child needed.

THERAPY

Since most diagnostic categories are not applicable to children, there is a growing trend to work with children on the basis of their behavior and their response to therapy.

Factors of critical importance that enter into a treatment plan for the child are those related to meeting his dependency and growth and developmental needs. This means an inclusion of the parents or guardians in the plan, a selection of methods that are within the scope of the child's ability to respond, and a therapist who understands the needs of well children throughout the life cycle.

Often the parents as well as the child enter into a therapeutic regimen. Sometimes the family is treated as a group. In other instances it is only the parent or parents who need to receive therapy in order for the child to benefit. In rarer instances it is only the child who receives help. Even when the parents are not themselves receiving insight therapy, they are usually given some form of counseling, even if it is only for supportive purposes.

Children are best treated on an outpatient basis such as in a child guidance center, specialized nursery or day center. In this way the child can continue to be a part of his family and community, which are so vital to his growth.

Whether the child is best treated in a group or on an individual basis often depends on his age and symptom manifestations. For a withdrawn child, a permissive small group setting might be more therapeutic, whereas a hyperactive child might better be seen individually at first in a setting with definite limits and reduced stimuli.

Individual therapy consists of establishing a therapeutic relationship between the therapist and the child within a prescribed time setting (usually one hour sessions two to four times a week). The method of therapy differs according to the therapist's school of thought. The traditional psychoanalytic approach is generally ineffective with children.

Anna Freud cites the underlying reasons for this failure as follows:[5]

There is an absence of free association in the child.

He does not enter analysis of his own free will.

Children do not take a long-term view of any situation; the present is more important than possible future gains.

The child acts in preference to talking.

Children, particularly the adolescent, feel more threatened than the adult by analysis.

Children tend to externalize their inner conflicts. They look for environmental solutions in preference to internal change.

The same factors that limit the use of verbal techniques make play therapy and behavior therapy particularly suited to the pediatric patient.

BEHAVIOR THERAPY

Behavior therapy has been gaining favor in recent years in the treatment of disturbed children. It is based on the concept of operant conditioning, which employs the use of negative and positive reinforcement. (See also pp. 182 to 189.) The aim of behavior therapy is toward the modification or erasure of undesirable symptoms rather than a complete cure.

In its simplest form, desirable behavior is rewarded with a wanted item such as candy, attention, affection or materials. Any undesirable behavior is ignored or reacted to with some form of disapproval. A simple example of this occurs in one center for disturbed preschool children where an expected behavior is that of sitting at the table to eat. In this setting the child who sits at the table during snack time is rewarded with juice and cookies as well as with approval. The child who chooses to stay away from the table is ignored and does not receive the treat. It is interesting to note that in this center even the most withdrawn child is found at the table during snack time.

Another form of operant conditioning involves the use of aversion techniques. Here undesirable behavior is followed by a negative stimulant producing an unpleasant experience. This can be of a chemical or physical nature, such as screaming at the child, electrical shock, production of an unwanted symptom or deprivation of a coveted prize. It is important to be sure that the negative reinforcer is one that is *unwanted by the child.* To some children physical abuse may be viewed as a positive reinforcer, since this may have been the child's only form of closeness to a parental figure.

The aim of this technique is to produce anticipatory avoidance learning. Thus, the child who receives a shock every time he bangs his head may soon learn to avoid this behavior. The inherent risk here is that he might substitute one form of unwanted behavior for another since the underlying disorder is still present, or that he may become hostile and aggressive. In general, aversion therapy is used only under controlled conditions and with children for whom other forms of therapy have been of no benefit. In some cases of lack of speech in autistic children, this has been the only form of treatment that has produced any results, even if on a very rudimentary level.

Another form of operant conditioning has been called the principle of negative practice. Under this technique the patient is asked to consciously practice the undesirable symptom or behavior manifestation. A child who grimaces, for example, may be asked to make this grimace over and over again. Instead of increasing the undesirable behavior, the conscious repetition tends to make the wrong responses disappear. This form of therapy has been most effective in the treatment of tics and stuttering.

The principal arguments against the use of operant conditioning are that the basic reason for the behavior has not been removed, and that it can only result in the substitution of one undesirable symptom for another. The behavior therapists contend that for the most part this fear has not been borne out and that conditioning is more effective in certain cases than the traditional psychoanalytically oriented approaches. The research to date is insufficient to prove if this form of therapy has any better results than other therapies.[10]

PLAY THERAPY

Play therapy is often mistakenly confused with free play. In free play the child is given toys and a place to play and left to his own devices. Although this may produce some therapeutic benefits such as enjoyment and a sense of achievement, for the disturbed child this is not enough. He needs to establish a meaningful relationship with people rather than with things. In fact, he may have been playing alone too long.

In play therapy play is the vehicle through which the child and the therapist can interact. The setting, although permissive, operates within certain well defined limits of time and space. These limits are often broad and differ from those of everyday life in that they permit the child to act out his feelings without fear of punishment or disapproval. The following is a description of one play therapy room.

> There was nothing about the room or the materials in it that would tend to restrain the activities of a child. Nothing seemed to be either too fragile or too good to touch or knock about. The room provided space and some materials that might lend themselves to the emergence of the personalities of the children who might spend some time there. The ingredients of experience would make the room uniquely different for each child. . . . Dibs stood in the middle of the room, his back toward me, twisting his hands together. I waited. We had an hour to spend in this room. There

was no urgency to get anything done. To play or not to play. To talk or to be silent. In here, it would make no difference. The room was very small. No matter where he went in here he couldn't get too far away. There was a table under which he could crawl, if he felt like hiding. There was a little chair beside the table if he felt like sitting down. There were the toys to play with if he so desired.[1]

In play therapy the child presents a microcosm of his own world which the therapist uses toward helping the child to grow. On the simplest level it enables the therapist to establish communication with the child.

Each time he named an object I made an attempt to communicate my recognition of his spoken word. I would say, "Yes. That is a bed," or, "I think it is a dresser," or "It does look like a rabbit." I tried to keep my response brief, in line with what he said and with enough variation to avoid monotony. When he picked up the father doll and said, "Papa?" I replied, "It could be Papa." And that is the way our conversation went with every item that he picked up and named. I thought that this was the way to begin verbal communication. Naming the objects seemed a safe enough beginning.[1]

Play therapy allows the child to express his feelings in the presence of a nonjudgmental adult.

He scooped up the sand with broad sweeps of his hands and built a hill over the grave he had made—over the grave of the buried toy soldier. When the hill was completed, he brushed the sand from his hands, sat there cross-legged looking at it. "That one was Papa," he said quietly, climbing out of the sandbox.
"It was Papa who got buried under the hill?"
"Yes," Dibs replied, "It was Papa."[1]

The therapy sessions are also reality testing situations for the child and permit the therapist to correct misconceptions.

THE NURSE'S ROLE IN WORKING WITH DISTURBED CHILDREN

Along with other health workers the nurse's goal in working with the disturbed child and his parents is that of maximizing the health potential. Her method of operation differs from other professional workers in that the nurse generally does not have a choice of client and patient contact is not limited to a precise time but often extends over a working day rather than a limited appointment. Also, the child is more apt to be seen in the company of others than alone. In institutional settings the nurse is responsible for the actual physical care of the child, introducing touch contact as a necessary part of her role. The nurse's functions often vary, depending on the setting.

THE NURSE'S ROLE IN PUBLIC HEALTH AND OUTPATIENT SERVICES

In public health agencies the nurse's role is more likely to center on prevention, education, case detection, referral to other agencies and parent counseling. In some instances the psychiatric nurse clinician may handle a child and/or his family for psychotherapy under the prescription and supervision of the referring psychiatrist.

Prevention

Prevention is accomplished through (1) giving anticipatory guidance relating to problems that many parents encounter, such as negativism in the two year old, (2) educating parents about growth and development and critical stages of growth, and (3) providing the parents with an opportunity to express their fears and fantasies about pregnancy, children, and so forth, particularly during times of family crisis. A good deal of prevention can be accomplished through classes.

Parent classes for prenatal couples are generally accepted as a needed service for the promotion of mental health and as a nursing responsibility. Unfortunately the same cannot be said for continuing education for parents. The need for knowledge concerning growth and development, particularly the critical periods of growth, and the prevention and management of behavior difficulties are topics of great importance to the parent as the child is about to go through these stages. Several agencies have recognized this need and provide classes in which mothers, and occasionally fathers, are able to gather at a time that is convenient to them. This can include such settings as local YM and YWCA's, shopping centers, child health stations, clinics, schools and private health centers. The classes may be sponsored by either private or public health agencies such as the local health department and group health insurance plans. They are also initiated by parent groups such as the PTA and by educational institutions such as a college of nursing.

Small group classes led by a discussion leader as opposed to a lecture-discussion seem to be most effective in drawing out group problems and in helping the group toward more effective problem solving. The discussion leader keeps the group on the topic, summarizes, helps to get everyone involved, helps the group to discuss those areas that are important to them and acts as a resource person when the group is lacking in information or in response to group needs. An example of a group discussion on sibling rivalry might go as follows:

Mrs. A.: Johnny was toilet trained, but now since the baby is born its like having two babies again. That boy is no end of trouble—I have to watch him every minute.

Mrs. B.: Have you tried giving him something special for being a big boy?

Mrs. A.: I've tried everything—bribery, punishment—nothing works. I'm at my wits' end.

Nurse: Does anyone else have a similar problem?

Mrs. C.: Billy was the same way when the baby came. Finally, I just gave up and let him be a baby. And then, miracle of miracles—the stage passed over and he became his old independent self again.

Mrs. D.: That sounds like my dog. Blackie was six when I had my first baby and he acted like a puppy—soiled all over the house and wanted to eat every time the baby ate. He's fine with the kids now. I let him smell the new ones when they come home.

Mrs. E.: I can remember when my sister was born. I couldn't understand everyone paying her so much attention. Here I was prettier than her and could walk and talk and everything. I went right over and hit her on the head. I can remember it to this day, and I was only two at the time.

Nurse: Any other comments? Does anyone wish to summarize?

Mrs. A: I guess maybe it's hard to be second when you've always been first. I'm sure I wouldn't want Jim (husband) to take a second wife. (Laughing.) Maybe I'll do what Esther did and just let Johnny be a baby again.

Case Finding

It is the usual practice of psychotherapists and child guidance centers to wait until patients are motivated to come to them. It is more often the nurse's responsibility to help patients to enter into this delivery system by referral and by discovering people who need the service.

Almost anyone can recognize a severely disturbed child. The identification of less serious problems requiring professional help may not be so clear-cut. It requires a working knowledge of growth and development and skill in patient observation and interviewing. Spot observation of the child and note of parents' comments of parent-child interactions can often give a clue that something might be amiss.

In a visit to the home of Mrs. T. the nurse noticed that the year old baby seemed malnourished and irritable. Mrs. T. seemed hesitant, but pleased that the nurse seemed genuinely interested in helping her. On inquiry, Mrs. T. explained that Kevin, in contrast to her three year old, was a difficult child to take care of. He was cranky, a feeding problem and didn't seem to be growing properly. She had been planning to take him to the clinic, but hadn't gotten around to it. The nurse's first thought was that there might be an undiscovered neurological impairment. In checking Kevin, the nurse found that the baby was indeed as described. He was unable to sit alone and cried in a whiny fashion when touched. His reflexes appeared to be normal. His color was pale, and his skin was flabby. The mother fed him during the visit by letting him lie on his back directly next to the rubber sheet, thrusting the bottle in his mouth and looking away from him. The mother commented that Kevin was mean like his father. Further examination revealed healed and healing lesions on his buttocks which the mother attributed to diaper rash. From the clues given by Kevin's mother, her approach to the baby and Kevin's skin condition, the nurse revised her first estimate. In addition to the retardation, malnutrition and irritability, there was also evidence of rejection by the mother.

Some of the questions that the nurse may wish to explore before deciding on a course of action are as follows:

1. Is the child's behavior deviant from the normal growth and development pattern for his age?

2. Does it represent a retardation? a regression? an unusual form of behavior? an uneven growth and development pattern?

3. Are there other areas of development that are also causing difficulty?

4. Is the deviant behavior of a single instance? repeated?

5. Does the behavior interfere with the child's ability to function?

6. Does the behavior change when the setting is changed?

7. Is there a physical defect that may be responsible for the behavior?

8. What are the parents' attitudes toward the behavior? Do they recognize his behavior as deviant?

9. What is the child's position within the family? Are there other family members with similar complaints?

At times the nurse may have to provide the incentive for the family to seek help. Sometimes a family may be unwilling or unable to accept the fact that there is something wrong with their child. Occasionally the family recognizes that there is a problem, but they are afraid or ashamed that others might find out. Also, they may have misconceptions about psychiatry, existing services, and so forth.

The first step after the nurse recognizes that there is a problem would be to find out if the family is aware of it, and how they see it. The nurse can approach the situation indirectly by taking a developmental history. This would include factors such as the type of birth (natural, prolonged labor, cesarean section), cry, sleep, sitting, standing, walking, speech, sociability, feeding, elimination and vision. She can find out how the parents view Johnny's development in comparison with other children in the family or with other children of his age. Another productive question is to ask the mother to describe a typical day for the child.

Sometimes the nurse might approach the situation directly by saying, "I notice that Bruce sits off by himself in the corner," and letting the mother take it from there.

In the case of Kevin cited earlier, the problem was to get the baby under medical supervision with his mother's cooperation and without threatening her. The nurse acknowledged Mrs. T's complaints about Kevin without comment. She evidenced no surprise or sign of disapproval when Mrs. T. stated that the baby's deceased father was taking revenge on her through the baby. Mrs. T. continued to open up and finally inquired if the nurse could get Kevin into a home for retarded children. At this point the nurse explained that Kevin would need a complete physical evaluation first. The nurse also confirmed the fact that the child's development was retarded for his age. She was then able to refer him directly to the pediatric clinic, which Mrs. T. found acceptable.

When parents object to taking the child for help, it is important to find out why. What is the parent's conception of what the condition of the child is, or of therapy? When, for example, a parent says, "I don't believe in head-shrinkers," the nurse can ask, "What do you think a head-shrinker is like?" or "What has been your experience with head-shrinkers?" In this way the nurse can clarify misinformation and misconceptions.

When the objection to seeking help is very strong, the family might need a gradient step, i.e., one that is socially acceptable to them at first. For example, a mother might state that there is nothing wrong with her child emotionally, she just has a speech problem. In that case the initial step of having the child's speech checked might be readily acceptable to the mother. In time and with help the family might come to accept the full reality of the problem and be more willing to seek psychiatric or other services as needed.

Referral

When the nurse makes a referral for mental health services and or diagnostic work-up, it is important that she not end her contact with the family until she is certain that the family is receiving help and that her services are no longer wanted or needed. Unfortunately in the United States waiting lists at most child guidance centers are long, and if the child does not present with an acute problem he may have to wait as long as a year or more. For preschool children there may be few or no available services, and in some parts of the country there is only inpatient service for the severely disturbed child. When the mental health services are inadequate in the community, it is important that the nurse in her professional capacity seek to correct this through such organizations as the local community health council, nurses' association or whatever channel seems most productive in getting results.

In the meantime the nurse can continue in her supportive role of listener, counselor and educator. In one clinic setting, for example, the nurse ran a group discussion and education session for all families on the waiting list for psychiatric services with some very interesting results.

Aside from mental health services, the family can be referred for other types of supportive help that are available in the particular community.

Parent Counseling

In addition to case detection and referral, the nurse may be asked to maintain a counseling relationship with the parent or parents of a disturbed child over a period of time. Unlike psychotherapy, the counseling situation tends to focus on handling the present rather than on working on uncovering and reevaluating the past. It aims to (1) help the parent to understand and to accept the therapeutic prescription, (2) detect and modify destructive parental attitudes, and (3) increase the level of parental functioning. Many of the principles of parental counseling are similar to those discussed under play therapy, except that with the adult the vehicle of communication is the interview rather than play. Successful counseling, therefore, depends on the nurse's attitudes and skills in interviewing techniques. As with the child, the nurse provides the climate for the parent, too, to express his feelings, fantasies and fears without disapproval.

Initially it is best to permit the parent to talk about whatever he wishes. The parent can talk about himself or the child—whatever he feels most comfortable with. This means that the nurse needs to be nonjudgmental and to guard against giving premature reassurances. If a parent says, for instance, "Oh, I'm a lousy mother," an answer of, "But, Mrs. X., you are an excellent mother," will only serve to cut the mother off. Mrs. X. now surmises that you disapprove of "lousy" mothers and that you probably wouldn't like her if you knew how really bad she was. A much better response would be to acknowledge the comment without giving any opinion, or to ask Mrs. X. to tell you why she feels as she does.

As the nurse gets to know the parent, his goals, his problems and his patterns of communication, the interviews can become more focused. The direction and depth of the interviews depend on agency policy, goals for the family, the preparation of the nurse and the amount and type of mental health consultation or psychiatric supervision that is available. Counseling sessions are particularly valuable during times of family crisis.

NURSE'S ROLE IN HOSPITALS AND INPATIENT SETTINGS

Inpatient services include specialized psychiatric hospitals, centers and schools for disturbed children where the child spends most of the day and may also spend nights. They also include psychiatric wards in general hospitals and pediatric services that admit disturbed children to their units. As noted earlier, the approach in many psychiatric child settings is to work with sick families; therefore, ambulatory mental-health types of services are provided for other family members.

In inservice institutions the nurse has the primary responsibility for the actual care of the sick child. Her role is that of a wise and understanding parental figure. She is responsible for (1) setting up and maintaining the therapeutic environment, (2) cooperative planning with the therapeutic team, (3) providing the caretaking needs of the child, and (4) carrying out her part of the therapeutic regimen for child and parents.

Therapeutic Milieu

The aim of the therapeutic milieu is to provide a setting that will permit the child to heal, to grow and to learn to become a functioning member of society. The therapeutic environment includes the underlying philosophy, operating procedures, level, training and ratio of personnel to children, as well as the physical environment.

To enhance the success of the therapeutic milieu, the setting should be one which a well child would seek out and thrive in. It needs to be a safe, happy, colorful place. It should provide for growth needs. Therefore, the equipment needs to be sturdy or expendable. Provision should be made for legitimate outlets for emotions, such as a punching bag or a hammer and saw. Toys and crafts should include those that make use of projective techniques, such as dolls with removable parts, puppets and a child-size doll house. There should be raw materials that could safely be used for destruction or construction, such as building blocks, clay and paints. Music and various expressions of the arts should be available in many forms to awaken the senses and to stimulate creativity.

Underlying the success of the therapeutic community is the philosophy that governs it. Major concepts, goals, policies and operating procedures are derived from the philosophy. Personnel are hired who subscribe to the philosophy and who are able to carry out the aims of the agency. The physical environment, including the equipment, is selected with a view toward implementing the goals. The following selected concepts relating to setting limits, and imposing restrictions, illustrate how the philosophy can serve as a guide to implementation.

One major concept of a therapeutic community is that it should aim to prepare its members to adapt to and to function as members of society. Toward this end, policies and procedures can be patterned after the society at large, but modified so as to be usable by the disturbed child. It might be beneficial to a specific child, for instance, if he could eat every three hours both day and night and could sleep for six hours and stay awake for six hours regardless of the time of day because he felt like it, or perhaps play a horn when he hears a rooster crowing. However, this pattern of behavior would hardly be one that he could continue outside the institutional setting, and it would eventually need to be modified.

A second important concept is that a therapeutic community should provide the greatest good for the greatest number of its members. Perhaps letting Paul relieve his hostility by striking out at others might help Paul, but how many other children has it injured? In addition, the help it would give the child who was doing the acting out would probably be short lived since he would now have evoked an avoidance or retaliatory behavior on the part of the other children toward him. It would be much better to remove Paul from the group and to find other outlets for his needs. To carry out the concept of the greatest good for the most numbers, there would be a need for imposing safety, geographical and time limits. How far can a child go before what he is doing is considered harmful to himself or to others? How much freedom of movement does a child have within the premises? Are all the rooms accessible to him? Is the child permitted off the grounds, and under what circumstances? Are there time limits for daily routines or, barring exceptions, is the child permitted to sleep, eat and play whenever the mood strikes him?

Nursing policies resulting from this concept would impose limitations when the child was (1) physically abusive to himself or others, (2) endangering his own health, such as by exposure to inclement weather with inadequate clothing, (3) destructive to other people's property, and (4) out of the supervision of an adult. It would give direction toward establishing daily routines and for job description.

Another major idea is that behavior is a manifestation of a need and is of itself neither good nor bad. Therefore, correction of an unwanted behavior should either aim at removing the need or redirecting the behavior into constructive channels. Punishment as a retaliation need not be resorted to, and when employed is usually an indication of inadequate staffing. Where there is a need for isolation, as in the example of Paul just given, the child could be sent to a special room, not for punishment, but to work out his problems with a therapeutic adult.

This concept indicates a need for a sufficient number of adequately trained personnel so a child could have a one-to-one relationship when needed without depriving the other children. It also has implications for continuing inservice education and staff meetings.

Therapeutic Team

The most important ingredient of the therapeutic milieu is the staff. In most agencies the personnel function as a team or a series of teams who cooperatively work together in the decision-making process. In small agencies or in single units, all the staff may be a single team. In such an instance, team meetings may consist of discussing more than one family unit at a session. Decisions affecting policy and other affairs of the agency may also be a part of the meeting or grow out of the agenda. When team members are chosen for a child and his family by case distribution rather than according to the unit the child is on, each team is apt to be of a different composition of staff members. In such instances the teams meet to discuss their particular family. Agency business is usually reserved for staff and administrative meetings.

The therapeutic team is composed of all the staff members involved with a specific family group or a specific group of children. This includes the psychiatrist, nurse, psychologist, social worker, teacher and occupational therapist. Nonprofessional help involved with the family care may also be included. The team holds periodic progress conferences to reassess and to modify the therapeutic regimen. If possible, a professional, preferably a psychiatrist, not involved in the treatment of any member of the family may participate in order to provide an objective outside opinion. As a member of the team, the nurse participates in all aspects and is responsible for presenting pertinent findings, participating in the formulation of and the carrying out of the treatment plan. These points will be elaborated on under the nurse's role with the child.

An important factor of the therapeutic team, particularly in relation to the child is that of consistency. It is important for the growth of the normal child that he have a parent or parent figure who cares about him, someone who loves him whether he has been bad or good, who is with him when he is ill or when he needs her at night. The child who has been emotionally deprived is particularly vulnerable to changes of significant adults. Sometimes months of work can be undone by the sudden departure of a staff member. Although it may be unrealistic to provide 24-hour parents or parent substitutes for every child, there are certain practices that can be established to minimize the trauma. For one thing children can be encouraged to go home whenever this is possible, or parents can come in for increasingly longer periods. Day hospitals from which the children and staff go home at night are becoming increasingly popular for this reason, as well as for purposes of economy. Short-term employment can be discouraged and staff assignments made so that each nursing service person has one or two children who are especially hers to relate to. Certainly the children can usually be prepared in advance for the termination of a relationship with any worker, including the cleaning help. When a staff member is leaving all the children need to be prepared well in advance with many individual and group discussions. The children can voice their feelings and be helped to adjust to the change.

In long-term institutions, a family system in which a group of children and several adults or a caretaking couple live in independent units as a family has proved helpful. The unit is managed like a household, with the children going off to school, therapies, and so forth.

Working with the Individual Child

Aside from being responsible for the therapeutic milieu, setting the limits and contributing to the team, the nurse works directly with the child, predominantly in the role of an understanding mother who helps the child toward developing his full potentials. She meets developmental and dependency needs, is the basis for reality testing, recognizes and encourages growth behavior and redirects nongrowth behavior. To be effective, the nurse needs to have an understanding of herself, including her ability to recognize the need for and to accept supervision. As noted earlier, she also needs to have a real grasp of the normal progression of growth and development and of psychotherapeutic techniques.

Anyone who works with the disturbed child undergoes an unusual amount of stress. The child constantly tests the worker to see if he really isn't like his parent, or parents, after all. As a therapeutic relationship is formed and the child begins to improve, his behavior may grow worse and more challenging from a management standpoint. The fact that the nurse is in close contact with the child for a good five to eight hours a day and that she becomes involved in his caretaking activities increases the stress for her. It is very important, therefore, that the nurse have supervisory help so that she can work out her own feelings and interactions as they relate to the children. It is also highly desirable that anyone working with disturbed children have some form of insight therapy for themselves. This will permit them to interact with the child without having their own engrams restimulated by the child's behavior. For example, Jane says to her nurse, "You don't want me at your house because you really don't care about me. My mother said you wouldn't take me home to visit with you." The nurse in question had her own problems with rejection and felt guilty. She was unable to answer the child truthfully or to help the child to look at her unusual request, and her interpretation of it. Instead, she became involved in explaining to Jane that there really wasn't enough room at her house. . . . Jane became concerned that the nurse really didn't want her. The end result was that both Jane and the nurse became more anxious.

Observations. In working with individual children it is helpful to correctly assess where they are on the developmental scale, their ability to communicate and to form a meaningful relationship and their pattern of behavior. This is important for two major reasons: First, the nurse as a member of the therapeutic team is responsible for aiding in the diagnosis. In general it is the nurse who has the most prolonged contact with the child, who sees him in the night as well as during the day and who carries out the activities of daily living. A second reason for assessment is to be able to intervene at a time when help is most beneficial to the child.

In addition to observation of growth and development, including the child's state of health, the following areas of deviation should be looked for according to the age of the child:

General Behavior. Are there bizarre manifestations, such as continuous hand waving? spinning? Is he aggressive toward self? toward others? compulsive? withdrawn? Does he have temper tantrums?

Activity. Is he hyperactive? passive? Is physical activity limited? Are his movements uncoordinated? unequal? What are his preferences for play activities? Is his attention span short? Does he focus on one activity to the exclusion of all others?

Communication. Is his communication verbal? non-verbal? understood by others? Is his speech infantile? retarded? Is he mute? Does he echo what others say? Does he communicate with people or with objects?

Eating. Does he have any bizarre eating habits? Is there evidence of pica? vomiting? Is there an excessive food intake? an inadequate food intake?

Sleeping. Is he restless? Does he have difficulty in falling asleep? Does he have nightmares? Is he a sleepwalker? Does he sleep excessively? very little?

Toilet Training. Is there a fear of toilets? fear of being soiled? actual soiling? Does he have enuresis? Abnormal interest in stool or urine?

Sex. Does he associate with his own sex? with the opposite sex? Would he like to be of the opposite sex? Are there any abnormal sex practices?

Social. Does he relate to his peers? to one other? to his parents? to other adults? to men? to women? Does he play alone? Does he have a preference for objects or for people?

Although a nurse may be assigned to a child on a one-to-one basis or have scheduled psychotherapeutic sessions with a child, in general she is usually assigned to work with a small group of children. The responsibility to the children is reality oriented and she interacts with the manifest behavior patterns of the child as they affect both the child and the group. Two types of behavior that need special recognition are those of the withdrawn child and the child exhibiting out-of-control behavior.

Withdrawn child. The first step in helping a severely withdrawn child is to establish communication. The lowest level on the social developmental scale is the child who is out of contact with reality and who cannot communicate effectively. The child needs to be observed to see what he can do, what he responds to and whether the response is negative or positive. Perhaps he watches a certain activity intently, or a specific person. Perhaps it is a color that fascinates or a certain food that will hold his attention. Note how he uses space. How close will the child permit another person to come to him before he moves away? These observations can give a clue as to how to establish contact.

The first contact with the child might be one of just being near or even in the same room with him. The nurse should indicate to the child that she is interested in him and in what he is doing even though to all outward appearances he seems to be unaware of what is going on. If he can tolerate it, she can sit next to him. As noted under play therapy, one way to help the child to establish contact with reality is to name the things that he touches or notices. The nurse can follow the child around and say, or even better still sing, what the child is doing as, "John is building a great big tower." Children, especially preschool youngsters, generally respond well to music and rhythms. If a child makes a response to music with his body, the nurse can try to duplicate the movement. For example, if the child is rocking forward, the nurse can also rock forward. When the nurse sees that she has the child's interest or attention, she can add a new movement to the rocking such as extending her arms. If the child imitates by extending his arms, nonverbal contact has been established.

Once contact has been made, and after the child can communicate, he is ready for a therapeutic relationship. It is important to remember that the child who is first learning to relate is easily hurt and is apt to withdraw back to his former behavior on the slightest provocation, such as lack of recognition, or attention paid to another child.

After communication has been established on a one-to-one basis, the nurse helps the child to go on to the next step in the social scale. It is sometimes difficult to remember that the sequence of development is the same regardless of the age of the child. For example, in the normal course of development the child first learns to follow directions before he can anticipate action in relation to a given event. The two year old needs to be asked to bring Daddy's slippers. The three year old, on the other hand, needs only to know that Daddy is coming to elicit the same response. A case in point is that of Bruce, age 7, an autistic child who had just learned to communicate at about the two year old level. When the nurse mentioned that Freddy couldn't see his picture, he took no action because it had no meaning for him. However, when asked to raise the picture higher so Freddy could see it, he did so eagerly.

Another sequential development is that parallel play precedes shared activities regardless of the age of the child. Therefore, group activities are helpful, such as those involving dancing or singing, where the child can join or not and where he need not be directly involved with others. Audience participation plays in which the members of the audience become the players is another form of parallel activity that has the additional advantage of allowing the child to make direct contact with another if he so desires. Establishing a relationship with another child is often very difficult for the withdrawn youngster even after he has made a good relationship with an adult. He often needs direct help from the nurse. With young children the use of communication games, such as using a telephone, playing store or delivering milk, are very helpful. At first the child will talk only to the nurse on the toy telephone or only deliver the milk to her house. To encourage inter-action with another child, the nurse can suggest that Henry would also like two quarts of milk or wishes to place an order. When the child is ready he can be made a part of the communication channel of the agency, such as by delivering messages or mail.

Out-of-control behavior. Behavior in and of itself is neither bad nor good. It is a manifestation of a need and may be effectual, in-effectual or harmful. When the behavior is out of the control of the child or when it is potentially dangerous to self or others, it needs to be prevented, stopped or redirected.

Out-of-control behavior is evidenced by temper tantrums, scream-ing, blind destructiveness, self-abuse and other evidence that the child is emotionally overwhelmed. When it occurs, and particularly when it is repeated, it is necessary to find out what triggers the response so that the nurse can intervene *before* the child goes out of control. For example, the nurse sees Mary wiping the sink in a circular motion. From the child's expression and from past experience the nurse knows that this type of activity is apt to cause Mary to go into a blind rage. The nurse interrupts this pattern by suggesting that Mary give the doll a bath.

When a child is being destructive he needs to be stopped even if physical means must be resorted to. However, the actions on the part of the nurse should be under her control and not be a reaction of anger or retaliation. Nor should there be any feeling of guilt attached to the actions. With a very young child, the nurse can take him in her arms and restrain him gently. She can rock him, sing to him, soothe him. It is amazing how very little actual physical pressure is needed to bring some children under control. They usually need and want to be stopped. As the nurse holds the child she can let him know by her touch and the tone of voice that she is trying to help him to gain control. In the case of a child who is striking out, she can hold his hands and say, "I can't let you hurt and I won't let anyone hurt you."

In order for the child to gain full mastery of himself, he needs to know what triggers his aberrant behavior, how to prevent it and how to solve his problems in a more productive manner. Therefore the child should be encouraged to talk about the events immediately preceding the out-of-control behavior. A statement like, "Don't hit, say it," might be sufficient to help him to verbalize. As he relives the incident, let him do so without invalidation or judgment. The important thing is not whether the child is telling the truth, but rather how the child sees the situation.

> When the teacher, Mrs. A., pointed at Jane in order to call her attention to something, Jane went into uncontrolled screaming. With some help, Jane was able to tell the nurse that Mrs. A. was a witch who was out to get her. If at this point the nurse had tried to convince Jane that the teacher was really a very nice lady who loved little children it would have done very little to alter the child's feelings about Mrs. A. To the contrary, it might have made Jane aware of the fact that it was somehow wrong to dislike Mrs. A. and that the nurse didn't believe her anyhow.
> Fortunately, the nurse caring for Jane simply let the child know that she heard what was said. After a time, Jane went on to describe how her mother always pointed her finger in the same manner as the teacher just before she was about to scream at her. Also that the teacher wore a pin that looked (to Jane) like the symbol for the Devil.

In the case of young children, and even with some older youngsters, it is easier to work out their problems through play. (See discussion on play therapy.) Of particular use are the projective media such as clay figures, dolls and puppets through which the child can relive an incident. Sometimes when one medium does not work, another can be tried.

> Brenda, age 6, a battered child, became hysterical whenever it came time for bed. The use of the doll family didn't seem to help too much. Brenda just couldn't bring herself to hurt the mother doll. However, when she played with clay it was a different story. Brenda made two figures. One she labeled the good mother and the other, the bad mother. As she worked with the clay figures Brenda pummeled and dismantled the bad mother until there was nothing left but the good mother. After this incident, Brenda was no longer afraid to go to sleep.
> Another case was that of Tim, a five year old hyperactive child with wild disruptive behavior. Tim was admitted to the pediatric ward for skin grafting over old burn areas. He became a management problem for the floor when he bit through the net restraint, went into other children's beds, rifled through their bedside stands, and so forth. One nurse discovered that drawing was the only thing that would hold his attention for more than a few minutes. Tim wouldn't draw a picture himself, but he delighted in telling the nurse what to draw and what colors to use. The nurse had no particular skill in drawing, but Tim seemed satisfied with whatever representations she made of his dictation. His favorite scene was of a house on fire with his parents looking out the window waiting to be rescued. This media was used with Tim in subsequent

therapy sessions to help him to work out his fire-setting and other aberrant behavior.

Destructive behavior can often be redirected into constructive channels. The child who likes to bang can be given a hammer and nails or a drum. The child who rips up things can be given paper to tear to be used later for stuffing a doll.

Working with the parents. In residential treatment centers the major responsibility for working with the parents rests with the social worker, psychiatrist or psychologist. The nurse generally works with the parents on an informal basis as an adjunct to working with the child. She sees the mother when the child is brought to and from the agency, at visiting times and at scheduled meetings, either individual or group. The aim in working with the parents is to obtain their cooperation and promote their understanding of the reasons for carrying out the therapeutic plan of care, and also to help them to become more effective parents. Informal parent-nurse meetings are held to discuss common problems and for educational programs. The method of conducting meetings and individual counseling is discussed under prevention and parent counseling.

In addition to seeing the parents at the agency, the nurse may occasionally be asked to make a home visit. The case of Ronny illustrates the value of seeing the family interaction at home.

> Mrs. T. complained that Ronny, age 4, was unmanageable and wouldn't listen to her. This particular behavior was not in evidence in the Day Center which Ronny was attending. On a visit to Mrs. T.'s home, the nurse noticed that when Ronny disobeyed his mother by climbing up a shaky ladder in his father's presence, Mr. T. did nothing to stop him. In fact, his expression of silent approval did not go unnoticed by Ronny. Later in the visit Mr. T. boasted that his mother couldn't manage him at Ronny's age either and that boys need to experiment. This visit gave an insight into family relationships that weeks of interviewing both parents had failed to uncover.

CHILD PSYCHIATRIC NURSE SPECIALIST

The status of the child psychiatric nurse specialist is just beginning to emerge. The preparation and job responsibilities vary with the specialist and how she sees it. Ideally the nurse specialist should be a therapist. Therefore, graduate education should include child development, pediatrics, child psychiatry and psychotherapeutic techniques. She should be prepared to carry selected children and their parents on a scheduled basis for psychotherapy either individually or in groups. In the general hospital the nurse specialist is an active participant in the inservice program for nurses and nursing personnel. She is usually responsible for consultation with other nurses and paramedical personnel.

The child psychiatric nursing supervisor generally works in a setting for disturbed children. As she is responsible for the supervision of the psychiatric nursing service personnel, she should have preparation beyond that of the nurse specialist in case supervision. Her role is to help the nurses to work out their problems relating to nursing service and to their interactions with the children to whom they are assigned. Individual process recordings in which the nurse records what was said and what went on, including the nurse's reactions to the session or incident, are reviewed jointly.

The supervisor is also responsible for the inservice education and staff sensitivity sessions for nursing personnel. These are in addition to the programs held for team members or all staff and focus on individual and group nursing management problems. At these meetings there is an examination of values and attitudes, as well as the decision-making process.

In the absence of adequately prepared nurses and in small institutions, these functions are often performed by members of other disciplines such as the social work supervisor, clinical psychologist or psychiatrist.

SPECIAL TYPES OF EMOTIONAL AND MENTAL DYSFUNCTION IN CHILDHOOD

THE BRAIN INJURED CHILD

Brain injuries in children occurring or present at birth or in early infancy are classified as severe, moderate or minimal. Children with severe or moderate brain injury exhibit neurological signs and have physical impairments of various degrees of severity. Those with motor involvement are classified as having cerebral palsy. Some have convulsive disorders, and some are mentally retarded. Speech and hearing impairments are frequent. Impaired judgments, learning disorders and emotional instability are also part of the picture. The child with brain damage often has a low threshold to stress, and any undue pressure can cause him to have a catastrophic reaction similar to a psychotic episode. Here we shall deal with the problems of the child who is minimally brain damaged.

Diagnosis and Characteristics

The child with minimal brain damage often goes undetected until after school age. Although he may have some awkwardness in locomotion and in performance of skilled activity, as in using scissors, he usually appears to be physically normal. Sometimes he exhibits difficulties in learning to speak, to skip, or to tell his left hand from the right. However, these signs usually do not cause any undue concern and are often thought to be because of his age. His hyperactivity and drive may even help him to excel in playground activities during the preschool years. The child is usually not recognized as having a problem until after he enters the first grade when, in spite of a normal or even superior IQ, he has difficulty in learning to read and to write. By this time his sudden bursts of wild behavior and his excessive activity make him a management problem for his parents and teachers.

In the absence of neurological signs, convulsions or mental retardation (children with these problems are considered to be more than minimally brain damaged), a diagnosis of brain damage is difficult to make. It needs to be based on the child's symptomatology and special psychological tests. He may or may not have an abnormal EEG. There may be a history pointing to brain trauma at or around birth, but this too may be lacking since subtle damage can occur without early visible evidence, as might be the case in anoxia to the fetus. The child may be left-handed in a family with right-handed dominance. Other characteristic features of a child who has sustained a minimal brain damage are as follows:

Hyperactivity. There is an inability to control physical activity. Although the child does not have conscious control of this, he can learn to exert some control by stopping movements when he notices them start.

Distractibility. He is easily distracted and has a short attention span. The normal child soon learns to screen out extraneous impulses and to focus on what is important in a given situation. The brain injured child is unable to do this and therefore can be easily distracted by a detail.

Perseveration and rigidity. The child may become fixed on one thing and repeat it over and over. He has difficulty in dragging his attention away from a task or train of thought.

Drive. A brain injured child working at a task will expend more energy than the task demands. Mental activities require a great deal of physical activity. This extra drive can be capitalized on by focusing it into a meaningful task.

Impulsiveness. The child acts before thinking. He often learns by simple trial and error and has difficulty analyzing a situation before doing something about it.

Perceptual difficulties. There are three components to perception: First, information is received through sensors and relayed over neural pathways to the brain. Then, in the brain it is interpreted, sorted, integrated and recorded for future reference. Third is the individual's response to the stimuli. Damage to any of the three components will result in difficulty in patterned behavior. The evidence of damage is in the manifested response the child makes to the stimulation. With minimal brain damage the response is apt to be one of distortion rather than of a lack of response; e.g., visual deficiencies seldom take the form of blindness, but rather of visual distortions. The child has figure-ground distortion so that he is unable to identify the foreground from a distracting background. He might describe a black and white picture of a girl standing in the rain as lines and circles. He sees letters and numbers upside down and backward (mirror reading) and has particular difficulty in transferring symbols to paper. His body image concepts are also distorted, so that it is not uncommon for him to draw a picture of a man with arms coming out of his head, to have difficulty distinguishing his left side from his right even though he is of school age. He has difficulty in concept formation and is often unable to tell a detail from a whole.

Receptive or expressive language problems. Another area of perceptual distortion is that of language. Although his end-organs are intact, the child may have difficulty in translating what he has heard, or in saying what he wants to say.

Emotional instability. There is often a low threshold of tolerance for excessive stimuli. This results in a sudden explosive-like behavior for a minor provocation. He is amazingly meticulous, and a wrinkle or anything out of place may cause anger. As he grows older he is apt to be overly concerned about his health and is subject to hypochondriasis. Even a sudden change in the weather may cause a negative response.

Complications

The response of the parents and teachers to the child often imposes additional problems for the child, resulting in increased emotional disturbances and learning difficulties. His seeming brightness in being able to figure out problems mentally, and then not being able to put them on paper, is often interpreted as stubbornness. His out-of-control behavior and lack of organization are seen as deliberate acts. In the absence of eye defects, his inability to learn to read or to perceive as the other children do is also not understood and the child may be labeled as stupid, inattentive or lazy. Without help the child soon develops a self-image of being "stupid" or "bad" or whatever he has been carelessly labeled by others. He, too, is unaware that he does not perceive things in the same way as the other children.

Older children who have not adjusted and have not received therapy often develop a block to all learning and many need psychiatric help in addition to a retraining program. The child needs to become aware of the fact that he misperceives, that it is not his fault and that with training the condition need not be a handicap.

Treatment

When the child is fortunate enough to be diagnosed before school age he can be helped, so that by the time he goes to first grade he can join his regular class. Even when the condition is not picked up until school age, many children can remain in their regular class while they receive additional tutoring instruction for two to three hours a week over a period of a year or two.

Medical management usually comes under the direction of a pediatric neurologist. Medications are prescribed on an individual basis and many of the children are able to progress without it. The child with a brain injury often has opposite reactions to drugs affecting the central nervous system, i.e., he can become hyperactive to the point of psychosis under the influence of diphenylhydantoin (Dilantin). Benzedrine, on the other hand, may have a quieting effect on him and may be prescribed to control his hyperactivity.

The major treatment of the brain damaged child is training or retraining. This can be in the area of speech, hearing, rhythms, perception, manual training and special education, depending on the need of the particular child.

Almost all the children with minimal brain damage need some form of individual special instruction. They need to be introduced into steps of learning that the normal child learns by acculturation. Some general principles that have proved to be effective in training the brain injured child are as follows:

1. Study the child's strengths and weaknesses. Find out which perceptual areas are left intact and can be worked with.

2. The child does best with a specific routine and orderliness. Disorganization is confusing and overstimulating. At first the child needs latitude in working off excess energy. Limitations can gradually be imposed as the child learns what to expect and as he gains control over his behavior. Habit formation is important. However, drills should be in the form of a process and not as memorization, since meaningless repetition will only set up an automatic circuit.

3. The child responds best to a system of immediate rewards. The child who is brain damaged has a low frustration tolerance and might give up with even a small amount of negative stimuli. Training should be in small graded steps that have a built-in victory, as in the Montessori method, Strauss method or an adaptation of teaching machines.

4. The child needs to learn to work independently. More and more learning aids are introduced so that the child can work alone.

5. There should be a multisensory approach which will involve as many as possible of the child's operant perceptual fields. Color and touch perceptions are usually intact. The use of color aids in organization of ground, form and space. The sense of touch is particularly useful as an aid in learning sizes, shapes and symbols when there are impaired visual perceptions.

Parents. The parents are an important part of the total rehabilitation program for the child. They are with him in his everyday activities.

Many of the parents are at a loss to know how to manage the child and feel that they are somehow to blame. This feeling of guilt is often unwittingly reinforced by teachers, physicians and other professionals who are not aware that the child's behavior is related to a physical defect. The parents need help in expressing their feelings and frustrations, in understanding the problem of the brain damaged child and in techniques of training him.

SCHOOL PHOBIA

The child with school phobia is apprehensive about going to school, and his anxiety is accompanied by physical distress such as abdominal pain, nausea and headaches. In spite of frequent absences from school he is usually an average or above average student. As is true of most phobias, the child is unable to explain what he is afraid of. It is not school itself that he fears, but the fear of leaving home. He has obsessional thinking around the area of being left by his mother. He imagines that his mother may fail to pick him up after school or that something terrible will have happened to her when he gets home or that she just won't be there. He feels rejected and unwanted.

There is usually a history of separation from the mother during the first years of life. This includes being left with baby sitters who are strangers to the infant. Events which threaten loss, or an actual loss or separation from a significant person, often act to restimulate the earlier separation experiences and to precipitate the symptoms.

When treated early, particularly if soon after the symptoms are noticed, the prognosis for an early and full recovery is excellent. Waldfogel et al. found that therapeutic counseling can be effective in as little as ten one half hour sessions spread over a period of ten weeks.[9] It is important that the child be made to attend school in spite of his and the family's discomfort during the period of treatment.

The longer treatment is delayed, the longer it takes to correct the underlying pathology. With children over ten it may take several years of therapy for both child and parents before there is relief of the separation anxiety. In some instances, residential treatment is indicated for a brief period of time, particularly when the family has been unsuccessful in getting the child to attend school.

BEHAVIOR DISORDERS

The term "acting-out behavior disorders" is a descriptive diagnosis for antisocial behavior in children. This includes lying, stealing, running away, truancy, fire-setting, alcoholism, drug addiction, sexual delinquency, destructiveness, vandalism and cruelty. To be classified as a behavior disorder the actions need to be part of the child's overall behavior pattern and severe enough to be of concern to parents, teachers and, at times, law enforcement officers. Minor mischievous acts of lying, stealing, and so forth, do not come under this category. When the acting-out behavior occurs in the adolescent and it comes to the attention of the legal authorities, it is designated as juvenile delinquency, which is both a legal and sociological term.

The chief motivating force behind the anti-social act is hostility. The hostility may be overt, as in cruelty and vandalism; it may be covert as in lying and stealing.

There are usually disturbed parent-child relationships or a history of little parent contact. In some instances it is the parent who gives the child a subtle message to act out the parents' own delinquent wish-fulfilling needs. They give the child a double-bind message; for example, saying, "Johnny, don't steal that bike," which at one time gives both the suggestion and their unspoken approval for Johnny to do so.

If the child is to live at home, the parents as well as the child should have therapy. Unfortunately many of the parents are resistant to any form of treatment. Often therapy is more successful if the child is away from his home environment. Since many antisocial acts involve group participation and approval, the problem is also sociological. For a further discussion of acting-out disorders as a sociological problem, see Chapter 12.

INFANTILE AUTISM AND CHILDHOOD SCHIZOPHRENIA

Infantile autism is a psychosis that becomes evident within the first few years of life. It is manifested by little or no communication with others, a lack of contact with reality, a lack of integration and irregular psychological and social development.

Some authors differentiate between infantile autism and childhood schizophrenia, whereas others feel that they are both part of the same illness, with schizophrenia being the less severe form of the two. A major differentiation is that the autistic child has a withdrawal psychosis that occurs early in life and before significant emotional growth has taken place. The schizophrenic child also has a withdrawal psychosis which occurs later in childhood, but before adolescence, and represents a regression in behavior. An inclusive name given to both conditions is the "atypical child."

Outstanding clinical features of the autistic and schizophrenic child are a withdrawal from people which may become noticeable in early infancy, identity with an inanimate object or animal, lack of speech or echolalic speech, bizarre postures and gestures, impassivity, violent outbursts, impulsiveness or excessive inhibitions.

The etiology is unknown and the causes are thought to be multiple. It is thought that heredity and biological factors play an important part. Extensive research indicates that psychological factors within the family structure support the theory that there are profound disturbances in the early mother-child and father-child relationships. In addition, there is usually a history of a family crisis which involved the separation of the child from the mother before the age of two. Pain may also be involved in the separation, such as a hospitalization experience.

The prognosis depends on the severity of the symptoms and the age of onset. Brown, in a 15-year follow-up study of children with atypical behavior, found that treatment variables had little significance in influencing the prognosis.[3] The most significant historical variable was that those children who made the best progress tended to have more siblings. There was also a significant difference between the initial behavior of the 20 most promising patients, who were doing well on follow-up, and the 20 worst, who were doing poorly. Those who entered treatment on a deeply regressed level failed to improve. Those who entered with some contact and a more mature level of functioning continued to improve.

Treatment usually involves the parents as well as the child and is often carried out over a period of years.

The child needs to develop some form of communication before any psychotherapeutic techniques can be effective. Suggested methods for reaching the child are discussed under behavior therapy and the withdrawn child.

If the child can be managed at home he can be treated in a Day Center and attend a special school within the center or a nursery. Many of the children are admitted to residential treatment centers, particularly when there are other children in the family.

SCHIZOPHRENIA IN ADOLESCENCE

Schizophrenia in adolescence is more like the adult form of the disease in symptomatology and methods of treatment. Unlike childhood schizophrenia, the onset is sudden and is characterized by a withdrawal into an inner world of fantasy and delusions. The patient shows a lack of affect toward stimuli; he has fragmented thinking with obscure use of language. The adolescent usually has the paranoid form of the psychosis, with delusions and hallucinations. The second most prominent form is that of the catatonic type with mutism, profound withdrawal, bizarre body postures, and so forth.

The schizophrenic adolescent is almost always treated as an inpatient, with follow-up on an outpatient basis on discharge. Methods of therapy are similar to those for adults, including the use of the interview, occupational and recreational therapies and, in some cases, shock therapy. Since the adolescent responds best to his peer group, group activities and group therapy are useful adjuncts to individual therapy. The prognosis for adolescent schizophrenia when treated early is good.

REFERENCES

1. Axline, V. M.: *Dibs: In Search of Self.* New York, Ballantine Books, Inc., 1964, p. 28.
2. Barsch, R. H.: Counseling the Parent of the Brain Damaged Child. *J. Rehabilitation,* 27 (No. 3):1-3, May-June, 1961.
3. Brown, J.: Prognosis from Presenting Symptoms of Preschool Children with Atypical Development. *Amer. J. Orthopsychiat.* 30 (No. 2):390, April, 1960.
4. *Diagnostic and Statistical Manual of Mental Disorders,* Washington, D.C., American Psychiatric Association, 1968.
5. Freud, A.: *Normality and Pathology in Childhood.* New York, International Universities Press, Inc. 1966. p. 34.
6. Mannoni, Mario: *The Child, His "Illness" and the Others.* New York, Pantheon Books, Random House, 1970.
7. Menninger Foundation, Children's Division: *Disturbed Children.* San Francisco, Jossey-Bass Inc., 1969.
8. Rank, B.: Intensive Study and Treatment of Preschool Children Who Show Marked Personality Deviations or "Atypical Development," and Their Parents. *In* Caplan, G. (ed.) : *Prevention of Mental Disorders in Children: Initial Exploration.* New York, Basic Books, Inc., 1961, pp. 492-494.
9. Waldfogel, S., et al.: A Program for Early Intervention in School Phobia. *Amer. J. Orthopsychiat.* 29 (No. 2):324-332, April, 1959.
10. World Health Organization Technical Report Series No. 381: Neurophysiological and Behavioral Research in Psychiatry. Geneva, W. H. O., 1968, p. 20.

SUGGESTED READINGS

Allen, F. H.: *Psychotherapy with Children,* New York, W. W. Norton and Company, 1952.

Alt, H.: *Residential Treatment for the Disturbed Child.* New York, International Universities Press, Inc., 1960.

Axline, V. M.: *Play Therapy.* Boston, Houghton-Mifflin Co., 1947.

Axline, V. M.: *Dibs: In Search of Self.* New York, Ballantine Books, Inc., 1964.

Bakwin, H., and Bakwin, R. M.: *Clinical Management of Behavior Disorders in Children.* Philadelphia, W. B. Saunders Company, 1972.

Bettelheim, B.: *Love Is Not Enough,* Chicago, Ill., Free Press of Glencoe, 1950.

Bettelheim, B.: *Truants from Life,* Chicago, Ill., Free Press of Glencoe, 1955.

Birch, H. G. (ed.) : *Brain Damage in Children: Biological and Social Aspects.* Baltimore, The Williams & Wilkins Co., 1964.

Caplan, G. (ed.) : *Prevention of Mental Disorders in Children: Initial Exploration.* New York, Basic Books, Inc., 1961.

Chapman, A. H.: *Management of Emotional Problems of Children and Adolescents.* Philadelphia, J. B. Lippincott Company, 1965.

Coles, R.: *Children of Crisis.* Boston, Little, Brown and Company, 1967.

Daniels and Wiswell: *Handbook for Leading Group Discussions with Young People.* New York, Child Study Association of America, 1969.

Finch, S. M.: *Fundamentals of Child Psychiatry.* New York, W. W. Norton and Company, 1960.

Freud, A.: *Normality and Pathology in Childhood.* New York, International Universities Press, Inc., 1966.

Hammer, M. and Kaplan, A. M.: *The Practice of Psychotherapy with Children.* Homewood, Illinois, Dorsey Press, 1967.

Lippman, H.: Treatment of the Child in Emotional Conflict. New York, Blakiston Division, McGraw-Hill Book Co., Inc., 1962.

Moustakas, C. E.: *Psychotherapy with Children.* New York, Harper and Brothers, 1959.

Parad, H. J. (ed.) : *Crisis Intervention: Selected Readings.* New York, Family Service Association of America, 1965.

chapter 15

MENTAL RETARDATION

Dear Miss Campbell:

I'm not sure you will even remember me. Jody and I first came to your attention three months ago when we came to ————— for evaluation of Jody's developmental level. I was worried then, but my thoughts were taken up with concern for Jody's health. Friends, neighbors, and relatives had all spent chilling hours telling me about the many diseases they had heard of in which children had acted like Jody. Frankly, when I first came to your desk, I was almost certain that the eventual verdict on Jody would entail some strange neurological disease that would end in her death. I'm sure that was why I was curt and unfriendly. You didn't seem to notice though. You offered me a cup of coffee, asked me gently about Jody's past, and then went over the details of her next two weeks' appointments with me. That's the first thing I remember about you. Later, you comforted me when I thought they were hurting my daughter or being unkind to her. You were particularly wonderful to me in that trying period when they tapped her spine. Finally, the last day when you sat with me at the conference table while the team went over their findings with me, I was so grateful to you for holding my hand. I really needed that. I'm sorry I made such a scene. . . . I've made quite a few since, but they've all been in the privacy of my own bedroom! It isn't easy to get used to, knowing your child can't be like other kids; knowing that she'll always be slow. You stay awake nights wondering what you did. You wonder why it happened to you and if you did something that hurt your baby. You try to remember what medicines you took during the pregnancy that the doctor didn't know about. Finally, when you put all those thoughts away for good you wonder what is to become of your child when you die. It's been a tough three months, but we all feel better now. Frank and I have been looking around for a home for Jody when she gets too big to live with us. We have not made up our minds yet, though we think we've found the one. The gentleman who interviewed us there was a very wise person. He explained his philosophy about the care of retarded children by telling us that the best thing in the world for anyone to do is that which he does best because then the person feels useful and that is happiness.[2] That meant a lot to me. It helped me put my life in perspective and Jody's too. In a way we are very lucky: Jody will always be our child. She will never have to go off on her own and suffer the stings of the world. Instead, we shall have the opportunity to find what brings her childish happiness and supply it to her as long as we live. That thought helps me at night sometimes when I have trouble sleeping. Well, that's about it. I just wanted you to know that things looked better since we left ————— and you really helped us more than I can ever tell you.

Jody's mother

The writer is the mother of a newly diagnosed retardate. Jody is more than a "retardate," however; she is a three year old who is handicapped in the area of learning. She is a little girl who will never grow up. Jody's mother's letter of thanks went to the nurse who coordinated her daughter's work-up.

To Jody, her mother and her father, mental retardation is a new and unique concept. For the little girl it may mean no more than the slightly disquieting feeling she gets when her mother seems sad and cries. To her parents, mental retardation has been, in kaleidoscopic sequence, a curse, a punishment, a sign of their parental guilt, a disease and a label that finally explained why Jody is not yet toilet trained, why she clings to mother rather than joining in the play of other children, and why she has been particularly difficult to raise from time to time. The tinge of horror is just leaving the consciousness of Jody's parents as they begin to realize that mental retardation does not necessarily mean drooling, unseeing, half-human forms on long wooden benches in state hospitals. The parents are only beginning to find out that communities and states are interested in the retardate and ready to explore the best means of enhancing the retardate's potential for development. Because of the increased financial support from the federal level of government, research on the medical, educational and adaptational problems of the mental retardate has accrued, offering greater opportunity than ever before to such individuals.

DEFINITION

There are basically two ways of looking at mental retardation, and out of those models are derived two types of intervention and philosophy of care. The first and more traditional model is the biomedical.

Workers who utilize this model regard mental retardation as a condition that arises from medical abnormalities. They regard the retardate as a "patient," a person who is sick and needs treatment. The medical model "appears to reinforce and augment the dehumanization" of the mentally retarded.[13] It encourages such workers as the nurse, doctor and psychologist to use a clinical label to hide the humanness of the retardate.

The second model, which reflects a more recent outlook and one that encompasses the multidisciplinary approach, is sociocultural adaptational. This frame of reference is utilized by doctors, nurses, psychologists, teachers and social workers who acknowledge the retardate's deviancy from norms, but who focus beyond the immediate physiological abnormalities to the potential for adaptation. These workers are more concerned with habilitation; their focus is on encouraging the development of personal adequacy, social competency and economic efficiency.[13] In other words, those workers who utilize the adaptational model focus on the task of helping the retarded individual to adapt to society, rather than relegating him to the abandoned heap of the diagnosed and forgotten.

A general definition is that mental deficiency is a condition of arrested or retarded mental development which occurs before adolescence and arises from genetic cause or is induced by disease or injury.[10] Another definition, published by the American Association on Mental Deficiency, states that mental retardation is subaverage general intellectual functioning which originates during the developmental period and is associated with impairment in adaptive behavior.[8] The first definition is highly suggestive of the biomedical model. The second one reflects the sociocultural adaptational model which concerns itself with the individual's potential for adaptation.

INCIDENCE

Mental retardation is by no means a rare condition. It has been estimated that there are 6,000,000 mentally deficient individuals in the United States today. From these statistics it is known that approximately three out of every 100 births will produce a retarded child.[3]

ETIOLOGY

The causes of mental retardation are many. Children who are born deficient may have inherited this condition from mentally deficient parents. This is the least complex cause.

More complicated are the different types of chromosomal abnormalities that result in retardation. One such condition is the *trisome,* or the presence of a single additional chromosome; the *monosome* is the absence of a chromosome. Another abnormality found to produce retardation is the deletion or absence of part of a chromosome. Sometimes a translocation of part of a chromosome from one chromosome to another occurs. Finally, *triploidy,* a condition in which the individual has one half again as many chromosomes as he should, occurs. From this condition "Down's disease," or mongoloidism,* results. Other diseases that are carried through the chromosomes, and thus inherited, are Tay-Sachs* and Hurler's* diseases. All these conditions involve multiple defects, including mental retardation.

Prenatal

The prenatal period is significant in the development of mental retardation. Exposure of the mother to certain drugs, x-rays and infections contributes to the fetus' abnormal development. Such illnesses as syphilis, German measles, toxemia and uncontrolled maternal diabetes have also been implicated. Some developmental anomalies of the prenatal period may result in retardation. Hydrocephaly,* microcephaly,* anencephaly* and macrocephaly* are usually accompanied by abnormalities in intellectual functioning.

Postnatal

Injuries to the brain inflicted through trauma, infection or anoxia may result in retardation. Also implicated are metabolic dysfunctional diseases such as phenylketonuria (PKU)* and hypothyroidism.* There are actually many metabolic disorders that produce mental retardation, but the majority of them, if diagnosed early enough, may be successfully treated with special diet and replacement therapy so that intellectual functioning is not impaired. Finally, retardation may develop in the face of cultural, sensory or maternal deprivation. In such cases physiological pathology is absent. Adequate treatment requires more stimulating input.

CARE OF THE RETARDATE

CHILDHOOD

There is a growing trend toward keeping the retarded child in the home and the community. Except for the individual who is so handicapped that institutional care is absolutely necessary, parents and helping professionals are coming to realize that the retardate thrives best in the home, surrounded by a warm, loving environment where he is encouraged

---

* See glossary.

to reach his maximum potential. In the early years the child-rearing practices do not vary appreciably from child to child, whether retarded or not. The intellectually handicapped baby will show his problem by learning more slowly. His ego also develops more slowly, which means a longer period of clinging to the mothering one, an extended period of bottle or breast feeding, and even an extended period of time before this child recognizes the mother as a familiar face. Because the ego emerges less quickly, the retardate is likely to be more demanding, more negativistic at times and more needful of the mother's attentions. Such a child may cry more and longer. He may be less easily soothed. These behaviors occur because such a child reflects his id impulses. It takes him longer than the normal child to modify his perception of himself in relation to the world around him. The retardate tends, as a youngster, to want what he wants when he wants it. These are difficult months and years for the mother. She is called upon to do more for her child and to do it longer.

During this period the public health nurse or the nurse employed in a pediatric clinic or doctor's office can assist the mother of a retardate by helping her to understand why her child acts as he does. The nurse can encourage the mother to get away from the house for short periods to relax. The nurse may assist both parents by planning with them a schedule that permits one parent to relieve the other so that prescribed periods of change and relaxation are possible. One agency has organized this type of counseling on a formal basis. In order to prevent a parental pattern of hopelessness and despair, the Pacific State Hospital in Pomona, California, developed a program in 1968 to support parents of retardates who are kept at home. Staffed by public health nurses and a social worker, and assisted by other community agencies, the Pomona group assist parents to train their child and they support the parents during the trying periods of waiting for hospitalization.

When the child is three to seven years of age, there are further problems which emerge. The retardate is slow in learning to dress, to tie his shoes and to feed himself. His differentness becomes more obvious to other children as he grows. Children who can sit, walk and run will be included in the games of the other young children in the neighborhood, but he is not likely to feel fulfilled by such activities because he is not sufficiently inventive or creative. As he approaches school age, the retardate is very likely to be exposed to increasing amounts of rejection from his peer group because he cannot function adequately in the games played, because his behavior may be poor as a result of his inadequate impulse control or because he does not evince a reciprocal interest in others. For any or all of these reasons the retarded child soon tastes the bitterness of rejection. He feels different from the others and he knows that he is different. Slowly the young child's image of himself begins to form as one who is inadequate, as the dumb one, the different one. The mentally deficient youngster learns to devalue himself.

In these years there is heartbreak for the loving parents. It is devastating for the mother, or father, who wishes to protect the child from pain, to see him exposed to the thoughtless rejection of his peer group. Yet there is little they can do to offset this situation. Curious neighbors, helpless relatives, well meaning strangers and not so well meaning individuals look, ask questions or shun the child. In these years the parents often overprotect the retardate to the point of babying him, keeping him an infant and dependent on them.

The nurse who maintains contact with the family may sometimes need to point out areas in which the child should be expected to develop self-reliance and autonomy. Indeed, it is the nurse who sometimes first suspects retardation in these early years of the child's life. When this happens, she refers the mother and child to pediatricians, clinics or centers where the diagnostic studies can be carried out to determine if the child is developing abnormally and, if so, to what extent.

The school years may be fraught with difficulty, or they may provide the basis for the individualized planning that will help the retardate to develop to his fullest potential. For the child who has not been tested and evaluated, the early years of elementary education can be a nightmare. The undiagnosed child may attempt to keep up with his class, though he does not really understand the demands of those teaching him. He may fail repeatedly in his inept attempts to do the required work. Soon he is labeled as stupid. This is the child who sits in the back of the room. He may sleep from boredom or be disruptive in an effort to get some kind of attention, even if it is negative. Usually the retardate is eventually tested and his real limitations come to light. The results are controversial. Where special classes are available, or even special schools, the retarded child is usually reassigned. Those who advocate such segregation believe the slower child is happiest in this type of specialized environment because he is now in a group of his equals; he no longer must suffer the stigma of being different. Also, he is not asked to master more than he is capable of doing. Supporters of special education believe that the retardate does best in an environment where he can learn those skills that will help him to adapt to society's demands after the learning years; special education endows the child with those skills that will enable him to be economically self-sufficient as an adult.

Those who oppose special schools think that this type of segregation only reinforces the differentness the retardate has been exposed to since he was old enough to compare himself with and be compared with his peer group. They contend that the limited child should re-

main with other children so that he might become more like them in the
ways that he is capable of emulating and that his limitations should be
taken into account by those teaching.

ADOLESCENCE AND ADULTHOOD

By the time the retardate reaches adolescence, his limitations are
usually acknowledged by parents, medical resource people and teachers.
If the retarded individual is profoundly retarded (IQ 0 to 24) he is likely
to require institutional care, for such people may have the intellect of
the very, very young, but their bodies continue to grow and mature.
Eventually their physical care requires the combined strength of several
adults. The severely retarded (IQ 25 to 39) are also likely to require
institutionalization. Those who are moderately deficient (IQ 40 to 54),
or mildly so (IQ 55 to 69), may be trainable if appropriate placements
are found. The borderline individual (IQ 70 to 84) is usually capable
of completing a modified course of education. For the borderline as
well as some mildly retarded persons, jobs are feasible after vocational
training. Such individuals can usually care for themselves and be
financially independent. For others who fall within the limits of the
mildly retarded and those of moderate retardation, work can also be
found. Such people may be trained to do jobs under close supervision
within the confines of sheltered workshops. Here they may find happiness by being effective, productive individuals and receiving recognition
for jobs well done.

For those retardates, both children and adults, who require institutional care or specialized training, there are schools organized to meet
their needs. Some are private; others are state operated. Though the
private institutions are generally smaller, with more attractive ratios
of staff to retardates, some state institutions are particularly good.
Parents must visit many agencies and examine the facilities in order to
make wise choices. A practical feature of the state institution is the
lower cost and the assurance that the child's care will continue after
the parents are deceased. Aspects of this latter problem are handled
by the establishment of trust funds to care for the child's continuing
needs. In regard to this problem, parents selecting a private institution
should choose one that is administered by a board, insuring that the
school will not close after the current administrator dies. In this way
the retardate's future welfare is secured.

One institution established to educate and train the retardate is the
Sunland Training Center, a publicly supported agency in Miami,
Florida. In this school there is an opportunity for growth through many
services. Among them are diagnostic, evaluation, medical and health
treatment, recreation, training, education, and focus on habilitation.
The physical plant contains 36 cottages with 20 children in each, except

for the nursery which contains 60. On the grounds are a shopping center, a chapel, two schools, a sheltered workshop, an infirmary, a gym, facilities for swimming, a ball field, picnic areas, a day care center and a farm. In 1965 the institution was reorganized along new administrative lines. Now there are four program divisions, each staffed by a director and interdisciplinary team with professional and subprofessional members. The divisions focus on (1) development and training, (2) independent living, (3) education and training, and (4) vocational rehabilitation. Each resident in the institution is placed in that program which most nearly meets his needs. Each division is responsible for certain cottages, and residents are assigned to them according to age, sex (after 12 years of age), functioning level, estimated potential and specific management problems.

In the Development and Training Division are the severely retarded children of school age. They are taught the rudimentary skills of daily living, i.e., feeding of self, toileting, dressing, locomotion, communication and brushing of teeth. Included in their curriculum are "clusters of appropriate activities" around mealtime, arising, bedtime, simple recreation and occupational activities.

The Independent Living Division contains residents of 17 years or older who will not be able to seek competitive employment but who can function adequately in a sheltered workshop. These individuals are taught the necessary skills to permit them to care sufficiently for themselves so that they can go to workshops.

The Education and Training Division of Sunland Training Center has a nursery for the preschooler and facilities for children from seven to 16 years of age. The curriculum in this division emphasizes development and use of language, motor skills, skills in reading, writing and arithmetic and social competency. Here, also, is dispensed information about jobs, prevocational training, homemaking and vocational guidance.

Finally, the center offers vocation rehabilitation for residents over 16 who demonstrate a potential for competitive employment. In a center of this kind there are ample facilities for diagnosing and meeting the needs of the retardate and equipping him to obtain his most effective level of functioning.

ROLES FOR THE NURSE

IN AN INSTITUTION

It is difficult to pinpoint discrete functions in the care of the mentally retarded that might be called nursing. Instead, it is useful to identify those tasks which might, more effectively, be carried out by the nurse. In a residential treatment facility, the nurse's education and training equip her to evaluate the behavior of retardates. The nurse can assess the retardate's abilities in relation to his physical and developmental needs; she may participate in the development and implementation of nursing plans for training and habilitation. The nurse is eminently qualified to act as a role model for others who care for the retarded. She may train and supervise such personnel. For the nurse who is so prepared, study of group structure and its impact on behavior may lead to alteration of the environment so that the retardate can be better trained and educated. Finally, the nurse observes and assesses staff approaches to the residents and types of relations which are fostered between them. Through her own behavior the nurse can influence the work of her colleagues.

SPECIAL THERAPY FOR THE RETARDATE

Because of his retarded development, the mentally deficient child is prone to psychological problems associated with anxiety and frustration. Such children are likely to have markedly devalued images of self which often result in behaviors that are considered inappropriate. Such behaviors may represent cries for attention, security and love. The psychiatric nurse who is particularly interested in long-term, complex problems may enjoy treating the retardate and attempting to supply his dependency needs.

As the retardate grows up, his lessened adaptability interferes with socialization processes which require cooperation, compromise and a capacity to give. The child is ostracized, and his self-image is badly distorted. Here, the nurse therapist may be instrumental in devising situations in which the retardate can achieve and be sincerely praised by her. The theme is always acceptance and affection.

Puberty is very difficult for the retardate. Not only does he have to undergo the same changes, bewilderment and periods of anxiety as his normally developing peers, but he must cope with the limitations imposed by his intellectual handicap. "He may be regarded as a man by society but he is totally unable to accept the responsibility of his new role. The weak ego of the retarded child is not strong enough to cope with this, and he is therefore frequently overcome by strong emotional states."[9] During this time the retarded child may not have the opportunity to release his tension through increased activity as his peers do, for the latter no longer accept him in their groups. The informal dances and the afternoon football and basketball games are usually not open to him as avenues of release. To compound his problems is the recognition that younger siblings and their friends have passed him in school. Thus, the adolescent retardate sees himself as more and more defective. On the one hand he feels tense and unable to release his anxieties arising from the many emotional and physiological changes in his body; on the other hand his problems are compounded by a self-image which is growing more worthless as he matures. Such individuals may develop acute anxiety states, usually accompanied by depression or physical complaints. In severe trauma, with disintegration of ego defenses, schizophrenia may develop. In any case, the adolescent retardate is usually a very unhappy, ill adjusted person. His basic problems are feelings of rejection and worthlessness. The nurse who attempts to modify such situations will develop relationships with retardates in which they can feel accepted and valued. To do this will require much time and ingenuity on the nurse's part.

INTERVENTION IN FAMILY PROBLEMS RELATED TO THE RETARDATE

Probably the severest blow to the family of a retarded child is the discovery of the child's limitations. If the child is so handicapped that his condition is known from birth, the postnatal care of the mother will differ from that of other patients in the unit. The new mother has recently undergone enormous changes in both her physiology and her thought processes. She has finally expelled the fetus that she has anticipated for many months as her body has swelled and changed shape. Now, in what should have been a moment of triumph and happiness, the mother has been delivered of an abnormal child. For the majority of women this is a cruel blow and one that is not easily absorbed. In the postnatal period there should be a period of mourning for the lost (normal) baby. At this time the mother needs physical rest which will increase the energy she has available for coping with the tragedy. Regression and dependency needs increase in the face of anxiety. This mother is one who needs to be cared for. She needs to see the nurse care for her baby not only to learn how to care for it herself, but also to see that the nurse is genuinely interested in the child. Psychologically a newborn baby is still an extension of the mother, and by caring for the infant the nurse indicates her acceptance of the mother and her imperfect child. Through observation of the accepting nurse, the mother can become more comfortable about herself. Though she will doubtlessly be hounded by suspicions about herself and her ability to produce a normal child, she will become more accepting of herself as the nurse cares for her and her infant.

The obstetrical nurse may help considerably by not pushing the new mother to care for her infant, by supporting the mother as she reconstructs her self-image, and by helping the father to become part of the mother-infant dyad and support them both.

In the developing years of the retardate, the pediatric or public health nurse may find opportunities to help families of retardates. The nurse may observe families that are too protective of their retarded member, or too aggressive in pressuring him to learn. Both types of observations should be brought to the attention of the parents and modifications implemented. Sometimes normal siblings are slighted unintentionally as the parents' attentions become focused completely on the retardate. Again that kind of observation needs to be brought to the parents so they might have the opportunity to share themselves more with their other children.

Finally, the nurse may be in a position to help families of retardates when they must decide on future placements for their handicapped children. Home, foster care and institutional care are the possible choices. Sometimes a decision for home care must be changed for institutional placement or foster care. These decisions are difficult, and though the nurse never tries to make them for her clients, she can help families to look at the pros and cons for each and then support the families when the decisions, no matter how painful, are made. If institutional care is sought, the parents should be helped to recognize that it is not the end of their relationship with the retarded child. Indeed, it is their responsibility to visit the child, to observe the persons caring for the child and to see that the atmosphere of the institution is a hopeful one. If the institution's care of the child declines in any way, the parents must take an active part in having the standard of care returned to its former level, or they may search for an agency that offers more appropriate care.

HELPING TO PREVENT
MENTAL RETARDATION

The nurse has an urgent role in the primary prevention of mental retardation. She may prevent countless incidences of defective births by disseminating information to the public. One of the most notable causes of retardation in the fetus seems to be related to poor socioeconomic standards and resultant poor prenatal care. If pregnant women can be urged to seek medical attention throughout their pregnancies, such causal factors as Rh incompatibilities, poor nutrition, maternal diabetes, syphilis and toxemia of pregnancy might be greatly reduced. Elimination of these complications alone would decrease the incidence of mental retardation. Also, the nurse who promotes genetic counseling for prospective parents may sometimes prevent the birth of a defective child. Many of the syndromes involving retardation are inherited. If men and women knew they could consult doctors who would test them quite painlessly and determine if they carried the genes which result in defective offspring, such births could be averted. Through genetic counseling such familial diseases as Tay-Sachs and Hurler's can be predicted. Parents and prospective parents need this information.

Secondary prevention can also be a reality. The public health nurse and the pediatric nurse can reach families of suspected retarded children and urge them to attend clinics where early detection and treatment of hereditary disorders such as PKU,* maple syrup urine disease,* galactosemia,* and hypothyroidism* are possible. In some of these conditions, medical or surgical treatment may prevent the complication of retardation.

The public health nurse can also help to prevent mental retardation by warning her clients of the dangers of lead poisoning. She can urge the mothers whose children chew paint and plaster to take them to the doctor for treatment so that such complications as mental retardation and even death do not ensue. For ghetto children, early detection of cultural deprivation is a means of preventing retardation, because enrichment programs may be found and utilized to prevent retardation.

The treatment of behavioral and personality difficulties is possible through tertiary prevention. Nurses who know their clients and children can counsel the parents to relate very concretely, to be very practical and flexible with their retarded children. Nurses can teach the parents that meaningful relationships grow out of shared activity as well as verbal and nonverbal reassurance. Finally, the nurse can set up group counseling for the parents of retardates so that they may have an opportunity for catharsis and for asking questions about management and institutionalization, and so that these people can have the opportunity to meet as a group with a mutual problem in order to draw support from one another.

REFERENCES

1. Baumeister, A. (ed.) : *Mental Retardation, Appraisal, Education, and Rehabilitation*. Chicago, Aldine Publishing Co., 1967.
2. Buck, P.: *The Child Who Never Grew*. N. Y., John Day Co., 1960.
3. Carter, C.: *Handbook on Mental Retardation Syndromes*. Springfield, Ill., Charles C Thomas, 1970.
4. Clarke, A. M., and Clark, A. D.: *Mental Deficiency*. New York, Free Press Division, The Macmillan Co., 1965.
5. Cortazzo, A., Bradtke, L., Kirkpatrick, L., Jr., and Rosenblatt, K.: Innovations to Improve Care in an Institution for the Mentally Retarded. *Children*, 18 (No. 4): 149-154, 1971.
6. Cytryn, L., and Lourie, R.: Mental Retardation. *In* Freedman, A., and Kaplan, H. (eds.) : *Comprehensive Textbook of Psychiatry*. Baltimore, The Williams & Wilkins Co., 1967.
7. Diedrick, G.: *Continuity of Care on a Continuum*. American Nurses Association Clinical Conference, 1969. New York, Appleton-Century-Crofts, Inc., 1969.
8. Heber, R.: *A Manual on Terminology and Classification in Mental Retardation*. Albany, N. Y., American Association on Mental Deficiency, 1961.
9. Hutt, M., and Gibby, R.: *The Mentally Retarded Child, Development, Education, and Guidance*. Boston, Allyn and Bacon, Inc., 1958.
10. Jervis, G.: The Mental Deficiencies. *In* Arieti, S.: *American Handbook of Psychiatry*. Vol. 11. New York, Basic Books, Inc., 1959.
11. Kanner, L.: Parents' Feelings about Retarded Children. *Amer. J. Ment. Defic.*, 57:375-383, 1952-1953.

---

* See glossary.

12. Maxwell, J.: Home Care for the Retarded Child. *Nursing Outlook,* 19 (No. 2): February, 1971.
13. Patterson, E., and Rowland, G.: Toward a Theory of Mental Retardation Nursing, an Educational Model. *Am. J. Nursing,* 70 (No. 3):534, 1970.
14. Steigman, M.: Community Services for the Mentally Retarded. *Hospital and Community Psychiatry,* 19 (No. 5):142-144, May, 1968.
15. Waechter, E.: The Birth of an Exceptional Child. *Nursing Forum,* 9 (No. 2): 202-216, 1970.

SUGGESTED READINGS

There is an extensive library pertaining to the retardate, and the suggestions listed here are not intended to cover the whole field; the books and articles presented are merely a beginning. For the student who is particularly interested in this topic, further reading in human development is recommended, especially the work of Piaget. Another area of significance is special education and learning theory. Finally, the *Journal of Mental Retardation* and *Children* are highly recommended for their current presentations on the topic of retardation.

Buck, P.: *The Child Who Never Grew.* N. Y., John Day Co., 1960.

The noted author has written a 62-page story of herself and her retarded daughter. This is a very readable little book which is packed full of the human aspects of a mother-child relationship. Almost effortlessly the reader learns much about the problems of the retardate and his family.

Fraiberg, S.: *The Magic Years.* N. Y., Charles Scribners' Sons, 1959.

Though this book does not concern itself with the retardate per se, it does focus on therapy of disturbed children. The author, who is a children's analyst, has written a widely acclaimed account of the treatment of children. It is suggested in order to give the interested reader a picture of how psychotherapy with the child may proceed.

Gregg, G.: Comprehensive Professional Help for the Retarded Child and His Family. *Hospital and Community Psychiatry,* 19 (No. 4):122-124, April, 1968.

The article offers a capsule version of much pertinent information that will help the nursing student to understand the problems of the retardate.

Gunzberg, H.: Educational Problems in Mental Deficiency. *In* Clarke, A. M., and Clark, A. D.: *Mental Deficiency.* New York, Free Press Division, The Macmillan Company, 1965, pp. 328-355.

The author discusses Piaget's contributions to the testing and understanding of the retardate. Though the general topic, i.e., maturation of thought processes, is a difficult one for the basic student, the writer presents this material in a manner which is easily understood.

Hutt, M., and Gibby, R.: *The Mentally Retarded Child, Development, Education, and Guidance.* Boston, Allyn and Bacon, Inc., 1958.

Though this book is over 10 years old it is still one of the most practical and readable accounts of the management of the problems associated with mental deficiency. It is a very dynamic text and offers invaluable suggestions to the practitioner.

Noble, M.: Nursing's Concern for the Mentally Retarded Is Overdue. *Nursing Forum,* 9 (No. 2):192-200, 1970.

This is another condensation of much information which is necessary for the nurse who will care for retardates and their families. This article is current and reflects the most up-to-date thoughts and philosophy involving mental deficiency.

Olshansky, S.: Chronic Sorrow: A Response to Having a Mentally Defective Child. *Social Casework,* 43:190-193, April, 1962.

An excellent discussion is presented about the ill-chosen term "acceptance" as the primary focus in counseling parents of retardates. The thoughtfulness of the writer and his conclusions offer a worthwhile model. It will remind the reader of past struggles with the also much used term "support."

Patterson, E., and Rowland, G.: Toward a Theory of Mental Retardation Nursing, an Educational Model. *Am. J. Nursing,* 70 (No. 3):531-535, 1970.

The authors present a practical, no nonsense discussion of mental retardation and the possible functions of the nurse.

Smolock, M.: The Nurse's Role in Rehabilitation of the Handicapped Child. *Nurs. Clin. N. Amer.,* 5 (No. 3):411-420, September, 1970.

The writer does not discuss the mentally deficient child exclusively; however, she does point out that all children, no matter what their handicap, have a great deal in common. She then continues an interesting account of the nurse's role in rehabilitation of all children with handicaps. There is not much material concerning the retardate per se, but the whole article puts the retardate's problems in perspective.

Waechter, E.: The Birth of an Exceptional Child. *Nursing Forum,* 9 (No. 2):202-216, 1970.

If the reader were limited to only one outside reading on retardation, I would recommend this one without reservation. It is a beautifully written paper that is filled with information about the problems of the mother who has just given birth to a defective child. The article is highly technical and yet it is highly practical. Every nurse practitioner should make this article a must!

chapter 16

THE FUTURE

Time is one of the most frustrating elements with which man must live. During childhood it moves too slowly; by adulthood it is too fleeting. Time is completely elusive; it can be measured but not observed; there is no known way to stop it or start it.

Time presents ever-increasing difficulties as technology and science join together to produce change in the latter half of the twentieth century. Man has invented and discovered so much in the past 50 years that he is in danger of being unable to assimilate the fruits of his wisdom. The possible outcome of this dilemma is obsolescence and extinction.

Because man is the only animal who can predict his future, he has a means of preventing such an end. The need to change is basic. What will be the directions of change for psychiatric nursing? We can only begin to identify the determinants of those directions. Professionalism is one; structure of the health institution is another. Social issues such as poverty, drugs and alienation provide still others.

The psychiatric nurse of the future will be the product of a different type of education. It is likely that she will assume a professional identity which is different from that of the nurse of the seventies. There are signs, even now, that the nurse of the future will be a more independent practitioner who will expect a colleagual relationship. He or she will be educated to provide care within an agency or on a private contractual basis. The psychiatric nurse who is part of a therapeutic team will participate in evaluating the individual who seeks help. The nurse will then take an assertive role in planning that necessary intervention and may or may not take part in the psychotherapeutic program based on the patient's needs, rather than the availability of other kinds of therapists or the ability of the patient to finance his treatment.

It is likely that the future psychiatric nurse will develop expertise in specific treatment modalities. Theoretical knowledge concerning psychotherapy is increasing at such a rate that it is almost a certainty that the psychiatric nurse of tomorrow, prepared at an advanced level, will have to focus in one narrow area in order to master the quantity of data available.

The structure of health institutions will also influence psychiatric nursing. Because of the ever-increasing human population there will be need for a different kind of nursing care. Emphasis will be placed on prevention. Large institutions may be replaced by small "first aid" units within the community. The nurse's task will involve less patient contact and more supervision of community members who will act as primary supporters. Psychiatric nurses may become "mental health engineers," entering communities to plan educational and social programs to enhance mental hygiene and to act in concert with community leaders to develop their plans.

It is likely that there will be increased consultations at state and federal levels as third party payment and government funding provide the financial means of continuing health services. Psychiatric nurses, like all professionals, will have to study sociology, anthropology, history and government in order to understand as professionals and citizens what is required of them and to meet those expectations.

The major health problems will be likely to involve masses, because individuals become closer as communication, transportation and population growth draw them into tighter proximity. Psychiatric nursing will be expected to join in the fight against poverty, which will be eradicated only after apathy is fought and overcome. Family structures will be altered with the decline of poverty. The change in family relations will be accompanied by problems of identity. All these factors will present a multitude of challenges.

Drugs and social alienation now and in the future will lay claim to the country's greatest pool of human resources—the young. Psychiatric nursing will be called upon to join in exploring the problem and providing this segment of society with less destructive means of expression and reaction. As data accumulate concerning the developmental needs of the young in a society and time that exerts overwhelming pressure on them, psychiatric nursing will be called upon to find constructive means of altering these forces.

There will doubtless be machinery to aid us. There will be manpower, also, who can assume selected parts of the work. The psychiatric nurse will have to identify what tasks can be assumed by the machines and which can be appropriately delegated to paraprofessional help. The characteristics that will aid in this decision-making and in therapeutic intervention will be technological knowledge of tomorrow coupled with the sensitivity, theoretical bases and social conscience of today.

REFERENCES

Mellow, J.: Professional Identity? *ANA Clinical Conferences, 1969.* New York, Appleton-Century-Crofts, Inc., 1970.
Levine, M.: Dilemma. Ibid.
Reinkemeyer, A.: Nursing's Need: Commitment to an Ideology of Change. *Nursing Forum,* 9 (No. 4):340-355, 1970.
Toffler, A.: *Future Shock.* New York, Random House, 1970.

GLOSSARY

abreaction—A release of pent-up emotion which occurs when an individual mentally relives or recalls abruptly a painful experience that had been deeply repressed. This form of therapy may be induced by the psychiatrist through the use of Sodium Amytal or Pentothal.

acting out—A pattern of socially unacceptable behavior in which the person unconsciously expresses emotional conflicts. Hostile or loving feelings may be expressed in some concealed form. The person thus expressing himself is unaware of the meaning of his behavior, which may be recognized by others or may escape their observation. Acting out is usually considered a neurotic behavior pattern, and the patient in therapy is prevailed upon not to use this mode of defensive behavior.

addiction—A strong emotional and/or physiologic dependence upon alcohol or some other drug or substance which has progressed to the point that the individual utilizing the substance can no longer limit its use.

adjustment—The continuous efforts of the individual to maintain his state of homeostasis, both physiological and psychological. Adjustment is never stationary because both the environment of the individual and his psyche are always in flux.

affect—The emotional feeling tone of the individual. A strong affect is an emotion; mood may be thought of as a prolonged affect.

affective psychosis—A psychotic disorder in which there is a predominance of severe mood or emotional disorder, i.e., the excited state in the manic phase of the manic-depressive psychosis.

aggression—An assertive force which may be expressed through attitude or behavior and is usually directed to external objects, though it may be turned inward, as is reflected in self-destructive behavior. Aggression is a healthy force which sometimes needs to be channeled. Psychiatric patients often have difficulty expressing basic aggressive feelings.

agitation—A state of restlessness or activity without purpose; a means of releasing nervous tension. Patients who pace up and down, wringing their hands and/or crying are usually described as being agitated.

ambivalence—The presence of mixed feelings toward an object. The feelings are usually opposite in character and may be conscious or unconscious, or only one of the opposing feelings may be in awareness.

anencephaly—One of the most common congenital brain malformations. There is an absence of the cranial vault and most of the central nervous system,

331

or at least the absence of both cerebral hemispheres. The anencephalic fetus usually dies during delivery or shortly thereafter.

apathy—A state of absence of emotions that is usually experienced as lethargy by the individual but is actually a defense against unacceptable feelings which lurk in the preconscious or unconscious.

attitude—An established manner or pattern of thought, which the individual develops from prior expectations and/or experiences about some object, place or person.

attitude therapy—A type of therapy used in residential treatment centers. Usually a component of milieu therapy in which the staff assume prescribed attitudes which are expected to have an identified effect on the patient.

basic drive—Urge; motivation; powerful because it reflects the homeostatic imbalance of the individual, who strives instinctively to decrease the bodily tension associated with it. Basic drives that motivate the individual are concerned with hunger, sex, thirst and security.

behavior—Any activity of the individual, either mental or physical. Some can be observed, but other behavior can only be inferred by the observer via physical activity *resulting* from mental behavior.

blocking—An inability to remember or an interruption of a train of thought or speech. The cause of blocking is usually emotional, except in the organically ill, and it is generally defensive in nature.

borderline state—Sometimes referred to as borderline psychosis. A diagnostic term used to denote the difficulty of determining whether the patient is basically neurotic or psychotic. The patient's symptoms may shift from one state to the other.

catatonia—A condition associated with schizophrenia in which the patient is characteristically immobile. The muscles are rigid and the limbs may be placed in various positions by the examiner, with the patient maintaining that stance indefinitely. It is not unusual for the patient to display alternating periods of hyperactivity and excitability. The catatonic patient is very difficult to communicate with and he is considered extremely sick.

catharsis—A process of releasing pent-up feelings by talking out ideas and thoughts. If appropriate emotions are experienced concurrent with the talking out, the patient is likely to feel great relief and calm afterward. If the process is characterized by discussion only (intellectualization), the patient usually experiences additional tension.

cathexis—The attachment of emotion and significance to an idea, person or object. Through cathexis, the object becomes invested with increased importance. The degree of cathexis is measured by the amount of interest in the object, the frequency with which it is in awareness (or is associated with other thoughts or objects) and the amount of influence which the cathected object has upon the individual's thinking or behavior. One of the first objects cathected by the infant is mother.

cerea flexibilitas—See *Catatonia*.

character—The total of the individual's attributes except those which are physical. The social, emotional and intellectual qualities of a person influence his character.

character disorder—An unhealthy and often socially unacceptable pattern of behavior and emotional response which is associated with a minimum of anxiety.

coma—A state of complete loss of consciousness. The individual experiences no perception nor is voluntary movement possible.

commitment—The legal process for hospitalization of patients who are unwilling, or too sick, to admit themselves to residential treatment facilities. Because of the bottleneck often created in general hospitals while qualified physicians are sought to sign papers, some states are passing legislation making it possible for other health professionals, such as the public health nurse, to initiate the commitment on an emergency basis until doctors can be located at the treatment facility itself.

complex—A group of associated ideas which have a strong emotional quality and which influence an individual's attitudes and behavior. Some of the more often mentioned complexes are the *castration complex,* associated with the child's fear of losing his genitalia or other multilating fantasies which stand for loss of the genital organs; the *inferiority complex* which is associated with feelings of inferiority and which may be based on actual inadequacies or felt inadequacies. The individual usually experiences anxiety as a result and may try to compensate for his feelings through the development of special skill.

compulsion—An involuntary urge from within to perform an act that may be rational or irrational. The completion of the act prevents anxiety from emerging.

conflict—The clash between opposing forces; may be conscious or unconscious; may be intrapersonal, as in the case of an instinctual wish which is opposed by a contradictory striving, or may be interpersonal when another individual is involved in the struggle.

conversion reaction—A neurotic disorder in which anxiety is expressed symbolically through the loss or alteration of a sensory or motor function.

convulsion—Seizure; referred to in folk language as a fit; generalized involuntary muscular contractions or spasms. Associated with brain trauma, epilepsy or, sometimes, toxicity.

convulsive disorders—Include grand mal, petit mal, Jacksonian and psychomotor seizures. Included also are certain minor or equivalent states: prolonged drowsiness, torpor, stupor, coma and twilight states.

countertransference—The emotional response of the therapist to his patient. Like transference, countertransference is influenced by the therapist's perception of the patient as being like significant people in his past. Because of the sometimes unconscious nature of the therapist's response to his patient, it is very important for the therapist to consult with a colleague from time to time about his caseload. This process is equivalent to the supervisory experience of the nursing student in psychiatry. Whereas she focuses primarily on learning new skills, the therapist reviews his work with a colleague to insure that his responses to patients are as therapeutic as possible, rather than emotionally based and primarily gratifying to him.

cretinism—Hypothyroidism in a young child.

culture—Those qualities that characterize a group of people and which are transmitted from one generation to the next. Culture includes all technological achievements, values, customs, institutions and social organizations.

daydream—Idle thoughts, usually characterized by indulgence and wish fulfillment. Daydreaming may be quite harmless as an escape from boredom, or it may reflect underlying psychopathology if the individual uses it habitually to escape the rigors of daily life.

decompensation, emotional—The breakdown of previously effective adjustment mechanisms.

dependency needs—Vital needs for mothering, love, affection, shelter, protection, security, food and warmth. Though originating in the newborn, these needs may continue in later years in overt or latent forms. The amount of dependency needs expressed may increase as a sign of pathology, i.e., regression, or these needs may increase under stress, such as overwhelming sickness or a catastrophe, in which case psychopathology is not necessarily reflected.

deterioration—In mental illness deterioration refers to the chronic downhill course which is exemplified by disintegration of intellectual and/or emotional functions. Emotional deterioration describes the apathy, loss of interest in appearance and environment and poor social adjustment seen in psychotic patients.

Down's syndrome—Mongolism; a disorder caused by changes in the chromosomes. The incidence of Down's syndrome is approximately one in every 700 births. In a middle-aged mother (over 32 years) the risk of having a mongoloid child is about one in 100. The mongoloid may have abnormalities in the anatomy of the brain and heart. There are over 100 other signs described in Down's syndrome, but they are rarely all found in one child. Mental retardation is the overriding feature of Down's syndrome. The majority of mongoloids are moderately or severely retarded. They tend to be placid, cheerful and cooperative until adolescence, when a variety of emotional difficulties may occur.

dynamics—A determination of the forces that have influenced behavior (s). If the dynamics are correctly identified, they may be used as predictors of future behavior. Suppose a patient is assaultive. If the staff correctly identify the behavior as the result of fear because the patient was approached by a male attendant, then they may assume that the patient will be assaultive again under the same circumstances. Staff may modify the assaultive behavior by trying to assuage the patient's fear or by keeping male attendants away from that patient.

echolalia—The automatic repetition by patients of words or phrases spoken to them. Seen in schizophrenic patients as a defensive behavior to avoid meaningful communication.

echopraxia—An automatic and repetitive imitation of the movements of others. This defensive behavior, like echolalia, is not meant to be hostile, as is the defiant behavior of mimicry. The schizophrenic's goal is not to hurt the other, but to protect himself.

ego ideal—The conscious aspirations, goals and qualities which are lauded by the individual; the existence that the individual would like to have.

egocentric—Having an overwhelming interest in oneself; self-centered. Unlike narcissism, egocentricity does not imply a high opinion of self.

egoism—Overevaluation of the self.

emotion—A subjective feeling which may be conscious or out of awareness, but which influences behavior.

epilepsy—A disorder characterized by periodic convulsions accompanied by a loss of consciousness or by other manifestations of interrupted brain waves. (See *Convulsive disorders* for further classification.)

extravert—The personality type which is highly sociable, outgoing, impulsive and emotionally expressive.

fantasy—Like daydream, though more vivid; a sequence of mental images. The fantasy may be an attempt by the individual to resolve an emotional conflict. Fantasies often occur when the mind is not occupied, such as just prior to sleep.

fetish—An object endowed with special meaning. A symbol or article which stands for a person or part of a person. The fetish often has sensual properties and is sometimes a source of sexual stimulation.

fetishism—The process of imbuing an inanimate object with special meaning.

folie à deux—A psychosis which is shared by two people. The people are usually related or have lived together long enough to have learned to share mutual delusions.

functional illness—An illness of emotional origin in which there is no demonstrable change in organs or systems. A functional psychosis is one that occurs in the absence of any lesions in the brain.

galactosemia—A disorder of carbohydrate metabolism which if untreated may lead to progressive mental deterioration. Diagnosis is through detection of the presence of galactose in the urine. A galactose-free diet, instituted early, prevents all clinical symptoms and permits normal physical and mental development.

gargoylism—See *Hurler's disease.*

guilt—An unpleasant, subjective feeling of self-criticism that results from acts, thoughts or impulses which are contrary to the individual's conscience. The amount of guilt an individual feels does not necessarily reflect the real amount of damage perpetrated by the guilty-feeling individual, but is likely to be a rough measure of the individual's conscience or superego. Psychopathologic feelings of guilt result from unconscious conflicts.

habit—A characteristic manner of response. Habits are developed through practice and are reflected in skillful performance.

halfway house—A treatment facility for patients who no longer need complete hospitalization, but who are not yet ready to return to their homes. Another type of care which is more protective than the halfway house, but less so than the hospital, is found at a quarterway house.

homosexual panic—An acute anxiety attack based on unconscious conflict of a homosexual nature. Such episodes sometimes occur when an individual is forced into close contact with others of the same sex, such as when a person is imprisoned or sent to boot camp or even hospitalized on a ward.

homosexuality—Sexual attraction or relationship between two individuals of the same sex; not always conscious. Homosexual relationships until quite recently were kept hidden, except in public places such as "gay bars" that were designated as social gathering spots for such individuals. Today there is increasing focus on the homosexual and his legal right to live in the style that he chooses so long as he does not harm others.

hospitalitis—A term used to describe patients who have become too comfortable living in the hospital and who are no longer motivated to get well and be discharged. When this situation arises the patient has regressed too far and focuses too exclusively on having his dependency needs met.

Hurler's disease—Gargoylism; this metabolic disorder causes multiple abnormalities including mental retardation. The clinical course of the disease is slow and progressive. It starts at a young age, leading to death before adolescence. The facial characteristics include bushy eyebrows that grow together, thick lips, large tongue and coarse features. No treatment is available for this disorder.

hydrocephaly—This term describes a number of conditions having in common an increase in the cerebrospinal fluid, resulting in enlargement of the head or ventricles. There are many neurological findings in this condition, and mental deterioration occurs. In milder cases the condition may be arrested spontaneously and the child may be only mildly retarded. Surgical intervention is sometimes performed successfully to shunt the fluid from the ventricles to the kidneys.

hypothyroidism—In a child, the absence of sufficient thyroid is known as cretinism. There are many clinical symptoms associated with this disorder if it is congenital and mental retardation is part of the picture if the condition is not diagnosed and treated in infancy.

hysteria—A form of neurosis characterized by either involuntary loss of physical function (conversion type) or by alterations in consciousness or identity (e.g., amnesia, sleepwalking) (dissociative type). Hysterical behavior is seen more frequently in women than in men. When it occurs in children, it is theorized to be a regressive behavior characteristic of the pre-oedipal child who expresses himself physically, rather than verbally, since the later skills are not yet fully developed.

ideas of influence—The delusion that one's feelings, thoughts or actions are under the control of external forces or persons. This delusion is observed in the schizophrenic, who may regard that influence as benevolent or malevolent.

ideas of persecution—The delusion that one is being threatened, discriminated against or mistreated. Ideas of persecution are often observed in the paranoid schizophrenic patient.

ideas of reference—The interpretation of external events as being relevant to the individual, i.e., as having direct reference to him. The delusional patient may be convinced that he is the object of thoughts, talk or action of others around him.

idiot—An individual with the lowest level of intellect. The tested IQ falls below 20.

imago—An unconscious mental image of significant persons in the life of the individual. The retained memory of the loved person is an idealized version.

imbecile—The intermediate level of below-normal intellect, between the moron and the idiot. Such an individual is usually trainable. The IQ tests between 20 and 50.

impulse—An urge; usually an abruptly felt motivation toward some object or person.

inadequate personality—The individual who responds less than adequately to intellectual, emotional, physical and social stress. This individual usually adapts poorly and is unable to integrate in new social situations.

inhibition—The restraint of urges, thoughts or behaviors. The inhibiting force is usually the superego.

insanity—A legal term indicating that the individual is so severely mentally ill that he is incapable of taking responsibility for his own actions and, as such, must be protected and cared for by others.

insight—A type of self-understanding that encompasses an intellectual and an emotional awareness of the origin, nature and mechanisms of one's attitudes and behavior. The beginning of insight is reflected in awareness, but is observed operationally when the individual modifies his dysfunctional behavior as a result of that awareness.

instinct—An innate impulse or drive that is characteristic of all members of a species, i.e., all human beings. Human instincts are self-preservation, sexuality, the ego and the herd or social.

integration—The organization of knowledge, experience and emotion into a useful whole personality which permits the individual to function effectively.

intelligence—The potential ability to acquire and to apply understanding, knowledge, experience and judgment, and the potential for gaining new knowledge in the problem-solving situation.

introvert—The personality type which is shy, withdrawn, emotionally reserved and self-absorbed.

investment, emotional—The attachment of significance to some object or person by an individual. When one is dedicated to some task or project he has usually made a substantial emotional investment in that project.

IQ—Intelligence quotient; an arithmetical figure which symbolizes one's attainment on various psychological tests. The tests ask the respondent to perform tasks which are then graded against standardized norms for the testee's age group. The IQ is determined by dividing the mental age (as determined by the various tests) by the chronological age, and multiplying by 100. Normal IQ is taken as 100. The outer limits of normality are 90 and 110.

la belle indifference—"The beautiful" or "the grand indifference," as translated from the French. The indifference characterizing some patients' attitudes toward somatic symptoms when the individuals are neurotic with conversion symptoms.

labile—Readily changeable; usually refers to emotions which are unstable.

latent—Hidden; inactive or dormant.

lesbian—A homosexual female.

logorrhea—Excessive talking or constant chatter.

macrocephaly—A congenital anomaly in which the brain is unusually large. Mental retardation is one of several complications found in the macrocephalic infant.

mannerism—Any kind of expression or activity which is peculiar to the individual. A mannerism may be bizarre and extremely pathological or it may be within the range of normalcy.

maple syrup urine disease—A metabolic disorder which causes amino and keto acids to accumulate in the blood and cause overflow of amino acids into the urine. Their presence in the urine causes a characteristic odor similar to that of maple syrup. One of the complications of this disorder is mental retardation. The disease is responsive to a modified diet in which the involved amino acids are kept quite low.

masochism—Pleasure obtained from the suffering of physical or psychological pain. The pleasure may have a sexual basis.

masturbation—Sexual stimulation or gratification of the self, by the self, usually obtained by stimulation of the genitalia.

melancholia—An antiquated term that is synonymous with depression, usually of psychotic proportions.

memory—The recollection of a past event; the reservoir of all past experience that may be recalled or recollected.

mental age—A term used to describe an individual's ability to perform intellectually as compared with others of comparable age; as contrasted with chronological age which is an absolute predetermined by the birth date.

microcephaly—This term covers a variety of disorders whose main feature is a small, peculiarly shaped head and mental retardation.

mongolism—See *Down's syndrome.*

mongoloidism—See *Down's syndrome.*

moron—The highest level of mental retardation, the IQ ranging from 50 to 69. Morons are usually educable and can be taught to do simple work so that gainful employment under close supervision is possible.

mutism—The absence of speech; may represent an organically based problem or one that develops as the result of negativism, perverseness or fear.

negative feeling—Unfriendliness, hatred, dislike or any feeling which can be classified as lacking warmth.

negativism—Behavior which opposes that which is sought; opposition, contrariness and resistance.

nervous breakdown—A lay term designating emotional illness. One must beware that the user has not defined the severity of the illness when this term is utilized.

neurosis—Also called psychoneurosis. Mild to moderately severe illness in which the individual attempts unconsciously to cope with levels of anxiety that are not readily controllable. Reality testing is not impaired. Neurotic disorders include depressive reactions, hypochondriasis, obsessive-compulsive reactions, conversion reactions, phobias and dissociative reactions.

nymphomania—A condition found in females who have a pathological abundance of sexual drive. The counterpart in the male is termed "satyriasis."

obsession—A repetitive thought that intrudes into the individual's awareness involuntarily.

organ language—An expression of intrapsychic conflict through alteration in the physiology. Similar to process of conversion reaction, except that an actual physical lesion is demonstrable. The psychosomatic diseases, i.e., functional hypertension, peptic ulcer, rheumatoid arthritis, ulcerative colitis and a variety of skin conditions, may be expressions of intrapsychic-conflict.

overt—Observable, out in the open; as distinct from latent, which is hidden.

passive-aggressive personality—An immature personality that is characterized by expression of aggression through passive maneuvers such as pouting, procrastination and obstructiveness.

passive-dependent personality—An immature personality that is characterized by expression of dependency needs through helplessness, lack of self-reliance, lack of self-confidence, indecisiveness and compliance.

perception—The process through which sensory stimuli are transmitted into awareness in the individual; thus, objects, persons and animals are recognized.

personality—The total of one's character traits, i.e., attributes, drives, aspirations, inhibitions, strengths, weaknesses and all patterns of reaction.

personality disorder—See *Character disorder.*

perversion—A personality disorder in which normal aims and strivings are altered or the normal drives remain but the *objects* of the drives are altered. Sadism, masochism and sodomy are considered perversions.

phenylketonuria (PKU)—An abnormality of metabolism. The majority of PKU patients are severely retarded unless the dysfunction is diagnosed early and treatment instituted. Typical PKU children are hyperactive and exhibit erratic, unpredictable behavior. A simple test utilizes the wet diaper and a drop of ferric chloride solution. If the abnormality is present, the spot turns a vivid green color. The test does not become positive until the infant is five to six weeks old. This disorder responds to dietary treatment, which must be continued until the child is five to six years old.

pleasure principle—A theory developed by Freud to explain the behavior of infants and others who are grossly immature. The theory states that such an individual automatically seeks gratification and the avoidance of displeasure.

positive feelings—Warm feelings of affection, love, or friendliness. Such feelings are constructive as opposed to the destructive nature of negative feelings.

power struggle—A psychological contest between two or more individuals to see who will be dominant.

psychopath—Synonymous with sociopath. An individual with a character disorder, whose illness is reflected in behavior which is asocial and antisocial. Such individuals are usually impulsive and irresponsible. They are often in trouble with the law.

psychosomatic disorder—Also called psychophysiologic disorder; a physical illness that is strongly influenced by psychological problems. This type of disorder demonstrates the coequality and mutual interaction of mind and body. Included in this group of disorders are such illnesses as chronic ulcerative colitis, asthma, urticaria, neurodermatitis and some instances of obesity.

psychosis—Severe mental illness in which thinking, acting and feeling patterns of the individual may become distorted. Loss of contact with reality also may occur. Hospitalization is often necessary to protect the patient.

rapport—A bond; in psychotherapy, rapport between the therapist and patient implies mutual feelings of comfort, acceptance, understanding, confidence and warmth.

rational—Sensible, reasonable.

reality testing—The process of determining subjective validity for an individual. That which is true, or valid, for anyone is determined by his subjective perceptions plus demands and requirements of the external world. The newborn does not test reality nor does he live by the reality principle. Instead, the infant and young child live by the pleasure principle, which means that they want (and expect) what they want, when they want it, no matter what the environmental situation is.

regressive therapy—This rarely used technique encourages the psychotic patient to give up his more mature levels of behavior in order to become more dependent and childlike. The theory behind the therapy is that when the patient is permitted to regress, and after his dependency needs have been met satisfactorily, he will reintegrate more effectively and as a result become emotionally healthier.

resistance—A defensive reluctance to cooperate in therapeutic work; is not voluntary, but occurs when the therapist uncovers material that is highly significant to the individual so that its acceptance would generate sizeable changes in that individual's perception.

retrograde amnesia—A loss of memory which begins at the time of the crisis that precipitates the failure to recall. Thus, a person who falls from a horse and develops retrograde amnesia would be unable to recall anything that happened to him prior to his fall.

Rorschach test—A psychological test consisting of ten cards with inkblots on them. The testee is requested to describe what he sees in each card. He may have as many interpretations as he wishes. The testee's responses disclose personality traits and emotional conflicts.

sadism—Pleasure obtained from inflicting physical or psychological pain on others. This term is used more broadly to connote the enjoyment of any cruelty.

schizophrenia—A group of psychotic disorders that often emerge in late adolescence or young adulthood. Individuals diagnosed as schizophrenic are usually withdrawn and seemingly afraid. There are loss of contact with reality, regressed behavior and inappropriate affect. Hallucinations and delusions are often demonstrated.

sensation—The perception of stimuli via the sensory end-organs, i.e., visual, auditory, taste, touch or olfactory.

sensorium—An abstract term describing the integration in the brain of the sensory perceptive faculties. The term "clear sensorium" is used to describe the presence of an accurate memory together with the correct orientation for time, place and persons.

sociopath—See *Psychopath.*

sodomy—Anal intercourse, usually between males or between men and animals. A legal term which may include other perversions.

status epilepticus—A severe condition in which there are more or less continuous epileptic convulsions.

stress—Any circumstance, biological or psychological, that taxes the coping or adjusting mechanisms of the individual.

stupor—A state of lethargy and irresponsiveness in which the sensorium is clouded and the individual seems unaware of his surroundings.

subconscious—A lay term for the preconscious.

Tay-Sachs disease—A metabolic disorder in which lipids accumulate throughout the central nervous system, causing progressive physical and mental deterioration and leading to death in two to four years. The disease is transmitted through the genes and occurs chiefly among Jewish infants. There is no known cure; however, the disease can be prevented through genetic counseling whereby it may be determined if the parents carry the recessive gene causing the disease.

thinking—The process of reasoning which is carried on in the mind. Thinking is not directly observable but must be inferred from observation of activity which results from thinking.

toxic psychosis—A psychosis brought on by the action of some toxin which has entered the body and interfered with normal metabolic activity.

transference—The unconscious attribution by an individual of his feelings and attitudes toward some significant person of the past to a person in the current interpersonal situation. In psychoanalysis transference is considered a necessity for cure. The person being analyzed works through his conflicts with significant figures in his childhood by transferring the feelings generated by them to the analyst and working them through in the analytic situation.

transvestism—Symptom of a perversion in which the individual gains gratification through dressing and sometimes masquerading in the clothes of the opposite sex.

trauma—Severe physical or psychological injury.

voyeurism—A perversion in which the individual gains sexual gratification from looking at others. The most common type of voyeur is the "peeping Tom."

withdrawal—A behavior in which the individual retreats from external relationships, social situations and painful conflicts. Withdrawal may be symptomatic of mental illness or it may be a normal defensive behavior after such trauma as catastrophic stress.

INDEX